Metabolic Care

D.E.F. Tweedle
MB ChB FRCS (Ed) ChM
Senior Lecturer in Surgery, University of Manchester
and Honorary Consultant Surgeon,
University Hospital of South Manchester

With contributions by

F. Cockburn
MB ChB DCH RFPS FRCP (Ed) FRCP (Glas) MD
Samson Gemmell Professor of Child Health, University of Glasgow

J. C. Stoddart
MB BS FFA RCS MD
Consultant Anaesthetist and Consultant-in-Charge
of the Intensive Therapy Unit, Royal Victoria Infirmary,
Newcastle upon Tyne

CHURCHILL LIVINGSTONE
EDINBURGH LONDON MELBOURNE AND NEW YORK 1982

CHURCHILL LIVINGSTONE
Medical Divison of Longman Group Limited

Distributed in the United States of America by
Churchill Livingstone Inc., 19 West 44th Street, New
York, N.Y. 10036, and by associated companies,
branches and representatives throughout the world.

First published 1982

ISBN 0 443 01867 7

British Library Cataloguing in Publication Data
Tweedle, D.E.F.
    Metabolic care.
    1. Metabolism, Disorders of
    I. Title   II. Cockburn, F.   III. Stoddart, J.C.
    616.3'9   RC627.54

Library of Congress Catalog Card Number 81–70268

Printed in Singapore by Huntsmen Offset Printing Pte Ltd

Preface

'The basic components of medical knowledge are water, electrolytes, oxygen, lipids, protein and carbohydrates'.

Irvine Page

Many patients have serious metabolic abnormalities, whose correction is essential for a successful outcome. In some these are readily apparent: in others they are recognised only by careful clinical and biochemical assessment. Several large texts are available which present in detail the complex alterations of physiology and biochemistry involved. This book attempts to present these problems in straightforward terms for the clinical practitioner.

I have been particularly fortunate in persuading two colleagues of international distinction to provide chapters on topics of which they have an exceptional experience. Professor F. Cockburn is the Samson Gemmell Professor of Child Health in the University of Glasgow. His knowledge and expertise in the field of neonatal nutrition is unique. Dr J.C. Stoddart is a Consultant Anaesthetist and the Consultant–in–Charge of a busy intensive therapy unit in the Royal Victoria Infirmary in Newcastle upon Tyne. Few clinicians have gained his experience of the day-to-day management of seriously ill patients. I am very grateful to them both.

As a young surgeon my interest in problems of surgical metabolism was stimulated by my late chief Mr A.M. Loughran, who as Consultant Surgeon at the West Cumberland Hospital provided a surgical education in its very broadest sense. Later, I was fortunate to spend four years in the Department of Surgery in Newcastle upon Tyne with Professor I.D.A. Johnston and a year in the Department of Surgery of Harvard University under Professor F.D. Moore. My attitude to metabolic care has been particularly influenced by these men and their help and encouragement has been of enormous value.

The manuscript was painstakingly typed by my wife, Dr I. Tweedle, with generous assistance from my secretary, Miss L. Shaughnessy. The illustrations were drawn by Mrs M. Harrison and the photographs were taken by Mr E. Hartles. Figure 4.1 was reproduced with the kind permission of Radiometer A/V and Professor Siggaard-Andersen. I am grateful to Messrs Churchill Livingstone, who have given invaluable advice and help during the preparation of the manuscript.

Manchester, 1982   D.E.F.T.

Contents

1

Body composition and homeostasis

It can be frustrating and frequently unrewarding to become embroiled in an argument about the relative merits of different forms of nutritional therapy with an expert on body composition, particularly if the latter has little contact with clinical medicine. The discussion will often be interspersed with arguments about the precise extent of the compartments under consideration and doubts concerning the methods used to measure their contents, and experts tend to be obsessed with their own particular narrow field of interest. Nevertheless, even experts will agree about certain basic facts concerning body composition and an elementary knowledge of these is an essential requirement to any attempt to maintain or to restore body composition. Although body composition varies considerably according to race, sex, age, weight and height, estimations of certain components provide valuable indices upon which to base individual requirements.

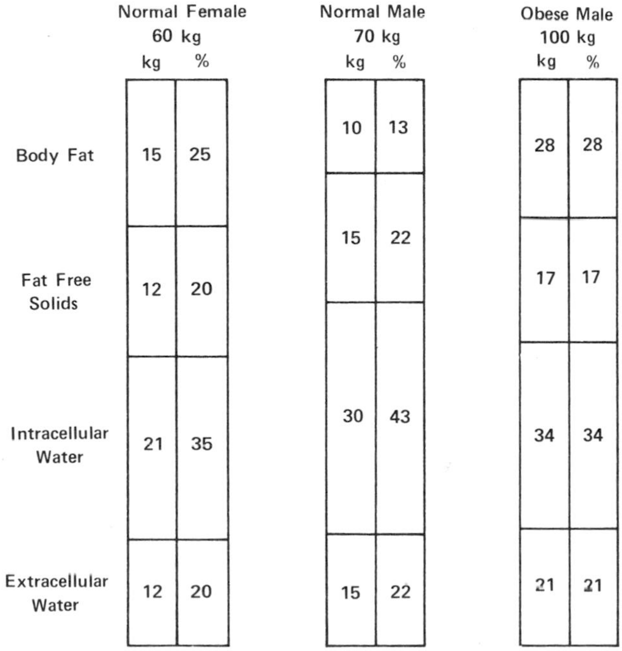

	Normal Female 60 kg		Normal Male 70 kg		Obese Male 100 kg	
	kg	%	kg	%	kg	%
Body Fat	15	25	10	13	28	28
Fat Free Solids	12	20	15	22	17	17
Intracellular Water	21	35	30	43	34	34
Extracellular Water	12	20	15	22	21	21

Fig. 1.1 Body composition

The body can be divided into two broad subdivisions, the body fat which may vary greatly and the lean body mass which is relatively constant in subjects of the same sex and height (Behnke 1942). As well as being convenient for descriptive purposes, this concept is important from a functional aspect. The body fat is to a great extent unnecessary for immediate survival, but the lean body mass is in effect the living body, responsible for synthesis of essential body components, energy exchange, excretion of waste products and defence. Any deficiency in the quality or quantity of the lean body mass has far–reaching consequences for survival and well–being.

The typical distribution of body fat, the fat–free solids and body water of a healthy 60 kg female and 70 kg male and a moderately obese 100 kg male is shown in Figure 1.1.

BODY FAT

This is predominantly neutral triglyceride (esters of glycerol and fatty acids) stored in the fat depots and amounting to about 10 kg in the 70 kg male. When energy intake exceeds requirements, the excess is stored as fat. When energy intake is insufficient to meet requirements, the fat stores are mobilised and oxidised. Being anhydrous with a calorific value of 39 kJ/g (9.3 kcal/g), fat is an ideal storage material (Fig. 1.2), and as these stores contain very little intracellular and extracellular water they have a calorific value of 33.6 kJ/g (8 kcal/g).

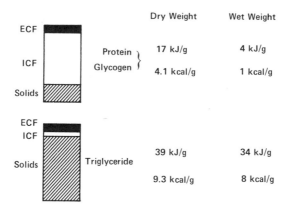

Fig. 1.2 Energy content of body substrates

Although these stores are unnecessary for immediate survival, they form a vital component of the defence against prolonged starvation, providing the major portion of endogenous energy supply and thereby reducing the draft on the protein of the lean body mass. Synthesis of vital components is not a function of this tissue but it is wrong to consider it inactive, for there is a continual synthesis and breakdown of triglyceride within it.

Fat also exists in the body as free fatty acids (that is, free from combination with other compounds) and as compound lipids (fatty acids combined with various substances such as choline, glycerol and phosphate). Although the amount is very small when compared with the triglycerides of the fat stores, this portion of the body fat is vital as it forms the major component of the membranes of cells and their intracellular organelles (see Ch. 8).

The intake of fat varies considerably from country to country and from individual to individual, influenced to a certain extent by economic status but mainly by taste or religious belief. Studies of an Indian aboriginal tribe have suggested that the minimum daily requirement may be extremely small, probably of the order of 4 g (Mitra 1942) which might be sufficient to provide 1 g of essential fatty acids (see Ch. 8 for further details). The recommended daily energy intake of healthy adult males is about 11 MJ (2600 kcal) for those in sedentary occupations and about 15 MJ (3600 kcal) for those in extremely active occupations (DHSS 1969). Although, as emphasised on many occasions in this book, protein should not be considered as a source of energy, these recommended intakes include the calorific value of protein which contributes at least 10% and in many diets as much as 20% of the total. Thus 80–90% of the total energy requirement must be provided in the form of fat and carbohydrate and in most Western diets the contribution of the two substrates is about equal.

LEAN BODY MASS

The fat–free mass consists of skeletal and cardiac muscle, the protein of the gastro–intestinal tract (including its smooth muscle), the skeleton and the body fluids with their mineral content. The term lean body mass is usually used to denote a component that is smaller than the fat–free mass and excludes the skeleton. It can be considered to be soft, cellular and predominantly protein in nature and it is the metabolically active portion of the body that determines energy requirements, oxygen consumption, carbon dioxide production, creatinine excretion and many other commonly measured indices of body metabolism. A healthy 70 kg male will contain 6–7 kg of protein and a healthy 60 kg female 4.5–5 kg. The mineral content of the lean body mass is very small (a few grams) but, as discussed later in this chapter, has a crucial role in the distribution of water within the body.

Man and other animals can synthesise some amino acids by condensation of the carboxyl group of α keto acids and an amine radicle (NH_2):

$$2\ RCOOH\ +\ CO\ (NH_2)_2\ \longrightarrow\ 2\ RCONH\ +\ H_2O\ +\ CO_2$$

α keto acid   urea   amino acid   water   carbon dioxide

However, neither animals nor the vast majority of plants are able to use the large amount of nitrogen in the air (about 80% by volume) to form amine radicals. The fixation of large quantities of nitrogen from the air is essential to the continuing existence of all plant and animal life on earth. Only a few plants are capable of such fixation and they require the help of various bacteria particularly those of the genus Clostridium, Pseudomonas and Aerobacter. It is fascinating to reflect that man could not exist without the help of these organisms, which in other circumstances are the harbingers of death.

The rate at which breakdown and resynthesis of protein occurs in the components of the lean body mass varies considerably. The epithelia of the gastro–intestinal mucosa is replaced every two or three days but the half–life of collagen may be measured in months. Like fat, the intake of protein varies considerably from country to country and from individual to individual, usually corresponding to economic status. A daily intake of 50 g is sufficient for a healthy 70 kg male providing that the protein is of good quality (see Ch. 8 for further details). The average diet of many Western countries contains twice this quantity. Although the nitrogen content of individual amino acids varies, mixed protein contains 16% nitrogen and this measurement is commonly used to determine protein content by multiplying the nitrogen values by 6.25. Body protein consists of 75% water and thus 1 g of nitrogen is equivalent to 30 g of hydrated protein. In the body, protein can only be partially catabolised and has a calorific value of 17.2 kJ/g (4.1 kcal/g). Consequently skeletal muscle and gastro-intestinal protein are poor sources of energy, releasing only 4 k J/g (1 kcal/g) of hydrated tissue (Fig. 1.2).

The lean body mass contains the body's meagre stores of carbohydrate, mainly in the form of glycogen in the liver and the muscle. The normal 70 kg male contains no more than 400 g. Oxidation of carbohydrate in the body will also yield 17.2 kJ/g (4.1 kcal/g), but, like protein, glycogen consists of 75% water and is also a poor source of energy, yielding the same 4 kJ/g of tissue. If carbohydrate intake exceeds immediate needs, the glycogen stores are rapidly repleted and the excess is converted into triglyceride.

This important difference in the function of the two basic subdivisions of the body, the fat stores and the lean body mass, is particularly evident during starvation and after injury as discussed in detail in Chapter 3. The concept of nitrogen balance is well known and accepted. Less commonly appreciated is the concept that the body's energy balance can be equated in a similar manner in terms of carbon balance (Kinney & Moore 1956). Thus nitrogen and carbon balance may be used to indicate changes in lean body mass and body fat respectively. Measurement of the former is relatively simple and may be done at the bedside. Measurement of the latter with any meaningful degree of accuracy requires sophisticated, expensive equipment. It is usually performed in special units and even then only for purposes of clinical research. Fortunately, body fat can be estimated relatively simply by calculation from skinfold thickness obtained with calipers (Durnin & Womersley 1974).

A more detailed consideration of the content, function and regulation of the individual components of these subdivisions is given below.

WATER

The major constituent of the body and the prime nutritional requirement is water, which comprises 50–80% of the body weight. The contribution of total body water is lower in females than in males of the same weight and in the obese. Its contribution to body weight decreases with age and the values shown in Figure 1.1 are useful working approximations. Thus a middle–aged man of average build weighing 70 kg has a total body water of 45 l and a middle-aged female of average build weighing 60 kg has a total body water of 33 l. Total body water is divided into two major compartments, the intracellular and extracellular water (ICW and ECW) by the semi-permeable cell wall (Figs 1.1 and 1.3) which is freely permeable to water but less so to electrolytes. The intracellular compartment is

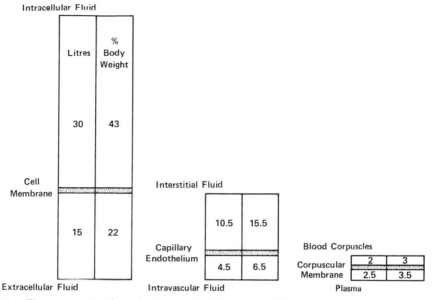

Fig. 1.3 The components of total body water (healthy 70 kg male)

greater and the intracellular fluid (ICF) of the 70 kg man is about 15 l. The extracellular fluid is further subdivided into interstitial fluid (IF) between the cells and intravascular fluid (IVF) separated by capillary endothelium which in health is permeable to water and electrolytes but not to protein (Fig. 1.3). The interstitial fluid compartment is the larger, comprising about 10.5 l. However, unlike other fluid compartments in the body, there is a portion (about 10%) of the interstitial fluid in some connective tissue that is relatively unavailable for equilibration. Finally the intravascular fluid volume of 4.5 l is subdivided into a red cell volume of 2 l and a plasma volume of 2.5 l.

This division of the total body water into compartments separated by membranes of varying permeability to solutes such as protein and electrolytes is a vital factor in homeostasis and changes in membrane permeability induced by disease processes have profoundly deleterious effects as will be discussed later. The function of these membranes and the mechanisms involved in the control of the flow of water and solutes between these compartments will now be considered in more detail.

Diffusion
The particles of a substance in solution are usually continually moving and if they are particularly concentrated in one area, they collide frequently. Consequently, they tend to disperse to areas of low concentration until uniformity of concentration is reached. If a solution of sodium chloride (NaCl) is separated from water by a membrane that is permeable to sodium (Na^+) and chloride (Cl^-), hydrogen (H^+) and hydroxyl (OH^-) ions, then these ions will pass through the membrane until the concentration of each ion is the same in both compartments (Fig. 1.4). The rate of diffusion will depend upon the difference in the concentration of the ions on either side of the membrane and its permeability.

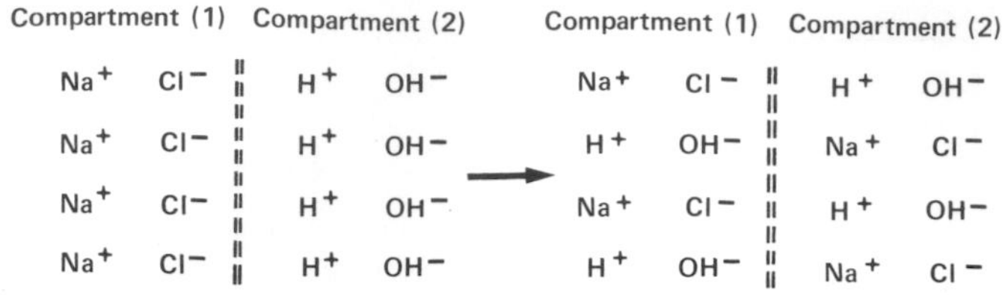

Compartment (1)		Compartment (2)		Compartment (1)		Compartment (2)	
Na$^+$	Cl$^-$	H$^+$	OH$^-$	Na$^+$	Cl$^-$	H$^+$	OH$^-$
Na$^+$	Cl$^-$	H$^+$	OH$^-$	H$^+$	OH$^-$	Na$^+$	Cl$^-$
Na$^+$	Cl$^-$	H$^+$	OH$^-$	Na$^+$	Cl$^-$	H$^+$	OH$^-$
Na$^+$	Cl$^-$	H$^+$	OH$^-$	H$^+$	OH$^-$	Na$^+$	Cl$^-$

Fig. 1.4 Ionic diffusion across a permeable membrane determined by the concentration gradient

The Donnan equilibrium and electrical neutrality

If a solution of sodium chloride is separated from a solution of the sodium salt of a protein (NaR) by a semi-permeable membrane that will allow the passage of sodium and chloride ions but not the protein ions (R$^-$) then an equilibrium is reached when the product of the concentrations of the sodium and chloride ions is the same on either side of the membrane (Fig. 1.5):

$$\text{Compartment (1)} \qquad\qquad \text{Compartment (2)}$$
$$2\text{Na}^+ \quad \times \quad 2\text{Cl}^- \quad = \quad 4\text{Na}^+ \quad \times \quad 1\text{Cl}^-$$

This equilibrium is named after its discoverer, the British physicist Donnan. The ionic concentration in each compartment is also influenced by the need for electrical neutrality in each compartment. Thus in Figure 1.5 the concentration of sodium ions in compartment (1) must be the same as the concentration of chloride ions, but in compartment (2) the concentration of sodium ions must be the same as the sum of the concentrations of the chloride and protein ions. As the products of the concentrations of sodium and chloride are the same on both sides of the membrane, it follows that the concentration of sodium ions is greater in compartment (2) than in compartment (1) and the converse holds for the concentration of chloride ions. It also follows that the concentration of osmotically active particles is greater in compartment (2).

Compartment (1)		Compartment (2)		Compartment (1)		Compartment (2)	
Na$^+$	Cl$^-$	Na$^+$	R$^-$			Na$^+$	R$^-$
				Na$^+$	Cl$^-$	Na$^+$	R$^-$
Na$^+$	Cl$^-$	Na$^+$	R$^-$			Na$^+$	R$^-$
				Na$^+$	Cl$^-$		
Na$^+$	Cl$^-$	Na$^+$	R$^-$			Na$^+$	Cl$^-$

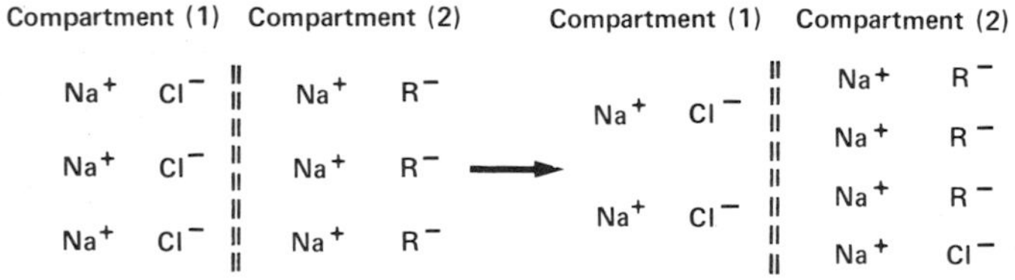

Fig. 1.5 Ionic diffusion across a semi–permeable membrane determined by the Donnan effect

This is the situation that exists in the body, the concentration of sodium in the plasma being slightly higher than in the interstitial fluid, the converse being the case for the chloride ion and, most important of all, the concentration of osmotically active particles is greater in the plasma. These features explain why the osmotic influence of the plasma proteins is greater than the 1–2 mosmol/l that they would be expected to exert.

Osmosis

With the exception of water in connective tissue, water may move rapidly between the various compartments through the cell membranes and vascular endothelium. Although hydrostatic pressure (arterial and venous blood pressure) influences fluid movement between the intravascular and interstitial compartments, the major force which determines fluid movement in the body is osmosis, (particularly between the intracellular and extracellular compartments). Osmosis is the attraction of particles for water which flows through a semi-permeable membrane such as the cell wall into the compartment containing the greater concentration of particles. Osmotic pressure is the number of osmotically active particles per unit volume and is usually expressed in milliosmoles per litre (mosmol/l), one millimole (mmol) of a substance in solution exerting one milliosmole of osmotic pressure. The osmolarity of body fluids can be determined in the laboratory by measuring the depression of freezing point, 1000 mosmol/l lowering freezing point by 1.86°C. Plasma, extracellular fluid and intracellular fluid osmolarities are the same and the normal range is 280–300 mosmol/l. Solutions within this range are termed isotonic and those of greater or lesser osmolarity are termed hypertonic or hypotonic accordingly. Osmotically active particles may be ionised (such as sodium) or non-ionised (such as glucose).

The composition of extracellular and intracellular fluid is shown in Figure 1.6 (modified from Gamble 1954). The concentrations of the cations and anions are shown in both mEq/l as originally defined by Gamble and in mmol/l as defined in the Système internationale. As discussed above, there must be electrical neutrality within each compartment. Consequently, when the concentrations of the substances in the compartments are expressed in mEq/l then the sum of the cations equals the sum of the anions. However, when the concentrations of these substances are expressed in mmol/l, then this convenient and understandable relationship apparently disappears, particularly in the intracellular compartment where the major ions are multivalent. The direction of this apparent distortion is reversed and of greater magnitude if the substances are expressed in mg/l when the contribution of protein to the anionic pool appears to be massive due to its large molecular weight.

The composition of the intracellular fluid varies according to the type and function of the cell and obtaining and analysing samples of pure intracellular fluid is a difficult procedure. The concentrations shown in Figure 1.6 should be considered to be approximate values only. The predominant osmotically active particles of the intracellular fluid are the ions potassium and phosphate, and of the extracellular fluid the ions sodium and chloride. However, osmotically active substances that cannot pass through membranes easily (if at all) have the greatest effect upon the intercompartmental movement of fluid between the intravascular and interstitial compartments. This factor is termed the oncotic or colloid osmotic pressure.

It can be seen from Figure 1.7 that at the arterial end of a capillary, the hydrostatic pressure acting in an outwards direction (32 mmHg) is greater than the oncotic pressure acting in an inwards direction (25 mmHg) and so water flows into the interstitial space. At the venous end of the capillary the hydrostatic pressure acting outwards (15 mmHg) is less than the oncotic pressure acting inwards (10 mmHg) and water flows into the capillary. This description ignores the usually trivial interstitial pressure (1 mmHg). Even the healthy capillary endothelium is not totally impermeable to protein and consequently small quantities of protein

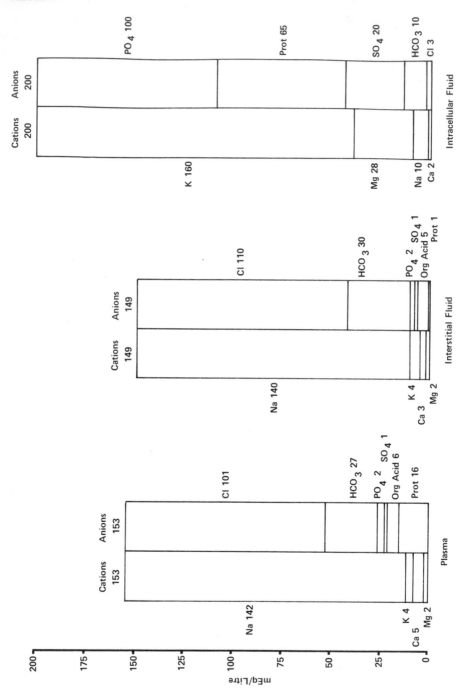

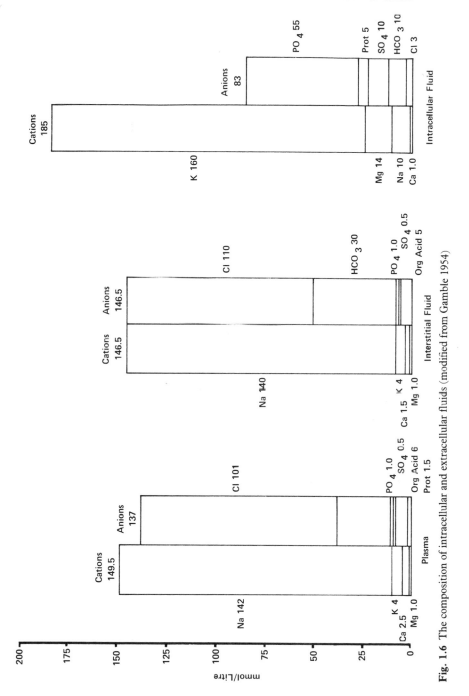

Fig. 1.6 The composition of intracellular and extracellular fluids (modified from Gamble 1954)

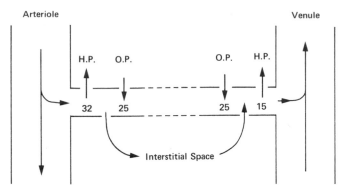

Fig. 1.7 The influence of hydrostatic pressure (H.P.) and oncotic pressure (O.P.) upon movement of fluid in the interstitial space (figures shown are in mmHg, for kPa divide by 7.52)

are continually extruded into the interstitial space. If it remained there, it would seriously impede the normal flow of fluid across the capillary endothelium by reducing the effect of the plasma oncotic pressure. However, under normal circumstances, such extruded protein is removed rapidly by lymphatic drainage. This scheme of fluid movement across the capillary wall was discovered by the physiologist Starling (1896) and extensively investigated by Guyton (1969). The clinical importance of osmosis is further emphasised by considering the effect of the addition of various fluids to body compartments (Fig. 1.8). Water is never infused intravenously as it may cause a fatal haemolytic anaemia. However, a similar effect is achieved by overinfusion of isotonic glucose solution (5%) which, upon metabolism of the carbohydrate, yields metabolic water in addition to that in the solution. The water is rapidly distributed through both the intercellular and intracellular compartments until they have the same osmolarity. Thus both the extracellular and intracellular spaces are increased in size. If an isotonic crystalloidal solution (such as 0.9% saline solution) is infused intravenously, the majority of the solution passes rapidly through the endothelium into the interstitial space. Cells contain very little sodium which is actively pumped through the cell membrane. As the solution is isotonic no water is withdrawn from the intracellu-

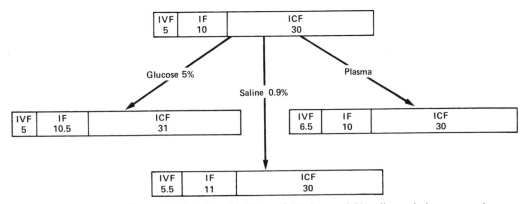

Fig. 1.8 The early effects of the infusion of 1.5 litres of 5% glucose, 0.9% saline and plasma upon the volume (litres) of the intravascular fluid (IVF), the interstitial fluid (IF) and the intracellular fluid (ICF)

lar space. Thus only the extracellular space is increased in size. If a colloidal solution (e.g. blood, plasma or dextran) is infused then very little escapes through the vascular endothelium so that expansion is confined to the intravascular compartment. These solutions usually increase oncotic pressure so that water is withdrawn from the interstitial space and eventually from the intracellular space. Thus infusions of colloidal solutions increase the intravascular space and usually decrease the interstitial and the intracellular spaces.

These three examples of the expansion of different fluid compartments by the infusion of different solutions emphasise that the possession of a thorough knowledge of basic medical science is an essential requirement for effective clinical therapy.

Water balance

In a healthy subject water intake and output vary considerably but usually water intake is determined by the need to cover requirements of water lost from four routes:

Water loss

a. Skin. Cutaneous loss of water vapour varies greatly, depending on body metabolism and the temperature and humidity of the environment. This environment is not only dependent on conditions existing in the room or ward but also upon clothing and bedding. In temperate climates cutaneous loss of water is about 600 ml/d (Table 1.1). This loss can be increased dramatically by sweating, particularly in tropical climates.

Table 1.1 The normal daily water intake and output in a temperate climate

Intake (ml)		Output (ml)	
Fluid	1400	Faeces	100
Solids	1000	Urine	400
Metabolism	200	Sweat	0
	2600	Skin	600
		Lungs	400
			2600

b. Lungs. Air entering the lungs is saturated with water vapour and some of this is lost to the atmosphere on exhalation. In health this loss amounts to about 400 ml/d (Table 1.1). This loss can increase to 1500 ml/d in a patient with a tracheostomy, particularly if the inspired air is unhumidified.

The combined loss from skin and lungs is sometimes termed 'insensible' or 'inevitable' and is close to 1000 ml/d which is the amount that is usually added to the measured losses on the daily fluid balance sheets on the ward.

c. Stomach and intestines. Faecal loss in health averages 100 ml/d but may be much greater in patients with diarrhoea. Gastric loss occurs only in disease but may be considerable due to vomiting or nasogastric aspiration. The typical volumes of fluid secreted into the gastro–intestinal tract and reabsorbed each day are shown in Table 1.2 and it is evident that fluid losses from this source by mouth, nasogastric tube, rectum or fistula may be considerable.

Table 1.2 The volume and electrolyte content of the daily intestinal secretions

Secretion	Volume (ml)	Concentration (mmol/l)			
		Na^+	K^+	Cl^-	HCO_3^-
Saliva	1500	15	30	10	30
Gastric	2000	50	15	120	–
Small bowel	3000	140	10	100	30
Bile	600	140	5	100	35
Pancreatic	700	140	5	70	100

d. Kidneys.   Water balance is usually determined by the volume of urine formed each day, the kidneys excreting any water in excess of requirements. In health 1100 litres of plasma flow through the kidneys each day of which 180 litres of fluid pass through the glomerular filters. Nearly all of this is reabsorbed, only 1500 ml/d being voided. As well as excreting excessive quantities of water, the kidneys must also excrete unwanted solutes. The kidneys are able to excrete these solutes in a small quantity of urine by their ability to transport solutes across a concentration gradient in the cell. However, there is a limit to this ability and consequently there is a minimal volume of urine in which the solute can be excreted and this is about 500 ml/d.

Water intake
Thus a healthy adult has a requirement of 2000–2500 ml of water per day which is met from three sources:
   1. Drinking water.   Although many subjects consume far greater volumes of fluid than required for urinary excretion of waste products, most individuals have an intake of about 1400 ml/day.
   2. Water in food.   It is frequently forgotten that food contains a large quantity of water and that intake in this form is almost as much as that in drink, amounting to about 1000 ml each day.
   3. Metabolic water.   Water is released by the oxidation of hydrogen atoms contained in energy substrates, particularly carbohydrates. Sometimes this is referred to as water of oxidation. In health the quantity is small, amounting to about 200 ml per day. However, if large volumes of isotonic glucose solution are infused, rapid utilisation produces carbon dioxide which is excreted by the lungs and water which, if not excreted by the kidneys as rapidly as it is formed, may cause overhydration and hypo–osmolarity.

MINERALS

The requirements, function and homeostasis of the major minerals of the body (sodium, potassium, calcium, magnesium, chlorine, phosphorus and sulphur) have been known for many years but it is only recently that requirements for at least 14 other minerals have been established. These minerals are usually referred to as the trace metals, as the trace quantities found in normal intake are sufficient. The content and extracellular and intracellular distribution of the major minerals are shown in Table 1.3.

Table 1.3 The mineral content of a healthy 70 kg male

| | Body content | | Concentration (mmol/kg) | |
	g	mmol	ECF	ICF
Sodium	90*	3900	142	5.0
Potassium	135	3400	4.5	130
Magnesium	25	1000	1.0	15
Calcium	1100	27 500	2.5	trace
Chloride	75	2100	103	5.0
Phosphorus	700	22 600	1.5	90
Bicarbonate	50	825	25	15
Sulphur	150	5500	1[†]	10[†]

* Only 63 g (2700 mmol) is freely exchangeable (see text)
[†] As sulphate

Sodium

A healthy 70 kg male contains approximately 90 g (3900 mmol) of sodium (Na), 45% being in the extracellular fluid, 10% in the intracellular fluid and 45% in bone. About 40% of the sodium in bone is freely exchangeable so that about 70% (63 g or 2700 mmol) of the sodium in the body is freely exchangeable.

Sodium is the predominant cation of the extracellular fluid (Fig. 1.6). As there must be electrical neutrality within each compartment, then the concentration of sodium in the extracellular fluid is also the major determinant of the anion concentration and the osmolarity of the extracellular fluid. The concentration of sodium in the extracellular fluid is 139–145 mmol/l, but only 10 mmol/l in the intracellular fluid. However, this difference in concentration and the converse difference in the concentration of potassium on either side of the cell membrane is not due to membrane impermeability. Sodium will pass quite readily from the extracellular fluid to the intracellular fluid, through the cell membrane, but the cell pumps it out again. There is some disagreement about whether potassium enters the cell by a similar mechanism to maintain electrical neutrality. This ionic pump requires energy and is one of the essential homeostatic mechanisms that determine basal metabolic energy requirements.

The major loss of sodium in a healthy adult is in the urine, but the kidney can retain large quantities if required. In the proximal tubules 80% of the sodium in the glomerular filtrate is reabsorbed passively and in the distal tubules a varying amount may be reabsorbed under the influence of aldosterone. Although 80% of sodium in the glomerular filtrate is reabsorbed regardless and only 20% is available for absorption or excretion according to requirements, 175 litres of glomerular filtrate are formed each day and the latter mechanism is an important factor in acid-base balance (see Ch. 4). Sweat is hypotonic and is an unimportant source of sodium loss in temperate climates and even in acclimatised patients undergoing surgery in the tropics (Tinckler 1966).

Sodium secretion into the gastro–intestinal tract averages some 700 mmol/d (Table 1.2) but nearly all this is reabsorbed and faecal loss of sodium is insignificant in the absence of diarrhoea. In a healthy individual, the major determinant of loss of sodium is the intake, 90 mmol being excreted in the urine and 10 mmol in the faeces and sweat with a daily intake of 100 mmol.

Potassium

A healthy 70 kg male contains approximately 135 g (3400 mmol) of potassium (K). The extracellular and intracellular distribution of potassium is the opposite to that of sodium and more uneven, 98% being in the intracellular fluid and only 2% in the extracellular fluid. Thus in the intracellular fluid, potassium with a concentration of 160 mmol/l has a corresponding role to sodium in the extracellular fluid, being the major determinant of the anion concentration and the osmolarity of the intracellular fluid. About 75% of the total body potassium is contained in skeletal muscle. Although the concentration of potassium in the extracellular fluid is low (3.5–4.5 mmol/l) its concentration is carefully regulated as it has profound effects upon neuromuscular conductivity, particularly upon the heart and intestines. As only 2% of the potassium in the body is in the extracellular fluid, plasma concentration is of little value as an index of the content in the body. In ill patients, balance studies provide a useful guide to therapeutic requirements but accurate information can be obtained under suitable conditions by radio–isotope dilution or whole–body scanning.

A healthy adult has a daily intake of about 60 mmol of which 55 mmol is excreted in the urine. Potassium excretion in the urine is determined partly by its concentration in the extracellular fluid, increases in concentration resulting in increased excretion. However renal conservation of potassium is not well developed and renal excretion of potassium continues in the face of intracellular depletion. Under normal conditions no more than 5 mmol/d are excreted in the faeces and sweat.

Calcium

A healthy 70 kg male contains approximately 1100 g (27 500 mmol) of calcium (Ca) of which 99% is contained in the skeleton as a complex salt, hydroxyapatite [$Ca_{10} (PO_4)_6 (OH)_2$]. Isotopic studies with ^{47}Ca suggest that only 5 g (125 mmol) of this is freely exchangeable. Although this is a very small quantity in terms of the total contained in the skeleton it is a very large quantity when compared with circulating calcium.

The calcium content in the plasma is 2.5–2.8 mmol/l and it exists in three forms:

a. As non-ionised protein-bound calcium — 50%
b. As calcium anion complexes — 5%
c. As divalent cations (Ca^{2+}) — 45%

It is the latter fraction, which is readily available, that is of major physiological importance, affecting neuromuscular conductivity, cell membrane function, enzyme activity, calcification and coagulation. Unfortunately the measurement of ionised calcium is a difficult process and routine estimation in the laboratory is usually of the total calcium content of the plasma. These analytical problems have clinical relevance, for biochemical hypocalcaemia may reflect hypoproteinaemia without disturbance of the homeostatic mechanisms requiring ionic calcium. The concentration of the serum proteins should be measured to allow adequate interpretation of total calcium content.

The concentration of calcium in the interstitial fluid is a little lower than that in the plasma as there is very little protein. The calcium in bone, although strictly extracellular, is not considered to be a part of the interstitial fluid as so little is readily available. The intracellular fluid contains only 1 mmol/l of calcium. The daily calcium intake is usually 1–2 g with an adult requirement of 600 mg in the diet. However, only 100–200 mg are excreted in the urine and the remainder, depending on intake, in the faeces. Although the major portion in the faeces is ingested calcium, some comes from intestinal secretions. The calcium content in sweat is unimportant in temperate climates.

Although parathormone and calcitonin indirectly influence calcium balance, the predominant function of these hormones is to maintain normal plasma concentration of ionic calcium. Parathormone is secreted by the parathyroid gland in response to hypocalcaemia, increasing resorption of calcium from bone, absorption in the duodenum and jejunum, and reabsorption in the kidney. Calcitonin is released rapidly in response to hypercalcaemia and inhibits resorption of calcium from bone.

Magnesium
A healthy 70 kg male contains approximately 25 g (1000 mmol) of magnesium (Mg) of which 50% is contained in bone. The concentration of magnesium in plasma is 0.8–1.2 mmol/l representing only 1% of the total body content. Magnesium is the second greatest contributor to the intracellular pool of cations with a concentration of approximately 15 mmol/l.

The normal daily intake of magnesium is 10–15 mmol of which 5 mmol are absorbed in the upper jejunum, 5 mmol excreted in the faeces and 5 mmol excreted in the urine. The control of magnesium concentration and balance is not clear but it may be influenced by parathormone. Magnesium content can now be measured in most laboratories by atomic absorption spectrophotometry.

Chloride ion
The chloride ion (Cl^-) is the principal anion of the extracellular fluid. A healthy 70 kg male contains approximately 2100 mmol with a concentration in the plasma of 97–102 mmol/l and a concentration in the intracellular fluid of 3 mmol/l. Its concentration and content in the body are determined principally by the concentration and content of sodium, but occasionally in some disease states the change in content of chloride is secondary to changes in the content of another ion (e.g. the hydrogen ion in pyloric stenosis).

Chloride is excreted predominantly in the urine. Like sodium it passes through the glomerular filter and 80% is reabsorbed in the proximal tubule. To a large extent, an equivalent quantity of chloride ions is reabsorbed to neutralise the quantity of sodium ions absorbed in the distal tubule. However, chloride reabsorption in the distal tubule is influenced by the acid–base status of the body as discussed in greater detail in Chapter 4. Thus bicarbonate ions may be reabsorbed and chloride ions excreted in the urine.

Bicarbonate ion
The bicarbonate ion (HCO_3^-) is the second largest component of the anion compartment of the extracellular fluid with a concentration of 24–28 mmol/l. Its intracellular concentration is lower, being about 10 mmol/l. Its concentration in

the body is determined to a great extent by the acid–base status and in general, the sum of the extracellular concentrations of chloride and bicarbonate ions is about 12 mmol/l less than the concentration of the sodium ions:

$$[Na^+] = [Cl^-] + [HCO_3^-] + 12 \text{ mmol/l}$$

Although bicarbonate ions may be ingested in various proprietary agents used in the treatment of indigestion, under usual circumstances oral intake is negligible, bicarbonate ions being formed in the body by the combination of water and carbon dioxide:

$$H_2O + CO_2 \rightleftharpoons H^+ + HCO_3^-$$

This reaction is reversible so that not only can bicarbonate ions be excreted by the kidney but they can also be excreted effectively by elimination of carbon dioxide through the lungs. These important mechanisms for the maintenance of acid–base homeostasis are discussed in detail in Chapter 4.

Protein ion

The macroscopic distribution of protein has been discussed above. Although not strictly a mineral, protein is considered here in view of its importance in electrolyte balance within the cell. Protein ions are zwitterions capable of acting as cations or anions, but in the acid environment of the body they act as anions. In the plasma, the many proteins that constitute the fraction called plasma protein have a concentration of 1.5 mmol/l (because of the analytical methods used in their estimation in the laboratory, plasma protein concentration is usually expressed as 60–80 g/l). As discussed above, the concentration of protein in the interstitial fluid is negligible. In the cells constituting the lean body mass of the body, the intracellular concentration of protein is 5 mmol/l.

Protein requirements and abnormal losses are discussed in detail in later chapters. A healthy adult requires 1 g/kg daily but many individuals in Western countries consume almost double this quantity and most of the excess is partly catabolised and the nitrogen excreted as urea in the urine. Protein loss in the faeces is usually 10–20 g/d and is a mixture of undigested protein enzymes and desquamated cells.

Phosphorus

A 70 kg male contains approximately 700 g of phosphorus which exists in the body in organic and inorganic forms. Organic phosphorus is combined with fat to form phospholipids that circulate in the plasma and form important components of the walls of cell membranes and intracellular organelles. The major portion of the phosphorus in the body is in the inorganic form as phosphate salts, approximately 80% being in the skeleton as hydroxyapatite (see above under Calcium).

Phosphorus is also an important component of metabolities such as adenosine triphosphate and creatinine phosphate, where the phosphate linkages yield a large quantity of energy upon breakdown. In theory the phosphate ion may be trivalent (PO_4^{3-}) but in the body it exists in divalent (HPO_4^{2-}) and monovalent ($H_2PO_4^-$) forms. At normal pH the divalent ion forms 80% and the monovalent ion forms 20% of the phosphate anion in the extracellular fluid. The ratio of these different forms is important in acid–base balance (see Ch. 4). The concentration of inorganic phosphorus in the plasma and interstitial fluid is only 1–3 mmol/l but it is the largest component of the intracellular anion compartment with a concentration of 55 mmol/l.

The absorption, extracellular concentration and excretion of phosphorus is determined mainly by the metabolism of calcium. The product of the plasma concentration of the two ions is constant so that an increase in the concentration of calcium results in a depression of the concentration of phosphorus and vice versa. Phosphorus is prevalent in the diet but is frequently deficient in intravenous feeding regimens.

Sulphur

A 70 kg male contains some 175 g of sulphur (5500 mmol). Although a small portion exists as inorganic sulphate in the body fluids and a larger quantity exists in a similar state in cartilage, sulphur occurs predominantly in the cell in proteins that incorporate the sulphur–containing amino acids, methionine and cystine. The concentration of the sulphate anion is also greater within the cell (Fig. 1.6 and Table 1.3). The major source of sulphur in the diet is from the amino acids methionine and cystine. Methionine cannot be synthesised in the body and must be included in the diet. A specific deficiency of this amino acid can be induced artificially but the normal diet usually contains ample quantities of this and of cystine and consequently a specific deficiency of sulphur in the body has not been observed. A daily requirement cannot be quantified but a daily amino acid intake of 1 g/kg body weight would supply a 70 kg male with approximately 25 mmol of sulphur.

Trace elements

This term is preferable to the more traditional term trace metals. A more recent term used to embrace these substances is essential biological elements. However, the term has nothing to commend it as elements such as sodium and potassium are also included in this category. The word 'trace' emphasises the distinguishing feature of these elements, namely that only trace quantities are required in the diet. The increasing recognition of trace element requirements is due in part to the increasing use of long–term parenteral nutrition with modern synthetic solutions. In the past electrolyte solutions were less pure and amino acid solutions were hydrolysates of protein so that trace quantities of these elements may have been contained in these solutions. Fourteen trace elements (chromium, cobalt, copper, fluorine, iodine, iron, manganese, molybdenum, nickel, selenium, silicon, tin, vanadium and zinc) are known to be required for normal growth and development of various animals (Underwood 1977) although a role for all of these has not been established in man. The major role of these metals is to act as an essential cofactor for effective function of specific enzymes. Until recently only seven of these elements (cobalt, copper, iron, fluorine, iodine, manganese and zinc) were considered to be important in the human but it has been suggested that trace quantities of chromium (Jeejeebhoy et al 1977) may also be required. Trace element deficiency is a rare occurrence in man and this account will be re-

Table 1.4 The weekly requirements of trace elements with an established role in man (μmol)

Cobalt	2 †
Copper	100
Iron	100*
Fluorine	100
Iodine	5
Manganese	200
Zinc	300

* The requirements of pre-menopausal females are higher (see text)
† This is usually given in the form of vitamin B_{12} (see text)

stricted to a brief consideration of the role of the seven established elements listed in Table 1.4. The figures given for daily requirements of cobalt, copper, fluorine, manganese and zinc should be considered as a rough guide only as precise data are extremely difficult to obtain due to difficulties of analysis.

Iron
Of all the trace elements, the metabolism of iron (Fe) is the most fully understood. As well as its major role in the formation of haemoglobin and myoglobin, iron is also an ingredient of many enzymes such as the cytochromes and peroxidases. The figure given in Table 1.4 is for males and post–menopausal females. Premenopausal females require approximately 250 μmol per week.

Iodine
Iodine (I) is required for the iodination of tyrosine to form the thyroid hormones, tri–iodothyronine and thyroxine.

Fluorine
The question of whether fluorine (F) is or is not an essential requirement for normal metabolism in man has provoked tremendous controversy. In spite of the violent emotional arguments raised against the fluoridation of water supplies, there can now be little doubt that trace quantities are required for the development of healthy teeth. Fluorine is also present in the skeleton.

Copper
Copper (Cu) is required for the normal maturation of red and white blood cells and the production of enzymes such as cytochrome oxidase and monoamine oxidase.

Zinc
If iron deficiency is the commonest deficiency of a trace element, zinc (Zn) deficiency is the next most common. Its distribution thoughout the body is widespread in enzymes such as carbonic anhydrase lactic acid dehydrogenase and carboxypeptidases.

Cobalt
Cobalt (Co) in the form of vitamin B_{12} is required for normal development of red and white blood cells and for normal neurological function. The weekly require-

ments of cobalt are more than covered by the intramuscular injection of 250 μg vitamin B_{12} (cyanocobalamine).

Manganese

Although manganese (Mn) is required for the formation or the activation of many enzymes such as pyruvate carboxylase involved in oxidative phosphorylation and deficiency syndromes have been described in experimental animals, deficiency of this element has not been described in man.

VITAMINS

When healthy animals were fed a chemically pure diet containing enough protein, carbohydrate, fat, minerals and water to meet their requirements, they died. It was evident that natural food contained some other constituent essential to sustain life. When it was shown that the disease beriberi could be prevented by the addition of 'unpolished' rice to the diet, the active ingredient in the rice 'polishings' was termed a vitamine (i.e. a vital amine). Subsequently, it became apparent that there was a number of such substances and that few of them were amines and so the word was respelt vitamin. Some vitamins are soluble in fat and some in water.

Vitamins are similar to trace elements. Both are required in very small quantities for highly specific functions within the body. They have high biological activity and cannot be replaced by other elements or vitamins, although some animals can synthesise certain vitamins (e.g. the rat can synthesise vitamin C).

It has not been customary to consider vitamins as a constituent of the body. However, these substances are stored in varying quantities, mainly in the liver and the kidney, and may therefore be considered to be components of the lean body mass. The extent to which vitamins are stored varies considerably from individual to individual and precise information of the intracellular and extracellular concentrations of individual vitamins is not available due to difficulties in measurement. Studies of the rate in which deficiency syndromes develop on a vitamin–free intake suggest that fat–soluble vitamins may be stored in considerable quantities, but that storage of water-soluble vitamins is much less extensive. Deficiencies of water–soluble vitamins may occur in three or four weeks but healthy individuals fed a diet lacking in vitamin A may only develop signs of deficiency after one year. However, abnormal haemostasis due to deficient intake of vitamin K in patients with obstructive jaundice may occur in two or three weeks. It is uncommon for a diet to be totally lacking in vitamin content, and mixed deficiencies are not uncommon.

As the precise measurement of vitamin content and concentration has only recently become available in special centres, the requirement for various vitamins in health and disease has been based upon studies involving the appearance and disappearance of clinical deficiency syndromes during known oral intakes. More is known about these requirements in health than in disease. The recommended oral intakes of vitamins are shown in Table 1.5 and are based predominantly upon those suggested for healthy, adult males by the Department of Health and Social Security (1969). The requirements of pregnant or lactating females are a

Table 1.5 Recommended oral intakes of fat-soluble and water-soluble vitamins (per day)

Vitamin A (retinol)	2500 iu
Vitamin D$_3$	100 iu
Vitamin E*	30 mg
Vitamin K$_1$ (phylloquinone)	0.3 mg
Thiamine	1.5 mg
Riboflavine	1.7 mg
Pyridoxine	2 mg
Folic acid	300 μg
Hydroxocobalamine	3 μg
Biotin	300 μg
Pantothenic acid	10 mg
Vitamin C	30 mg

* May not be required — see text

little greater, particularly for vitamins A, D and C. These intakes are recommended for maintenance and therapeutic requirements in disease or deficiency may be greater.

The requirements during intravenous feeding present a particularly confusing picture. It would appear that if large quantities of water-soluble vitamins are given intravenously by bolus injection, a large proportion of the infused vitamins are excreted in the urine as the plasma concentration exceeds the renal threshold. Some vitamins may be destroyed by sunlight and others may become inactive if stored in solution with amino acids. Consequently, intravenous supplements of water-soluble vitamins should be added to simple crystalloidal solutions immediately before infusion and the bottle protected from sunlight, if necessary by using a cloth or bag. The majority of patients requiring intravenous feeding are already nutritionally impoverished or have increased requirements and the recommended intravenous intakes shown in Table 1.6 are provisional suggestions based upon the knowledge available at the present time. Although the daily requirements are shown, it may prove satisfactory to give suitable quantities of the fat–soluble vitamins as a weekly supplement. Many patients requiring intravenous feeding are capable of ingesting and absorbing their vitamin requirements from the gastro – intestinal tract if the supplement is in the form of an elixir. If this route is unavailable, vitamin supplements may also be given by intramuscular injection.

Table 1.6 Recommended intravenous intakes of fat–soluble and water–soluble vitamins (per day)

Vitamin A (retinol)	3000 iu
Vitamin D$_3$	250 iu
Vitamin E*	30 mg
Vitamin K$_1$ (phylloquinone)	0.3 mg
Thiamine	3 mg
Riboflavine	3 mg
Nicotinic acid	30 mg
Pyridoxine	4 mg
Folic acid	600 μg
Hydroxocobalamine	5 μg
Biotin	300 μg
Pantothenic acid	15 mg
Vitamin C	60 mg

* May not be required — see text

Fat-soluble vitamins

Vitamins A, D and K are vital to the human. Although vitamin E is an essential component of the diet in many animals, an essential role in man is still uncertain. Being fat–soluble, these vitamins require bile to ensure normal intestinal absorption. When given by the intravenous route it may be satisfactory and is usually more convenient to provide these vitamins as a weekly supplement.

Vitamin A

Vitamin A (retinol) can be synthesised in the body from a precursor, carotene, but the latter is less well absorbed and has only half the biological activity of the vitamin. Both are yellow–red pigments necessary for normal vision (particularly for dark adaption) and for normal development of the epithelia of the eyes and the respiratory, gastro–intestinal and genito–urinary systems. Deficiency produces thickening, keratinisation and metaplasia of these epithelia. The recognition that deficiency of this enzyme renders experimental animals more susceptible to the development of malignancy has provoked interest in a possible role in human malignancies.

The daily requirements of vitamin A are not known but 2500 iu (equivalent to 0.75 mg retinol) or 5000 iu carotene orally are known to be sufficient to prevent the development of vitamin A deficiency in health and will not produce exfoliative dermatitis. Normal intake is 7500–10 000 iu daily and any excess is stored mainly in the liver. This store contains sufficient vitamin A to cover normal requirements for at least one year, but requirements are greatly increased by infection. In patients requiring intravenous feeding, vitamin A is preferable to carotene, and it is suggested that the daily intravenous provision should be 3000 iu.

Vitamin D

Vitamin D_3 is formed in the skin by the action of ultraviolet irradiation upon 7–dehydrocholesterol and is the naturally occurring vitamin found in egg-yolk, butter, and fish liver oils. Vitamin D_2 is formed by the action of ultraviolet irradiation on the provitamin ergosterol, which is present in certain plants such as yeast. Both vitamin D_2 and D_3 increase calcium and phosphorus absorption from the intestine and deposition of these minerals in bone. These functions are closely interdependent on those of parathormone and calcitonin.

It is evident that the daily requirements of vitamin D depend upon the amount of ultraviolet irradiation from sunlight received by the body and in normal circumstances synthesis of vitamin D_3 in the skin is sufficient to cover all needs. In patients receiving intravenous feeding 250 iu vitamin D_3 daily appears to be sufficient and will not produce hypercalcaemia.

Vitamin E

The tocopherols (vitamin E is α-tocopherol) are yellowish oils which are powerful anti–oxidants. Deficiency of vitamin E is associated with a number of clinical syndromes in many animals, the most well-known being the occurrence of sterility in rats. Deficiency of this vitamin has not been clearly established in man, although it has been suggested that muscular dystrophy and haemolytic anaemia may be associated with a deficient intake. Nevertheless, the Food and Nutrition Board of the National Academy of Sciences — National Research Council, Washington, USA recommends a daily intake of 10–30 mg depending on the intake of fatty acids. In patients receiving intravenous nutrients the required quantity is contained in the fat emulsion, Intralipid®. Patients receiving fat-free intravenous nutrients may not have any requirement for vitamin E.

Vitamin K

Vitamin K_1 (phylloquinone) is synthesised by green plants and contained in the diet. Vitamin K_2 and K_3 (menaquinone and naphthoquinone) are synthesised by intestinal bacteria in man and other animals. This synthesis can be disturbed by the use of oral antibiotics. Vitamin K is required for the formation of a number of blood coagulation factors, particularly prothrombin. The requirement is uncertain but 2 mg weekly appears to be sufficient to prevent abnormalities of haemostasis. Vitamin K_2 and K_3 should not be given intravenously as they may produce haemolysis and other toxic reactions.

Water–soluble vitamins

Vitamin B and vitamin C are the water–soluble vitamins. Vitamin B has been shown to consist of a number of closely related compounds referred to as the vitamin B complex, but each of these compounds is a separate vitamin with a specific action and a characteristic disease is associated with each deficiency. They are essential constituents of common enzyme systems and most of them can be synthesised by intestinal bacteria. Consequently, like vitamin K, exogenous requirement may be increased by the use of oral antibiotics.

Thiamine

Thiamine (vitamin B, B_1, or aneurin as it was known formerly) is the vitamin that is contained in the husk of rice and beriberi is the disease associated with the eating of polished rice in the Far East where thiamine deficiency is still endemic in some areas. Thiamine acts as a coenzyme that is required for many of the stages in the oxidation of carbohydrates. Its deficiency is associated with anorexia, weakness, confusion, paraesthesiae and ultimately in loss of sensation and paralysis. A daily oral intake of 1.5 mg is sufficient to cover requirements in the adult, and 3 mg should be given if the vitamin is infused intravenously.

Riboflavine

Riboflavine (vitamin B_2) forms the active group of the flavoproteins which act as carriers of hydrogen released by oxidation reactions. Deficiency of riboflavine is associated with recurrent lesions of the epithelia, particularly angular stomatitis. In view of the importance of the flavoproteins it is surprising that the clinical features of deficiency are less dramatic than might be expected. A daily oral intake of 1.7 mg or intravenous intake of 3 mg should be sufficient to meet adult requirements.

Nicotinic acid

Nicotinic acid (niacin or nicotinamide) can be produced from tryptophan by intestinal bacteria but the normal diet contains more than enough in the form of cereals, vegetables and meat. Nicotinamide is a component of the coenzymes NAD and NADP which are essential for hydrogen transport in glycolysis and aerobic respiration. Deficiency of the vitamin produces metabolic disturbances in many of the tissues of the body but the nervous system is particularly involved. The disease pellagra is characterised by dermatitis, gastro–enteritis and delirium. A daily oral intake of 20 mg is sufficient to prevent deficiency in the adult and 30 mg should be sufficient for intravenous requirements.

Pyridoxine

Pyridoxine (vitamin B_6) and other substances such as pyridoxamine can also be synthesised by intestinal bacteria, but like nicotinic acid this is an unimportant source in man. The vitamin is a coenzyme required in transamination, deamination and decarboxylation reactions. The metabolism of tryptophan is particularly affected. Deficiency may produce various forms of dermatitis and abnormal function of the central nervous system. A daily oral intake of 2 mg is recommended for adults, and 4 mg should be sufficient for intravenous requirements.

Folic acid

Folic acid is a coenzyme required for the synthesis of purines and pyrimidines and hence plays a vital role in cell division and maturation. Deficiency of this vitamin probably produces abnormalities in all tissues of the body where there is a high turnover of cells, but it is the red and white blood cells that are particularly affected with macrocytic anaemia and hypersegmentation of leucocytes being the characteristic features. A daily oral intake of 300 μg is suitable for adults.

Recent studies have shown that intravenous feeding with mixtures of amino acids, sorbitol, and ethanol produced rapid falls in red blood cell and plasma folate concentrations (Wardrop et al 1975). Although ethanol was originally implicated, similar falls have been observed in patients receiving intravenous nutrients without ethanol (Wardrop et al 1975, Ibbotson et al 1975). A daily intravenous supply of 600 μg should be sufficient to prevent this complication in all patients.

Hydroxocobalamine

Hydroxocobalamine (vitamin B_{12}) and closely related substances such as cyanocobalamine are important coenzymes located in the mitochondria but their precise role remains unknown. Like folic acid, deficiency of the vitamin produces abnormal haemopoiesis but in addition there is degeneration in the central nervous system. The vitamin requires a mucopolysaccharide (intrinsic factor) secreted by the stomach to facilitate its absorption in the distal ileum. Deficiency may occur in spite of a normal intake due to:

1. Lack of intrinsic factor (e.g. pernicious anaemia, carcinoma of stomach, partial gastrectomy)

2. Malabsorption (e.g. Crohn's disease, tuberculosis, ileal resection)

3. Bacterial overgrowth in the ileum (e.g. blind loop syndrome, intestinal diverticulosis).

The daily oral requirement for adults is 3 μg and 5 μg should be sufficient to meet intravenous requirements.

Biotin

Biotin is a coenzyme required for carboxylation and decarboxylation and deficiency in man may produce seborrhoeic dermatitis, lethargy and paraesthesia. The daily requirement is unknown but 300 μg has been suggested as adequate by the Food and Nutrition Board of the National Academy of Sciences (1979).

Pantothenic acid

Pantothenic acid is present in coenzyme A which is involved in the oxidation of carbohydrates and fatty acids and in the synthesis of cholesterol, steroid hormones and triglycerides. Deficiency is associated with fatigue and paraesthesiae but these clinical features only occur after many months. The diet contains 5–10 mg per day but the daily requirement is unknown and 15 mg is provisionally suggested for the intravenous requirement.

Vitamin C

Vitamin C (ascorbic acid) was isolated nearly 200 years after Captain Lind (1753) established that scurvy could be prevented by eating 'summer fruits and salads'. It is a strong reducing agent and easily oxidised by canning. Unlike man, many animals can synthesise this vitamin. The precise function of ascorbic acid is unknown but it is required for the hydroxylation of dopamine to noradrenaline and other steroid hormones. The daily intakes recommended for ascorbic acid vary greatly from country to country, but 30 mg orally should be sufficient to prevent deficiency, and 60 mg is suggested as the intravenous requirement.

2

Abnormalities of water and mineral metabolism

DEFICIENCY SYNDROMES

This chapter will be restricted to a consideration of the causes, effects and treatment of deficiency of water and minerals. The effects of starvation and injury, haemorrhage and deficiency of specific amino acids and fatty acids are discussed in Chapters 3, 5 and 8 respectively. The effects of deficiency of trace elements and of vitamins have been described in Chapter 1 and further details are given in Chapter 8.

In the majority of patients the maintenance of normal water and mineral balance is not difficult and may not tax the clinician unduly. The normal homeostatic mechanisms outlined briefly above may counteract minor abnormalities of intake, excretion or abnormal loss. However, in some patients these abnormalities may be so extensive as to require prompt correction or death will occur. In some of these patients there may be complex abnormalities with loss of water, sodium, potassium and magnesium combined with alterations in acid–base balance which will tax the clinician's skill to the limit, but most cases are more simple, involving only water or sodium deficiency.

A reduced extracellular or intracellular concentration of a mineral does not necessarily indicate a reduction in the total body content. Changes in concentration may be produced by changes in the content of water in these compartments without a corresponding change in the content of the mineral. A reduction in the compartmental concentration or the total body content of a mineral may be deleterious. Tetany may be produced by a reduction in the extracellular concentration of calcium without any change in the total body content. The total body content of calcium may be considerably reduced in patients with metabolic bone disease, but the extracellular concentration is normal.

Water depletion

The use of the term 'dehydration' should be confined to the lack of water alone, but it is more commonly used in clinical practice to describe the loss of sodium and water. When defined in this manner, combined deficiency of salt and water is one of the commonest problems observed in clinical practice and water depletion is less common. A relative lack of water can occur due to unavailability of a normal intake or, more commonly, due to excessive loss.

The maintenance of normal water balance is considered in Chapter 1. The common causes of water depletion are shown in Table 2.1.

Table 2.1 The causes of water depletion (these are often accompanied by sodium depletion — see text)

Inadequate intake	Excessive loss
Environment	Fever
Oropharyngeal and oesophageal disease	Hyperventilation
Coma	Artificial ventilation
Immobility	Intestinal obstruction
Apathy	Peritonitis
	Crush injury
	Burns
	Water–losing nephritis
	Diabetes insipidus
	Acute tubular necrosis (recovery phase)

Inadequate intake
The most dramatic but rare examples of dehydration due to deficient intake occur in individuals who are stranded at sea or on land without water, particularly when exposed to the sun (Gamble 1947). If those stranded at sea drink sea water, the excess salt is excreted by the kidneys with a susequent increase in the rate and extent of water loss. In hospital, some patients with lesions of the mouth, pharynx or oesophagus may have obvious difficulties in drinking sufficient water. There are many more patients, particularly on neurosurgical, geriatric and paediatric wards who, through apathy or disability, may suffer from an accumulating lack of water intake without doctors or nurses being aware of it.

Excessive loss
As with inadequate intake, the commonest causes of excessive water loss in hospital may be insidious. Artificial ventilation may rapidly increase water loss by evaporation if the inspired gases are insufficiently humidified and a similar loss may be produced by tracheostomy. It is often forgotten that simple hyperventilation and associated fever may have a similar effect. Fluid may be lost internally due to transcellular accumulation into the bowel lumen, into coelomic cavities such as the peritoneum or into the intercellular tissues following burns or crush injuries. This internal dislocation of extracellular fluid into the bowel lumen or coelomic spaces requires active transport across epithelial cells and is frequently referred to as 'third space loss'. The clinician must be aware of possible transcellular loss and of its potential magnitude as loss by this route cannot be assessed by normal clinical measurement. Loss of fluid into this third space invariably involves loss of sodium also. External loss of water and sodium accompanies the transcellular loss in patients with burns. Less common causes of water loss are lack of antidiuretic hormone (ADH) secreted by the posterior pituitary (diabetes insipidus) and water–losing nephritis. If recovery from acute tubular necrosis occurs, there is often a period of diuresis during which time the patient is unable to excrete a concentrated urine and large intakes of water and electrolytes may be required (see Ch. 7).

Clinical features
The fluid shifts and altered physiology induced by water and sodium depletion are compared in Figure 2.1. The initial effect of water depletion is to increase the

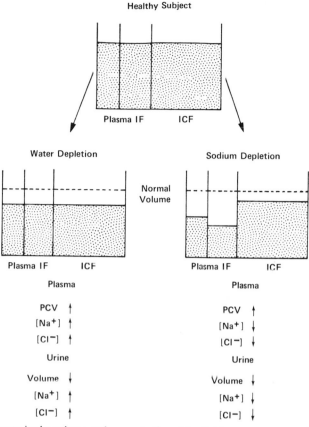

Fig. 2.1 The changes in the volume and concentration of the fluid compartments and urine output produced by water and sodium depletion

concentration and osmolarity of the extracellular fluid which provokes a shift of water from the intracellular space until there is the same tonicity on either side of the cell membrane. Thus, although there is a reduction in the extracellular space, the major effect of water deficiency is to produce an intracellular dehydration. The mechanism of this intracellular dehydration is shown in Table 2.2. If there is a sudden loss of 3 litres of water from the extracellular fluid without a corresponding loss of solute, then the osmolarity of the extracellular fluid increases con-

Table 2.2 The changes in the volume and concentration of the fluid compartments produced by water depletion

	Extracellular fluid		Intracellular fluid	
	Volume (l)	Osmolarity (mosmol/l)	Volume (l)	Osmolarity (mosmol/l)
Healthy subject	15	280	30	280
Initial extracellular water depletion	12	$\dfrac{280 \times 15}{12} = 350$	30	280
Subsequent extracellular and intracellular water depletion	14	$\dfrac{280 \times 15}{14} = 300$	28	$\dfrac{280 \times 30}{28} = 300$

siderably. Water is attracted from the intracellular space until the osmolarity is equal on both sides of the cell membrane which occurs at 300 mosmol/l when the extracellular volume is 14 litres and the intracellular volume is 28 litres. Thus the effect of a loss of 3 litres of water from the body is to reduce the extracellular volume by 1 litre and the intracellular volume by 2 litres. Although there is an absolute difference, the percentage reduction in the intracellular and extracellular compartments is the same. In practice the intracellular water loss keeps pace with the total body loss and initial extracellular water loss of the magnitude shown in this example does not occur. These changes should be compared with Table 2.9.

Although it is evident that the patient is not well, the clinical symptoms and signs of water loss are not very evident, particularly in the early stages. The sensation of thirst is poorly understood and is frequently influenced by psychological factors. Scientific studies of the mechanism of thirst have suggested that local reflexes in the pharynx (Cannon 1918) and distal reflexes in the hypothalamus (Anderson & McCann 1955) may be involved. A total lack of thirst usually accompanies combined water and sodium depletion, even when very severe. In severe dehydration thirst is accompanied by dryness of the mucous membrane, particularly in the mouth. Severe dehydration also produces a loss of skin turgor and sunken eyeballs but these signs are not evident in moderate dehydration. Eventually muscle weakness and mental depression may progress to coma and death. The increased concentration of the extracellular fluid is indicated by increased concentration of haemoglobin, packed cell volume and serum electrolytes and urea and the patient excretes a reduced volume of highly concentrated urine.

Treatment

The requirement is for water and the safest route is undoubtedly the gastro–intestinal tract as overloading by this route is almost impossible. In patients in whom the intravenous route must be used, either through the unavailability of the gastro–intestinal tract or because of the urgency of the clinical situation, hypotonic solutions may be infused. However, in most patients it is sufficient to infuse isotonic glucose solutions. One litre of isotonic glucose (5%) contains 53.3 g of glucose dissolved in 1000 g of water. Metabolism of the glucose will produce a further 32 g of water so that the net result of infusing 1 litre of isotonic glucose is to increase total body water by 1032 ml. If rapid correction is required in patients with cardiac or renal disease and there is concern lest the circulation be overloaded, the infusion rate should be regulated according to the response of the central venous pressure (see Ch. 5). The effectiveness of therapy can be gauged most accurately by serial measurement of the serum osmolarity. However, such precise measurement is unnecessary in the majority of patients and the technique is not available in every hospital. A decrease in serum osmolarity indicates satisfactory response to therapy. That the deficit has been fully restored can be ascertained by observing a return to normal values (or pre–dehydration values) of the serum electrolytes, urea, creatinine, total protein and albumin.

When starting treatment it is convenient to note that if thirst is present without clinical signs, a 70 kg male will usually require at least 1500 ml of water to restore his total body water to normal in addition to the 1500 ml or more that he requires to cover his losses for the coming day. If there are signs of a dry mouth and oliguria, the deficit will be at least 2 or 3 times as great. Some clinicians base their therapy upon the serum concentration of sodium e.g.

70 kg male; serum sodium concentration 154 mmol/l
TBW_1 = normal total body water (70×0.6 = 42 l)
Na_1 = normal serum sodium concentration
TBW_2 = actual total body water
Na_2 = actual serum sodium concentration

Then, assuming that there has been no loss of sodium

$$
\begin{aligned}
TBW_1 \times Na_1 &= TBW_2 \times Na_2 \\
42 \times 142 &= TBW_2 \times 154 \\
TBW_2 &= 38.7 \text{ litres} \\
\text{Deficit} &= 3.3 \text{ litres}
\end{aligned}
$$

Such calculations assume that only water and no sodium has been lost and that the serum concentration of sodium was 142 mmol/l before dehyration.

Sodium depletion

Loss of sodium is usually accompanied by loss of water also and, as the water and sodium are usually in the same proportion as in the extracellular fluid, the concentration of sodium in the extracellular fluid shows very little change. However, pure sodium depletion may also be observed. The common causes of sodium depletion are shown in Table 2.3.

Table 2.3 The causes of sodium depletion (these are often accompanied by water depletion — see text)

Inadequate intake	Excessive loss
Environment	Intestinal obstruction
Oropharyngeal or oesophageal disease	Peritonitis
Coma	Vomiting or aspiration
Immobility	Diarrhoea or fistulae
Apathy	Drainage of ascitic fluid
Saline–free infusion	Operation
	Lack of acclimatisation
	Crush injury
	Burns
	Diuretics
	Salt–losing nephritis
	Fibrocystic disease

Inadequate intake

All the causes of inadequate intake of water discussed above are usually associated with an inadequate intake of sodium. However, it is the water depletion that is of major importance. If a patient's fluid requirements are provided solely by intravenous dextrose solutions, then sodium depletion may occur. More often, such therapy induces little change in total body content of sodium but produces an extracellular and intracellular dilution of all the electrolytes (see overhydration).

Excessive loss

Loss of sodium and water is commonly observed in surgical practice due to intraluminal accumulation in obstruction of the gastro–intestinal tract and intraperitoneal accumulation in peritonitis. This internal, transcellular dislocation of sodium does not result in any true loss of sodium from the body, but the functional depletion of sodium induced in this way may be fatal. External loss of sodium may occur in obstruction or infection of the gastro-intestinal tract due to vomiting, nasogastric aspiration and diarrhoea. The sodium content of various gastro–intestinal secretions is shown in Table 1.2. Similar losses may be sustained as a consequence of drainage from fistulae according to the site in the bowel. Large quantities of sodium and water may be lost when ascitic fluid is drained from the abdominal cavity and as much as 1.5 litres of saline may be required to replace the extracellular fluid lost during extensive abdominal operations. Although an increased salt intake is always advised for those who are not acclimatised to a tropical environment to compensate for increased loss in sweat, studies of surgical patients in such surroundings have failed to demonstrate any increase in their requirements. Large quantities of sodium may be lost in patients with burns due to exudation. Diuretics including mercurials, thiazides, ethacrynic acid, furosemide and spironolactone may produce considerable sodium loss if given in excessive quantities over long periods of time. Salt–losing nephritis and fibrocystic disease of the pancreas (mucoviscidosis) are uncommon causes of severe loss of sodium.

Clinical features
The fluid shifts and altered physiology induced by water and sodium depletion are compared in Figure 2.1. The initial effect of sodium depletion may be a decrease in the concentration and osmolarity of the extracellular fluid. Some water may move into the intracellular space but the kidneys rapidly excrete more urine until extracellular tonicity is restored with a subsequent reduction in the extracellular volume. The oncotic pressure exerted by the plasma proteins usually ensures that there is little change in the intravascular compartment and it is the interstitial space that is reduced most. However, when sodium depletion is severe, the oncotic pressure is not sufficient to maintain the intravascular compartment which is also reduced in size. The signs and symptoms of sodium depletion are shown in Table 2.4. In contrast to the intracellular depletion produced by water deficiency, the extracellular depletion produced by sodium deficiency rarely causes thirst. The patient becomes weak and apathetic at a more early stage and may have cramps. Headache is common, particularly if the patient drinks water and his extracellular sodium concentration falls further, and as the condition

Table 2.4 The signs and symptoms of water and sodium depletion

Water depletion	Sodium depletion
Thirst present	Thirst absent
Skin turgor normal in early stages	Skin turgor reduced in early stages
Eyeballs normal in early stages	Eyeballs sunken in early stages
Venous filling normal in early stages	Venous filling reduced in early stages

progresses the patient may feel giddy and may faint due to the decrease in intra-vascular volume. Loss of skin turgor and sunken eyeballs are early signs and the tongue may be wrinkled. Later the patient may show the rapid, shallow pulse and cold clammy skin associated with hypotension. The veins are often collapsed making it difficult to insert the cannula required for intravenous infusion of saline. The changes in blood chemistry are determined to some extent by the cause and also depend on the extent of the deficit. In the early stages there will be little change but as the plasma volume falls the packed cell volume usually increases and as there is an intracellular shift of water the mean corpuscular volume increases also. The concentrations of plasma sodium and chloride are often normal, but may be low (hyponatraemia and hypochloraemia) in contrast to pure water depletion where they are increased (hypernatraemia and hyperchloraemia). The urine output is normal at first, but later falls and is of high specific gravity but containing little sodium or chloride.

Treatment

As loss of sodium is usually accompanied by loss of water, the requirement is for isotonic saline. Although this can be given orally in solution or in the form of salt tablets and water, most patients find this unpleasant. Saline can be infused through a nasogastric tube but many patients with large deficits of sodium have disordered function of their gastro–intestinal tract and consequently the intravenous route is used in nearly all cases.

A method of calculating the requirements for sodium based upon change in body weight may be used e.g.

$$\begin{aligned}
&\text{Acute weight loss of 4 kg}\\
&\text{Loss of sodium} \quad = 4 \times 142 \quad = 568 \text{ mmol}\\
&\phantom{\text{Loss of sodium} \quad} = 568 \times 6 \quad = 3408 \text{ ml } 0.9\% \text{ saline}
\end{aligned}$$

This method assumes that the acute weight loss was due to loss of isotonic saline alone and that the extracellular concentration of sodium was 142 mmol/l before the initial loss. The calculation also ignores completely the considerable functional loss of sodium that may occur into the 'third space' without change in body weight. Another method of calculation is based upon change in packed cell volume. However, packed cell volume varies widely from patient to patient and in many critically ill patients the packed cell volume may be altered by blood transfusion and haemodilution so that this method is often invalid. In the acute phase there may be little change in the extracellular sodium concentration, but when there has been a shift of water from the cells to partially restore the extracellular fluid volume, the fall in extracellular sodium concentration may be used to calculate the deficit e.g.

$$\begin{aligned}
&\text{60 kg female whose serum sodium concentration is 127 mmol/l}\\
&\text{Total body water} \quad = 60 \times 0.5 = 30 \text{ litres}\\
&\text{Sodium deficit} \quad = (142 - 127) \times 30 = 450 \text{ mmol}\\
&\phantom{\text{Sodium deficit} \quad} = 450 \times 6 = 2700 \text{ ml } 0.9\% \text{ saline}
\end{aligned}$$

In females the total body water is only 50% of body weight. This calculation will underestimate the deficit as the extracellular fluid volume is not totally restored by the shift of water from the cells so that the dilution of the extracellular sodium concentration is incomplete.

In clinical practice, the rapid infusion of such volumes will often produce hypervolaemia. However, it is unnecessary for usually the infusion of only 50% of the calculated deficit during the first day will, in the absence of renal disease, re-establish normal renal function which is always superior to the efforts of the clinician in restoring homeostasis. In patients with cardiac disease, rapid infusion should be controlled by regular measurement of central venous pressure (see Ch. 5). The response to treatment can be assessed by serial measurements of serum sodium concentration and the appearance of sodium in the urine. In patients who are shocked due to loss of sodium, a more rapid restoration of blood volume can be obtained by the use of artificial plasma expanders (see Ch. 5). These patients are often acidotic and the use of an appropriate quantity of isotonic sodium lactate solution (⅙M concentration) to replace a portion of the sodium deficit may be useful. However, such refinement is rarely necessary as restoration of blood volume and subsequent renal function is usually sufficient to correct this abnormality also.

Potassium depletion
Although it is the extracellular fluid with its predominant ion being sodium that provides a suitable environment in which the cell lives, the organism exists because of intracellular function which is inextricably linked with potassium content. As 98% of the body potassium is in the cells and the concentration of potassium in the extracellular fluid is carefully regulated by the kidneys, the concentration of potassium in the plasma bears little, if any, relation to the state of potassium balance in the body. Whole–body monitoring and isotopic exchange techniques have been used in research but are of little use in everyday clinical practice. As a consequence of the unavailability of a simple index of potassium metabolism, depletion of potassium may not be as obvious to clinicians as depletion of sodium, but the effects are just as profound.

Hypokalaemia without alteration in the total body content of potassium may occur in alkalosis from any cause due to a shift of potassium ions from the extracellular fluid into the cells with a corresponding movement of hydrogen ions in the opposite direction (see Ch. 4). As in hyponatraemia, hypokalaemia can also occur due to extracellular and intracellular dilution produced by the infusion of excessive quantities of glucose solutions. The dilutional hypokalaemia is also

Table 2.5 The causes of potassium depletion

Inadequate intake	*Excessive loss*
Environment	Starvation
Oropharyngeal or oesophageal disease	Metabolic response to injury
Coma	Vomiting or aspiration
Immobility	Diarrhoea or fistulae
Apathy	Protein–losing enteropathies
Potassium–free infusion	Villous adenoma of the rectum
	Potassium–losing nephritis
	Diuretics
	Cushing's syndrome
	Corticotrophin

compounded by an intracellular shift of potassium produced by the increased plasma concentration of insulin induced by the infusion of glucose. Fatal hypokalaemia has been produced by the infusion of concentrated solutions of glucose without adequate supplements of potassium. The causes of potassium depletion are shown in Table 2.5.

Inadequate intake
Obviously, an inadequate intake of potassium may accompany an inadequate intake of water and sodium in the conditions considered above. An inadequate intake of potassium is also a common feature of surgical practice, particularly after operation and in patients suffering from intestinal obstruction or peritonitis. These patients usually suffer from increased loss of potassium also. If intravenous replacement of fluid and electrolytes is restricted to isotonic solutions of saline, deficiency of potassium may be reflected by a reduction in the plasma concentration. This can be avoided by the routine use of Ringer's or Hartmann's solutions for replacement of crystalloid losses.

Excessive loss
The mechanism of the loss of potassium as a consequence of starvation will be discussed later. It has been emphasised that this loss is 'balanced' (Moore & Ball 1952) as there is a corresponding loss of the other constituents of the cell and consequently there is usually no alteration in the plasma concentration of potassium nor in the urinary potassium/nitrogen ratio — 3:1. It might be argued, therefore, that this loss cannot be considered to be excessive. Moore & Ball also described 'differential intracellular depletion' in which potassium is lost at a greater rate from the cell than the other cell constituents and 'extracellular depletion' in which the initial loss of potassium was from the extracellular fluid with subsequent intracellular loss due to transference. Both varieties of depletion produce an elevated urinary potassium/nitrogen ratio, but differential intracellular depletion is less likely to be associated with hypokalaemia which is inevitable in extracellular depletion. Differential intracellular depletion of potassium is a metabolic consequence of injury as discussed later and may be observed after operation. Extracellular depletion of potassium is commonly seen in patients with gastro–intestinal disease due to losses by vomiting, nasogastric aspiration, diarrhoea or from fistulae of the duodenum and proximal jejunum (Table 1.2). Large quantities of potassium may be lost in patients with protein–losing enteropathies (e.g. Crohn's disease) and in the mucus secreted by the comparatively uncommon mucus–secreting adenoma of the rectum or sigmoid colon. Renal loss of potassium may occur due to diuretics such as furosemide and in salt–losing nephritis. The use of diuretics and potassium supplements either singly or in combination has reduced the incidence of potassium depletion produced by this therapy but occasional cases of severe depletion may still be encountered. Potassium may be lost concomitantly with hydrogen ions as in pyloric stenosis but hypokalaemia may occur without such loss in both metabolic and respiratory alkalosis as will be discussed later. Patients with Cushing's syndrome and those receiving corticotrophin (ACTH) have an excessive loss of potassium in the urine due to increased adrenal secretion of mineralocorticoids.

Clinical features

Patients with severe potassium deficiency may present a varied clinical picture as the potassium depletion is usually only one part of the clinical problem. However, potassium depletion may occur without other complications and the major step in diagnosis is the consideration that the patient may be suffering from potassium depletion. Subsequently a careful history may be more helpful than the clinical examination. As might be expected from the distribution of potassium within the body, the major effects of depletion are seen in muscle and nervous tissue. The patient is usually apathetic and lethargic and may exhibit a total disinterest in his surroundings, but on occasions may complain of nausea, anorexia and cramps. The skeletal muscles are weak and hypotonic and ultimately there may be paralysis. These changes are usually more profound in the legs. The smooth muscle of the intestines becomes hypotonic and ileus and abdominal distension are commonly observed. Abnormal conduction and contractility in cardiac muscle is evident with decreased cardiac output and supraventricular cardiac arrhythmias. The electrocardiogram may show prolongation of the PR and QT intervals, depression of the ST segment, prolongation and depression or inversion of the T wave and, in severe cases, the appearance of the U wave. As discussed above, the concentration of potassium in the plasma may be normal, but hypokalaemia is usually observed in the later stages. Similarly the urine may contain large quantities of potassium. Cellular function in the kidney may be affected also with a decreased ability to concentrate the urine and ultimately oliguria or anuria.

Treatment

A deficit of potassium produced by disease is frequently accompanied by deficits of water and sodium and potassium replacement should be accompanied by replacement of these deficits. This concomitant replacement will lessen the risks of inducing hyperkalaemia in patients with reduced extracellular fluid volume and poor renal function. Due to its predominantly intracellular situation, the approximate quantity of potassium required to replace the deficit cannot be calculated by the methods discussed above in the treatment of water and sodium deficits. Studies involving measurement of total body potassium and the retention of potassium during replacement have shown deficits ranging from 200–1400 mmol, depending on the size of the patient, the disease from which he is suffering and the length of time the loss has been occurring. However, in the majority of patients, the deficit is between 200 and 500 mmol. Although a considerable quantity of potassium may be lost in one day, the simple administration of that quantity in addition to normal daily requirements over the next 24 hours may have no therapeutic effect whatsoever and in certain circumstances may be extremely dangerous. Continuing tissue catabolism will produce further loss of potassium into the extracellular fluid and ultimately into the urine. If potassium is infused intravenously in these patients, cellular uptake is negligible and fatal hyperkalaemia can be induced. Adequate restoration of the potassium deficit must await the effective treatment or natural cessation of the disease process when the cells will accept potassium avidly. Although a poor indicator of the potassium content of the body, the serum potassium concentraton must be measured frequently during replacement therapy. If the concentration remains within the normal range, there is no evidence of extracellular fluid overloading and if there is little potassium appearing in the urine, then it is evident that cellular uptake is occurring and therapy may continue at the same or an increased rate. It is advisable to stop all potassium replacement or maintenance therapy in patients whose serum concentration reaches 5 mmol/l. A few patients still die each year as a consequence of excessive administration of potassium. However, many more patients die from cellular failure associated with potassium loss. If the serum potassium concentration is 3 mmol/l or less, 150 mmol can be given during the first day without risk of producing hyperkalaemia. Patients undergoing elective operations of moderate severity do not require routine supplements. Undoubtedly, the safest method of giving potassium is by mouth. Although potassium chloride can be given as a 20% solution, potassium salts are bitter and are usually given in Great Britain in tablet form. The slow-release type of tablet has produced ulceration, perforation and benign strictures of the small intestine in a few patients and its use has been criticised (Baker et al 1964). There are numerous proprietary preparations containing potassium that can be added to nasogastric feeding regimens. Although orange juice is frequently stated to be a good source of potassium, 1 litre contains only 25 mmol.

The majority of ill patients require intravenous potassium supplements and the quantities are in excess of those contained in electrolyte replacement solutions such as Hartmann's or Ringer's solutions. The usual method of infusion is to add the required quantity from sterile ampoules of potassium chloride solution to bottles of saline or dextrose solutions. This is usually added by a doctor or senior nurse on the ward, but these additions are now being performed with increasing frequency under more sterile conditions in the pharmacy. In the average case, it is unwise to add more than 80 mmol of potassium to each litre; it is imperative to shake the container well (mixing may prove to be a difficult problem with the plastic bag type of container) and the infusion rate should not exceed 20 mmol/h at any part of the day. All patients receiving intravenous potassium supplements require at least daily measurements of their serum potassium concentration.

Patients recovering from devastating catabolic illnesses such as septicaemic shock may have large deficits that can be restored with therapeutic advantage in a more rapid manner by an experienced clinician. These patients may retain 200 mmol of potassium given over a period of 10 hours without any marked increase in their serum concentration. However, this form of therapy should not be attempted by the inexperienced. Rapid restoration of this nature requires measurement of the serum concentration every four hours, and constant display of the electrocardiogram and pulse rate. Many of these patients have been receiving digitalis and too rapid infusion of potassium may produce ventricular arrhythmias. This type of therapy should be confined to the intensive care unit.

Large quantities of intravenous potassium salts are also required in the treatment of diabetic acidosis and during intravenous feeding with hypertonic solutions of glucose when the exogenous provision of insulin stimulates cellular uptake with subsequent hypokalaemia. Such patients usually have an increased requirement for inorganic phosphorus and it is beneficial to supply part of the potassium supplement in the form of a mixture of the monohydrogen and dihydrogen phosphate salts.

Calcium depletion

The varied distribution of calcium in the skeleton, intracellular fluid and extracellular fluid have been discussed previously. It is apparent that calcium exists in the body in many forms each of which has a special function and a convenient index of calcium metabolism is not available. The common causes of calcium depletion are shown in Table 2.6.

Table 2.6 The causes of calcium depletion

Inadequate intake	Excessive loss
Dietary deficiency	Immobility
Deficiency of vitamin D	Skeletal metastases
Intestinal malabsorption	Hyperparathyroidism
Prolonged calcium–free infusion	

Inadequate intake

The diet of most Western countries contains adequate milk and milk products to ensure that sufficient calcium is ingested. However, there are many countries in the world where intake may be inadequate. Although sufficient calcium may be ingested, absorption may be inadequate due to lack of vitamin D, steatorrhoea with the formation of insoluble soaps from the saponification of fatty acids and calcium, or following massive resection of the small bowel. Calcium deficiency may also occur with prolonged intravenous feeding without calcium supplements.

Excessive loss

Excessive loss of calcium is relatively common, but rarely of great severity. Demineralisation of bone can occur due to disuse atrophy or to osteolytic metastases and, more rarely, due to hyperparathyroidism.

Clinical features

Calcium depletion may be manifest by metabolic bone disease or symptoms due to abnormally low concentrations of plasma calcium (hypocalcaemia).

Metabolic bone disease.   There are three basic varieties of bone disease due to calcium depletion. In osteomalacia or rickets there is failure of calcification of the bone matrix due to a lack of calcium or vitamin D in the diet. In the many varieties of osteoporosis there is loss of calcium from previously normal bone due to disuse atrophy or replacement, but in osteitis fibrosis cystica there is loss of calcium due to hyperparathyroidism.

Hypocalcaemia.   As discussed previously, a low concentration of plasma calcium may reflect hypoalbuminaemia and be relatively unimportant. It is the depression of the ionised fraction of the plasma calcium that has such a profound effect upon conduction in nervous and muscular tissue. The classical sign of tetany, the *main d'accoucheur* in which the hand is flexed at the wrist and meta-carpal–phalangeal joints and extended at the interphalangeal joints, may be apparent or induced in less severe cases by inflating a sphygmomanometer cuff round the upper arm (Trousseau's sign). A similar phenomenon can be demonstrated by tapping a branch of the facial nerve in the cheek which will produce twitching of the facial muscles (Chvostek's sign). In severe cases there may be paraesthesiae, carpopedal spasm, laryngospasm and spasm of the abdominal muscles.

Rarely the patient may have convulsions. Hypocalcaemia is usually accompanied by hyperphosphataemia and calcium is often absent from the urine as indicated by the Sulkowitch test. The electrocardiogram may show prolongation of the QT interval.

Treatment
The treatment of metabolic bone disease is beyond the scope of this book and hypocalcaemia is an uncommon event in everyday hospital practice. The hypocalcaemia observed in patients with acute pancreatitis usually reflects their hypoalbuminaemia and infusion of calcium rarely alters the serum concentration which reverts to normal levels with an improvement in the serum albumin concentration. Transient hypocalcaemia may follow the removal of parathyroid tumours and on occasion the fall in concentration may be profound. In these patients, the fall is in the ionised fraction and responds to treatment with calcium gluconate. Initially, this should be given intravenously and as much as 100 ml of a 10% solution may be required in the first 24 hours. Following this, calcium gluconate can be given orally in tablet form according to requirements. The routine need for infusion of 10 ml of 10% calcium gluconate solution with every 2 litres of blood during massive transfusion is controversial. If the rate of infusion is not rapid, the binding of ionised calcium by the citrate in the transfused blood may be easily overcome by mobilisation of calcium from bone without any major change in the serum concentration. Tetany may be produced by changes in the serum concentrations of other ions and in particular by alkalosis (see below) and some other form of therapy may be indicated.

Magnesium depletion
Although magnesium depletion had been recognised in a variety of patients in the previous two decades (Flink 1956, Booth et al 1963, Heaton et al 1967) it is only during the last decade that it has become apparent that magnesium depletion is a comparatively common event. Indeed, it would appear that some degree of magnesium depletion usually accompanies depletion of potassium by virtue of their intracellular situation. The common causes of magnesium depletion are shown in Table 2.7.

Table 2.7 The causes of magnesium depletion

Inadequate intake	*Excessive loss*
Intestinal malabsorption	Starvation
Prolonged magnesium–free infusion	Metabolic response to injury
	Diarrhoea or fistulae
	Protein–losing enteropathies

Inadequate intake
Magnesium is prevalent in many foods but particularly in grain and green vegetables. However, it is absorbed in the upper small bowel and patients with steatorrhoea due to biliary or pancreatic disease may absorb insufficient quantities for normal requirements. Intestinal malabsorption may also occur in patients with coeliac or Crohn's disease and in patients with high jejunal or duodenal fistulae, or after massive resection of the small bowel. It is uncommon to observe a low-

ered plasma concentration of magnesium (hypomagnesaemia) following a few days of infusion of magnesium−free fluids in the uncomplicated case, but hypomagnesaemia is a common complication of long−term intravenous feeding with magnesium-free solutions and may be aggravated if concomitant hypophosphataemia is treated by infusion of potassium dihydrogen phosphate.

Excessive loss

Magnesium is released from the cell as a consequence of injury (see below), and large quantities may be excreted in the urine in patients who have suffered severe or prolonged injury or sepsis. In addition to the poor absorption that may occur in Crohn's disease, such patients may lose excessive quantities by exudation from the bowel and so too may patients with ulcerative colitis.

Clinical features

Florid signs of magnesium deficiency are uncommon. As with potassium, the major effects of depletion are evident in the muscular and nervous systems. The skeletal muscles may show fasciculation and a positive Chvostek or Trousseau sign may precede frank tetany (see above, under hypocalcaemia). Mental depression, personality disorders, convulsions and delirium have accompanied hypomagnesaemia, and athetoid and choreiform movements are common.

Treatment

Although magnesium may be given orally, deficiency is frequently associated with disturbed function of the gastro−intestinal tract. However, 2 g (8 mmol) of magnesium sulphate may be given three times a day to patients with chronic deficiencies. It may also be given as an intramuscular injection of a 50% solution of magnesium sulphate, but the injection is painful and the volumes required to replace any major deficit make this an unattractive route. Severe deficiencies require prompt and adequate replacement by intravenous infusion. Ampoules containing 20 ml of a molar solution of magnesium chloride can be made in the pharmacy so that 1 ml of solution contains 1 mmol of magnesium. The addition of 20 ml of this solution each day to either a bottle of isotonic saline or glucose is usually sufficient to correct minor deficiencies, but 40 mmol/d may be required to correct major deficiencies, particularly if the patient is delirious. The dangers of infusion of large quantities of magnesium are very similar to those associated with hyperkalaemia and the same careful observation of the electrocardiogram and heart rate are required. The measurement of the serum concentration of magnesium is more difficult than that of potassium, but its concentration must be measured every 48 h in patients receiving 20 mmol/d and daily in patients receiving 40 mmol/d.

Tetany

It is convenient at this stage to consider the mechanism by which alterations in the extracellular concentration of the four cations discussed above may produce tetany. In general, the irritability of nerves and skeletal muscles is determined by the extracellular ionic concentration, according to the formula:

$$\frac{Na^+ + K^+ + OH^-}{Ca^{2+} + Mg^{2+} + H^+}$$

Thus, in general terms, hypotonia and paralysis is associated with low extracellular concentrations of sodium and potassium or high concentrations of calcium and magnesium. Conversely, hypertonia, or tetany, is associated with high concentrations of sodium and potassium or low concentrations of calcium and magnesium. Hypotonia is aggravated by acidosis and hypertonia by alkalosis. In many clinical conditions, changes in more than one of these ionic concentrations may occur and treatment will vary accordingly.

Phosphorus depletion

Phosphorus occurs in the body in organic and inorganic forms. Although in starvation the concentration of circulating phospholipids may fall, deficiency of organic phosphorus appears to be uncommon. Because of its predominantly skeletal and intracellular distributions, the study of changes in the phosphorus content of the body is difficult but phosphorus depletion may be encountered in the elderly and in infants where it is sometimes associated with osteomalacia. The common causes of phosphorus deficiency are shown in Table 2.8.

Table 2.8 The causes of phosphorus depletion

Inadequate intake	Excessive loss
Deficiency of vitamin D	Starvation
Malabsorption	Metabolic response to injury
Treatment with aluminium hydroxide	Hyperparathyroidism

Inadequate intake

Phosphorus is so abundant in food that a deficient intake is extremely rare, but absorption in the bowel may be impaired due to lack of vitamin D, steatorrhoea, or the intake of excessive quantities of aluminium hydroxide (an antacid) with the subsequent formation and excretion of insoluble aluminium phosphate.

Excessive loss

An increased urinary excretion of phosphorus after injury was one of the first observations to be recognised as part of the metabolic response to injury (Cuthbertson 1930). As might be expected from its intracellular distribution, phosphorus, like potassium, is lost in 'balanced' quantities during starvation, the increase in excretion being of the same magnitude as the increase in the excretion of the other intracellular components. Increased renal excretion of phosphorus is found in hyperparathyroidism.

Clinical features

Although a total body deficiency of phosphorus may occur, its clinical importance is far less than the consequences of a decreased concentration of serum inorganic phosphorus. Hypophosphataemia occurs as a consequence of total body depletion of phosphorus, but it may be produced in comparatively healthy individuals by infusion of large quantities of glucose, particularly if the infusion is accompanied

by intravenous or intramuscular insulin. The hypophosphataemia produces a reduction in the concentration of 2, 3–diphosphoglycerate and adenosine triphosphate in red blood cells which results in an increased affinity of haemoglobin for
oxygen, thus decreasing the release of oxygen in the tissues (Travis et al 1971).
Severe hypophosphataemia may also produce a haemolytic anaemia (Jacob &
Amsden 1971) and deaths have occurred (Silvis & Paragas 1972). Although serum
inorganic phosphorus may fall following elective operations (Gouillou et al 1976)
the concentrations of serum inorganic phosphorus and of 2, 3–diphosphoglycerate and adenosine triphosphate remain within normal limits (England et al 1979).
The fall in the concentration of serum inorganic phosphorus after operation
appears to be mainly due to dilution rather than increased excretion and would
appear to be a transient and self–limiting phenomenon of little clinical importance.

Treatment
The loss of phosphorus after injury reflects tissue catabolism and restoration follows naturally with the cessation of the traumatic insult and the resumption of a
normal dietary intake. Hypophosphataemia may be corrected by the infusion of
phosphate salts. As hypokalaemia frequently accompanies hypophosphataemia,
potassium salts are usually given. A convenient method is to ask the pharmacist
to prepare a ½ M solution of potassium dihydrogen phosphate (a molar solution
may show precipitation after a few weeks) and the addition of 20 ml of this solution to 500 ml of glucose or saline solution will provide 10 mmol of phosphorus.
Commercial solutions of 20% glucose with added phosphorus are now available
and the use of these solutions for intravenous feeding should reduce the incidence
of hypophosphataemia associated with infusion of large quantities of glucose. If
the solutions are being prepared in the pharmacy, 15 mmol of phosphorus should
be added to each 500 ml of 20% glucose.

EXCESS SYNDROMES

The problems of deficiency discussed above may often be prevented by adequate
therapy, but of necessity they are produced by disease or neglect. The problems
of excess discussed here may be produced by disease but frequently they are a
consequence of inappropriate therapy.

Excess water
The term overhydration is frequently used by clinicians to describe patients
whose underlying defect may be either too much sodium or too much water (see
dehydration in the preceding chapter). Some clinicians refer to excess water as
water 'intoxication'.

Excessive intake
It is almost impossible for a healthy individual to drink water over a prolonged
period at a greater rate than the kidney's maximal excretory rate (about 750 ml/h)
and consequently water overloading due to excessive drinking has only occurred
in psychiatric patients (Bewley 1964). Excess intake may be produced by the in-

fusion of hypotonic fluids, or by the infusion of isotonic glucose solution which when oxidised yields water and carbon dioxide which is excreted by the lungs. Thus infusion of 500 ml of isotonic glucose (5%) effectively provides 515 ml of water. Severe water overloading can result from the infusion of isotonic glucose solutions unless accompanied by sufficient sodium. The water intake of many patients may be greater than expected unless accurate records are kept as many patients who are receiving the major portion of their fluid intake by vein are also drinking 'sips' of water each hour that frequently amount to 500 ml or more each day. Occasionally, large quantities of water may be absorbed from the colon due to frequent enemata (Lancet 1959) and water may also be absorbed during transurethral resection of the prostate (Marx et al 1960).

Reduced loss

The major site of water loss is by the kidneys and patients with acute or chronic renal failure may rapidly become overloaded with water. In most cases there is a concomitant retention of sodium. However, water retention may occur due to excessive secretion of antidiuretic hormone in response to stress, pain, fear, or anaesthesia. It is evident that such secretion is commonly found after operation when the tendency to overloading may be compounded by the infusion of excessive quantities of isotonic dextrose solution (Zimmerman & Wangensteen 1954, Le Quesne 1954). Although this antidiuretic phase may be prolonged after severe injury or major operation, it usually lasts for only 24–48 hours after most operations. The fear of overloading the patient during this phase should not deter the clinician from infusing adequate quantities of fluid. Rarely, patients are seen who have inappropriate secretion of antidiuretic hormone (Goldberg 1963). The majority of these patients have malignant disease and in some cases the tumour secretes antidiuretic hormone. Patients suffering from cardiac failure may have excessive water retention due to failure of adequate renal filtration but many of them also have excessive retention of sodium.

It is important to recognise that the commonest cause of water overloading in surgical practice is excessive infusion in patients with temporary or permanent renal dysfunction. Although it may develop rapidly, it usually occurs over 24–48 hours and its development is frequently a reflection of inadequate medical care. The fluid requirements of patients with renal failure are discussed in Chapter 7.

Clinical features

The symptoms usually start slowly but may begin suddenly. In the early phase, the patient is weak, apathetic and may have nausea and vomiting. Later, there is mental confusion and the patient may become delirious. As the condition progresses the patient may twitch and suffer convulsions and ultimately he may become comatose and die. Physical examination may reveal very little other than muscle twitching. Oedema is not marked but an unusual gain in weight may have been recorded. The fluid shifts and altered physiology induced by excess water and sodium are compared in Figure 2.2. The initial effect of water retention is to increase the volume and to decrease the concentration and osmolarity of the extracellular fluid (Table 2.9). As the concentration of the extracellular compart-

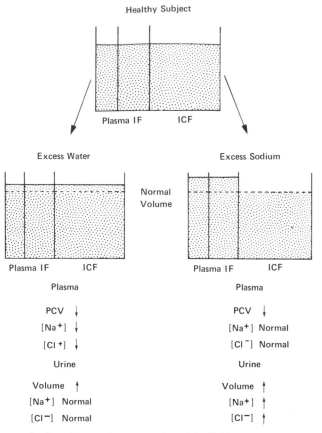

Fig. 2.2 The changes in the volume and concentration of the fluid compartments and urine output produced by excess water and sodium

ment falls, water flows into the intracellular compartment until tonicity is equalised. Thus there is a corresponding increase in the volume and decrease in the concentration of the intracellular compartment. This is the converse of the mechanism that occurs in water depletion and, although the increase in the intracellular compartment differs when compared in absolute terms, the percentage increase of the two compartments is the same as shown in Figure 2.2 which

Table 2.9 The changes in the volume and concentration of the fluid compartments produced by water excess

	Extracellular fluid		Intracellular fluid	
	Volume (l)	Osmolarity (mosmol/l)	Volume (l)	Osmolarity (mosmol/l)
Healthy subject	15	280	30	280
Initial extracellular water excess	18	$\frac{280 \times 15}{18} = 235$	30	280
Subsequent extracellular and intracellular water excess	16	$\frac{280 \times 15}{16} = 263$	32	$\frac{280 \times 30}{32} = 263$

should be compared with Figure 2.1. As is the case with water depletion, the intracellular accumulation of water keeps pace with the total body accumulation of water and initial extracellular accumulation of water of the magnitude shown in Table 2.9 does not occur. In both water depletion and excess the twofold changes in the volume of the intracellular compartment when compared with the extracellular compartment simply reflect that the volume of one is twice that of the other. The plasma concentrations of sodium and chloride and the packed cell volume are decreased and because of the intracellular accumulation of water, the mean corpuscular volume is also increased. Although the plasma concentration of sodium and chloride may be very low, the urine often contains sodium and chloride as aldosterone secretion is reduced by the expansion in the plasma volume.

Treatment

The treatment of water overloading depends upon the urgency of the clinical problem. In most patients it is sufficient to provide about 1 litre of water each day (including that contained in food) and normal renal function will restore total body water content to normal levels within 2–3 days. This process may be accelerated by the use of diuretics such as furosemide. In patients with congestive heart failure, digitalisation is usually required. Occasionally, patients will be encountered who are overhydrated but in whom a diuresis will not occur in spite of normal renal and cardiac function. These patients are usually hypoproteinaemic and consequently have a low oncotic pressure. Their water overloading is predominantly in the interstitial space and they are unable to mobilise this fluid due to their low oncotic pressure. An effective method of treatment is to infuse 500 ml of triple–strength plasma which increases the oncotic pressure and withdraws water into the intravascular space which can then be excreted by the kidneys.

In a few patients, the embarrassment to the circulation may be so acute and the response to the mode of treatment outlined above may be so slow that the clinician may decide that more urgent methods of treatment are required or the patient may succumb. A rapid removal of water from the circulation and ultimately from the body can be achieved by haemodialysis using hypertonic solutions. The removal of water from the circulation may be so rapid that it exceeds transcapillary refilling and hypovolaemia and hypotension may occur. If the necessary equipment and expertise is unavailable, peritoneal dialysis with hypertonic solutions provides a less dramatic rate of removal from the body.

Excess sodium

The concentration of plasma sodium shows very little correlation with either total body content of sodium or total exchangeable sodium content. Hypernatraemia is usually an indication of water depletion (see above).

Excessive intake

In the absence of renal disease, an excessive increase in total body sodium due to oral intake is most unlikely. However, rapid infusion of isotonic saline solution can result in overloading of sodium even in a healthy young adult.

Reduced loss

Following operation or injury there is an increased secretion of aldosterone resulting in sodium retention (Zimmermann et al 1955, Venning et al 1958). As with the secretion of antidiuretic hormone the length and degree of this secretion are determined by the severity of the injury, but after most elective operations this lasts for 36–48 hours. Before the mechanism of this post–traumatic retention of sodium had been discovered it was recognised that infusion of excessive quantities of isotonic saline solution was particularly likely to produce overloading with sodium during this period (Coller et al 1945). Even a healthy individual has a limited ability to excrete a saline load, a reflection of an evolutionary desire to conserve the *milieu intérieur* (see Ch. 3) and it is not surprising that this should be more pronounced after injury. Following this discovery, many doctors have emphasised the dangers of infusing excessive quantities of saline following operation. Nevertheless, the fear of overloading the patient with saline must not deter the clinician from infusing adequate quantities to replace extracellular fluid lost during or after operation. Excessive secretion of aldosterone also occurs in patients with congestive heart failure and cirrhosis of the liver and rarely as a consequence of aldosterone–producing tumours of the adrenal cortex (Conn's syndrome). Sodium retention may occur in acute or chronic failure and as patients with severe cardiac or renal disease are undergoing surgery more frequently now, careful monitoring of central venous pressure and urine output is essential in such situations. In some of these patients, particularly those with poor nutrition, there is an even greater retention of water and consequently hyponatraemia may be observed although total body sodium is considerably increased. This is commonly observed during the first two days following operation, when in spite of renal conservation of sodium and a strongly positive sodium balance, the serum sodium concentration falls slightly due to dilution in the extracellular space.

Clinical features

The predominant feature of excess sodium in the body is oedema. The initial effect of excess sodium is to produce an increase in the extracellular concentration but the resulting increase in osmolarity stimulates the osmoreceptors of the hypothalamus and antidiuretic hormone is promptly released so that a corresponding quantity of water is reabsorbed by the distal tubules in the kidney until osmolarity is restored. Thus the volume of the extracellular fluid is increased, but as sodium is predominantly extracellular there is no increase in the intracellular fluid volume. In the plasma the packed cell volume is decreased but the concentrations of sodium and chloride are usually normal. In patients who have received excessive quantities of sodium and have normal function, the urine volume is usually increased with a high concentration of sodium and chloride.

Treatment

Hypernatraemia due to water deficiency is treated simply by increasing the water given by mouth or nasogastric tube. If intake is restricted to the intravenous route, the same effect can be achieved by infusing isotonic glucose solution (5%) or half–strength (0.45%) solutions of sodium chloride.

The logical treatment of sodium excess is to restrict or stop sodium intake and to promote its excretion. In patients with congestive heart failure this may be achieved simply by stopping the addition of salt to food and prescribing diuretics that increase sodium excretion such as furosemide and ethacrynic acid. Digitalisation may also improve renal excretion of sodium by its effect on a failing circulation. The use of the aldosterone antagonist spironolactone may be effective in patients with cardiac and hepatic disease who are suffering from secondary aldosteronism.

There is no logic to infusing hypertonic solutions of saline in patients with hyponatraemia and excess total body sodium as has been suggested in the past. The major portion of the excess sodium is in the interstitial space and as the capillary barrier is freely permeable to sodium, the major portion of the infused sodium also passes into the interstitial space with very little effect upon the plasma volume as intended. Many of these patients are hypoproteinaemic and sodium retention is occurring due to the increased secretion of aldosterone in response to a reduction in circulating blood volume. The most effective treatment is to infuse concentrated solutions of plasma or albumin with a low content of sodium.

Oedema
It is convenient at this stage to discuss the ways in which oedema can be produced. Oedema is the accumulation of abnormal quantities of fluid in the interstitial tissues. The factors influencing the movement of water across the capillary endothelium have been discussed in Chapter 1 and the vital role of the oncotic pressure exerted by the plasma proteins has been emphasised above. Any condition in which there is reduction in the plasma proteins will be associated with oedema. Thus oedema may be observed in patients with long–standing malnutrition and in patients with burns or sepsis. A reduction in the concentration of the plasma proteins due to dilution rather than a true reduction in total content has a similar effect and excessive infusion of isotonic saline or retention of sodium as described above is the commonest cause of oedema. Not only is the volume of the extracellular fluid compartment increased, but there is a concomitant decrease in oncotic pressure. However, a considerable increase in the extracellular volume can occur before oedema develops. These mechanisms produce generalised oedema throughout the body, but the patient's posture and the effect of gravity will determine the site of maximum accumulation. Patients who are confined to bed may have no clinical evidence of oedema at the ankles, but gross pitting may be elicited over the sacrum. Pulmonary oedema may be evident on clinical or radiological examination. Local oedema affecting one limb suggests inadequate lymphatic drainage due to infection or malignant disease.

Excess potassium
Some 98% of the potassium in the body is contained within the cells and a clinical syndrome associated with an excess of total body potassium has not been described. It may be impossible to induce an intracellular overloading with this ion, because when the cell is replete excess potassium is excreted by the kidneys. However an excess of extracellular potassium may be easily produced by disease or inappropriate therapy and hyperkalaemia may be rapidly fatal.

Excessive intake

In the presence of normal renal function it is extremely uncommon to observe hyperkalaemia. Renal function must be considerably impaired before the ingestion of normal quantities of potassium produces hyperkalaemia. However, it may be produced in patients with normal renal function by intravenous infusion of excessive quantities of potassium salts and unfortunately such events still occur with distressing frequency. The plasma of blood preserved with acid–citrate–dextrose solution may contain high concentrations of potassium, particularly when stored for many days, and massive transfusion of this blood may produce a marked elevation of the serum potassium concentration. The life span of transfused cells is also reduced by storage and the subsequent in vivo haemolysis tends to exacerbate the condition.

Reduced loss

The commonest cause of hyperkalaemia is acute or chronic renal failure and this is discussed in greater detail in Chapter 7. The ingestion of normal quantities of potassium may produce hyperkalaemia in a patient whose renal output falls below 500 ml/d. In an anuric patient, hyperkalaemia may develop without any intake due to release of potassium by breakdown of protein and the development of acidosis.

Extracellular transference

Although potassium is lost in the urine following injury and total body content falls, moderate hyperkalaemia is a frequent consequence of the liberation of potassium by the damaged cell, particularly during the oliguric phase of the response to injury (see Ch. 3 for further details). It is a common observation that acidosis increases and alkalosis decreases the serum potassium concentration (see Ch. 4 for further details). The precise mechanism is not known but presumably potassium ions are released from cells containing an increased concentration of hydrogen ions in order to maintain electrical neutrality on either side of the cell membrane.

Clinical features

Unfortunately the initial signs of hyperkalaemia are not dramatic. The patient and the doctor may fail to appreciate muscle weakness until flaccid paralysis, which usually effects the lower limbs first, occurs when the serum potassium concentration is dangerously high. Often the first obvious indication of hyperkalaemia is the development of ventricular fibrillation. This arrhythmia is preceded by characteristic changes in the electrocardiogram. At first there are tall, peaked T waves and as the serum potassium rises the P waves disappear. Finally, the development of abnormal QRS complexes indicates that the development of ventricular fibrillation is imminent.

Treatment

Because of its potential danger, hyperkalaemia should never be ignored. Although it may be expected as a transient phenomenon during the oliguric phase after injury for example and no treatment is required, the serum concentration should be monitored carefully until it has returned to normal. Ideally, the treatment of chronic hyperkalaemia due to chronic renal failure should be supervised by a renal physician and may involve dietary control, regular haemodialysis or renal transplantation. Severe hyperkalaemia of rapid onset requires urgent treatment. The infusion of glucose and insulin stimulates potassium uptake by the cells and is probably the most rapid method of lowering the extracellular concentration over a period of few hours. If 500 ml of 20% glucose are infused with 20 units of insulin over a period of 30 minutes, a fall in the serum potassium concentration should be noted within one hour of starting the infusion. If the patient is acidotic, infusion of a solution of sodium bicarbonate may be effective (see Ch. 4 under hypokalaemic alkalosis). These methods produce a temporary but often life–saving fall in serum potassium concentration allowing more effective and permanent therapy to be organised. Cation exchange resins which exchange sodium for potassium ions in the gastro–intestinal tract (Knowles & Kaplan 1953) are now used infrequently as peritoneal dialysis or haemodialysis is available in most hospitals.

Excess magnesium
Although there have been very few reports of clinical problems ascribed to magnesium excess, the condition may be more common than has been previously considered and occasional deaths have occurred.

Excessive intake
Magnesium may be absorbed from the colon from magnesium sulphate enemata and this salt is also used as an oral purgative (Epsom salts). In some institutions magnesium chloride is used routinely in intravenous feeding regimens. The occasional infusion of this additive by those who are unfamiliar with its use requires careful attention to ensure correct dosage. Hypermagnesaemia without any increase (more probably a decrease) in total body magnesium may occur in patients with hyperparathyroidism due to mobilisation of magnesium from bone.

Reduced loss
The most common cause of magnesium excess is inadequate excretion in renal failure (Randall et al 1964).

Clinical features
The importance of the extracellular concentration of magnesium in determining electrical conductivity in nerve and skeletal muscle has been discussed above. Hypermagnesaemia is associated with muscular flaccidity and loss of tendon reflexes. The patient is lethargic and may lapse into coma. The electrocardiogram may show prolongation of the PR and QT intervals, peaked T waves, atrioventricular block and ventricular ectopic beats.

Treatment
The majority of patients have renal impairment and treatment should be directed to improving renal function and reducing the intake of magnesium. If an extremely large quantity of magnesium has been given intravenously by mistake and the patient's life is threatened, magnesium may be removed from the circulation by haemodialysis. In severe cases artificial ventilation may be required until

neuromuscular function returns to normal. If the equipment and expertise for urgent haemodialysis are unavailable, a temporary reduction in the serum magnesium concentration may be produced by the infusion of an isotonic solution of sodium sulphate in dextrose (Chakmakjian & Bethune 1966). This treatment also lowers the serum concentrations of potassium and calcium and supplements of these two ions may be required.

Excess calcium

An increase in the total body content of calcium is unusual and of less importance than increase in the plasma concentration of ionised calcium. The distribution of the different fractions of calcium within the plasma has been discussed in Chapter 1.

Excessive intake

Abnormal quantities of calcium may be absorbed from the bowel in hyperparathyroidism, sarcoidosis and with prolonged and excessive treatment of osteomalacia with vitamin D. The excessive ingestion of milk to control dyspeptic symptoms is now an uncommon cause as more effective control can be achieved with various drugs. Hypercalcaemia may also occur with increased release of calcium from bone due to immobilisation, Paget's disease or to osteolytic metastases. An increase in the protein–bound calcium (which has little clinical significance other than that associated with the primary disease) may be found in thyrotoxicosis, multiple myeloma and non–bony malignant disease.

Reduced loss

Although greater quantities of calcium are excreted in hyperparathyroidism as a consequence of mobilisation from bone, there is an increased reabsorption of calcium in the renal tubules.

Clinical features

The role of the extracellular concentration of calcium in the maintenance of normal conduction in nerve and skeletal muscle has been discussed in Chapter 1. Hypercalcaemia may be associated with psychiatric disturbances, lassitude, anorexia and vomiting and ultimately with coma. The electrocardiogram may show a shortened QT interval. The urine usually contains large quantities of calcium. Patients with hyperparathyroidism may have radiological changes in the bones and metastatic calcification.

Hypercalcaemic crisis is a rare condition occurring mainly in patients with metastatic disease or hyperparathyroidism, but occasionally it may also occur following excessive treatment with vitamin D. The patient may be disorientated and frankly psychotic in addition to exhibiting the neuromuscular abnormalities described above.

Treatment

The treatment of hypercalcaemia or excess calcium content in the body depends upon the aetiology. In patients with primary and tertiary hyperparathyroidism, surgical extirpation of one or more parathyroid glands is usually required. Patients with secondary hyperparathyroidism do not suffer initially from hypercalcacmia and treatment of the underlying renal disease may prevent progression to tertiary hyperparathyroidism. In all patients excessive intake of calcium, milk or vitamin D should be stopped.

Severe hypercalcaemia may require urgent and aggressive treatment. The diuretic furosemide increases renal excretion of calcium in addition to sodium and infusion of isotonic saline solution combined with intravenous administration of furosemide has a marked calciuric effect. Up to 4 litres of saline per day can be infused if renal function is adequate. However, many patients with hyperparathyroidism have impaired renal function and infusion of large quantities of sodium may produce fluid retention and overloading of the circulation. Severe hypercalcaemia has been treated by intravenous infusion of inorganic salts of phosphorus (Goldsmith & Ingbar 1966) and of sulphur (Chakmakjian & Bethune 1966) but injudicious use of this therapy may produce further disturbances of water and electrolyte distribution. The use of oral phosphates (Goldsmith & Ingbar 1966) produces a less dramatic fall in serum calcium concentration but is less likely to produce the disturbances of water and electrolyte distribution that may follow intravenous infusion. The sulphates have a calciuric effect but the phosphates probably deposit calcium in bone and other tissues. Cessation of therapy with both salts may be followed by rebound hypercalcaemia. Intravenous injection of mithramycin at a dose of $25-30$ μg/kg will lower the serum calcium concentration over a period of three to five days. If the hypercalcaemia is a consequence of metastatic bone disease, treatment with large doses of cortisol may be effective.

Excess phosphorus
Retention of phosphorus may occur in renal failure. There are no recognisable consequences of hyperphosphataemia per se, the important features being due to the secondary hypocalcaemia that ensues.

Excess trace elements
A chronic excess of some trace elements may occur as inborn errors of metabolism. An excess deposition of iron is the major feature of haemochromatosis and an excess deposition of copper is the major feature of hepatolenticular degeneration. It is inevitable that with increasing use of long–term intravenous feeding and trace metal additives, accidental infusion of excessive quantities of these elements will occur. Treatment with penicillamine or haemodialysis may be indicated and expert advice should be sought.

Excess vitamins
Some vitamins may be toxic when given in excessive quantities. Hypervitaminosis D produces hypercalcaemia and death due to renal failure may occur if the cause is unrecognised. The hypercalcaemia rapidly disappears when therapy with vitamin D is stopped. The treatment of severe hypercalcaemia is discussed above. Hypervitaminosis A is associated with epithelial dysplasia and abnormal development of bone with premature fusion of the epiphyses. The epithelial dysplasia will rapidly disappear on withdrawal of the vitamin but premature fusion of the epiphyses will remain as a legacy of ill-considered therapy.

3

Starvation and the effect of injury

The first records of the response of the animal kingdom to starvation or injury appear to be those of John Hunter (1791a) who noted that 'there is a circumstance attending accidental injury which does not belong to disease, namely that the injury done has, in all cases, a tendency and means of cure'. This and other observations concerning starvation and injury were made without any laboratory aids and have proved with time to be remarkably accurate.

Larrey, Napoleon's chief surgeon, first recorded traumatic glycosuria (1829) but it was many years later before major investigations of the biochemical changes following starvation and injury were made by Benedict (1915) and Cuthbertson (1930) respectively. Although severe injury, and in particular that involving the gastro—intestinal tract, is inevitably accompanied by varying degrees of starvation, it is now evident that the response to injury differs quantitatively from that due to simple starvation alone (Moore & Ball 1952, Wilkinson 1956, Cahill 1970).

Starvation, particularly for long periods, should not occur under medical supervision but many of the complex examinations performed in the investigation of the gastro—intestinal tract require a limited period of starvation before the procedure. It is not uncommon for a previously malnourished patient with defective gastro—intestinal function to receive only one meal each day over a five day period of investigation. In many hospitals, the patients now order their own food which is distributed and any residue collected by non—nursing staff. As a consequence the nursing staff may be unable to give an accurate account of the patient's intake. Unfortunately, suitable supervision of large numbers of patients by trained dietitians is rarely possible due to insufficient staff who are often employed elsewhere in the time-consuming and usually unnecessary chore of instructing obese patients how to lose weight. It is not surprising that there is a high incidence of malnutrition in general hospital populations (Bistrian et al 1974, Hill et al 1976).

STARVATION

As discussed in Chapter 1, the glycogen stored in liver and muscle amounts at the most to 400 g (1600 kcal, 6.7 MJ) and is rapidy exhausted. In total starvation of fluid and substrate all homeostatic requirements must be met by mobilisation of body protein and fat.

Water loss

The oxidation of body protein and fat in complete starvation will provide about 250 ml of water each day. The remaining requirement must be met by the water in the intracellular and extracellular fluid. If water loss continued at the normal rate of 2500 ml per day then it is evident that death would soon follow. However, as first observed in animals by Hunter and studied in detail in man during World War II by Gamble (1947), the body responds by reducing water output from all sources and in particular by excreting highly concentrated urine. In such circumstances, the obligatory urine volume (that is the minimum volume of urine in which the excretory solutes can be excreted by the kidneys functioning at their maximum concentrating capacity) can be as low as 350 ml per day. Unfortunately, there is little possible reduction in the insensible loss of water except that engendered by a fall in metabolic rate after prolonged starvation. Thus about 1500 ml of water per day are required of which 250 ml are produced by the oxidation of tissue and the remaining 1250 ml must come from body water.

Protein and fat loss

Although many tissues can utilise acids as an energy substrate, some tissues use predominantly glucose. Glucose can be produced from glycerol released by the hydrolysis of triglycerides in the fat stores. However, although this does occur during starvation, such a process is extremely inefficient, 8–10 g of depot fat being required to provide each gram of glucose. The major source of glucose during starvation is provided by gluconeogensis from protein.

As emphasised in Chapter 1, the body does not store protein. The free amino acids in the blood amount to a few grams and plasma proteins have a functional role rather than acting as a protein reserve. Although, in the face of inadequate intake, body protein may be partly broken down to meet a specific amino acid requirement or oxidised more extensively for energy, it should never be forgotten that this body protein had, like plasma protein, a functional role which will now be compromised to a varying extent. Although it is apparent that there is a limit to the extent of protein loss that the body can withstand, precise definition is not possible. The rapid loss of about 30% of body weight of total body protein is usually fatal (Moore et al 1963, Lawson 1965, Cahill 1970). Preoperative weight loss was found to have a profound influence upon survival following gastrectomy (Studley 1936), 12 out of 18 patients surviving who were more than 20% below their ideal weight compared with 27 out of 28 patients surviving who were less than 20% below their ideal weight. A major goal of nutritive therapy is to prevent or minimise the loss of lean body mass.

Fat is a highly efficient fuel that is stored by the body in large quantities whenever energy intake is in excess of requirements, regardless of the source of energy (fat, carbohydrate or protein). This is the only function of the fat stores although they have an insulating function that may also have survival value in cold climates. Body fat may contribute as much as 45% of the weight of an obese female and as little as 10% in a lean male.

From the above it is evident that the chances of survival from starvation will be improved if as much as possible of the energy requirements are met by oxidation of fat rather than protein. In 1915, in a meticulous scientific study, Benedict had investigated the effects of starvation in a healthy male volunteer for 30 days and demonstrated that such a mechanism did exist (although he was apparently unaware of why protein continued to be broken down). In this study, Benedict noted that as the subject lost weight there was a concomitant decrease in oxygen consumption, basal metabolic rate, respiratory quotient and urinary excretion of nitrogen and an increase in the urinary excretion of β hydroxybutyrate and aceto– acetate formed by the oxidation of fatty acids. These changes are indicative of a diminution in the contribution of protein and an increase in the contribution of fat to the metabolic fuel. In the established fasting state, protein contributes only 15% of the fuel. Subsequent studies of fasting using more sophisticated methods than those available to Benedict have confirmed these findings and indicated mechanisms by which this change is achieved (Cahill et al 1966, Owen et al 1967, Cahill 1970).

The concentration of blood glucose falls rapidly after the onset of fasting. On the fourth day it falls to about 3.8 mmol/1 and is maintained at that level, falling further just before death. In the plasma the gluconeogenic amino acids, and in particular alanine, show a progressive decline. These changes in the concentration of blood glucose and the gluconeogenic amino acids coincide with an increase in the concentration of plasma glucagon and decrease in the concentration of plasma insulin. Glucagon increases gluconeogenesis from protein in the liver and insulin has an inhibitory effect. Studies in normal subjects and mild diabetics suggested that the integrated changes in intermediary metabolism in response to starvation are initiated by the fall in concentration of serum insulin (Cahill et al 1966). Alanine is quantitatively the most important gluconeogenic amino acid but skeletal muscle contains only 7% alanine. However alanine may be formed in muscle by transamination of pyruvate (Fig. 3.1), the amine radicle being supplied by oxidation of the branched chain amino acids leucine, isoleucine and valine (Mallette et al 1969). The decrease in gluconeogenesis during fasting produces a corresponding fall in the excretion of urea and its concentration in the blood and the excretion of creatinine falls slightly.

The mobilisation of the fat stores is reflected by an increase in the concentration of free fatty acids and glycerol in the plasma. As well as using glucose for

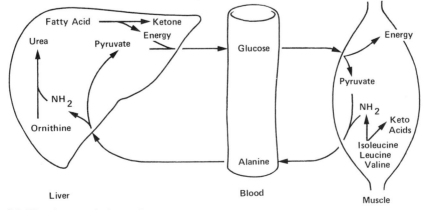

Fig. 3.1 The glucose–alanine cycle

fuel, skeletal muscle, cardiac muscle and the renal cortex can all utilise fatty acids. Oxidation of the fatty acids results in an increase in the plasma concentration and urinary excretion of aceto–acetate and β hydroxybutyrate. Cahill & Aoki (1970) have indicated that although the term ketone bodies is traditionally used to describe aceto–acetate and β hydroxybutyrate, neither substance is a ketone and β hydroxybutyrate is not a keto acid. The term probably arose because of the observation that acetone, a ketone, could be detected in the breath and urine of diabetics and fasting or fat–fed subjects.

As a consequence of the increase in the urinary excretion of these two keto acids, there is a concomitant increase in the urinary excretion of ammonia as there is a limit to the kidney's ability to excrete hydrogen ions (see Ch. 4). Ketone bodies are water–soluble and do not require insulin to enter the cell. Thus ketone bodies can easily cross the blood brain barrier and during prolonged fasting they may supply 80% of the fuel requirements of the brain, the remainder being supplied by gluconeogenesis from protein (Owen et al 1967). As might be expected, tissues such as skeletal and cardiac muscle which can use fatty acids as fuel can also use ketone bodies.

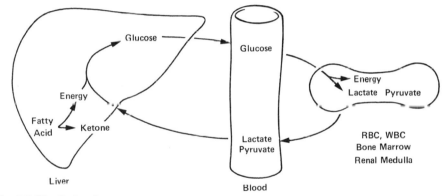

Fig. 3.2 The Cori cycle

Glucose may be only partly oxidised by tissues other than brain to lactate and puruvate. In muscle, as described above, the pyruvate may be converted to alanine using amine radicles from branched chain amino acids. In the liver, glucose can be resynthesised from alanine via pyruvate, the amine radicle being used for amination of a keto acid or excreted as ammonia. (Mallette et al 1969). Lactate and pyruvate formed by glycolysis in the renal medulla, bone marrow and blood cells may be transferred directly to the liver (Fig. 3.2) and used to resynthesise glucose (Cori 1931). The similarity of the Cori cycle and the glucose–alanine cycle are evident from Figures 3.1 and 3.2. These cycles enable energy produced by the oxidation of fatty acids in the liver to be transferred to the periphery in the form of readily usable glucose. Partial oxidation of this glucose yields pyruvate which is transported to the liver (as alanine in the glucose–alanine cycle) where it is used to synthesise glucose. These cycles reduce gluconeogenic demands from protein during starvation.

The predominant metabolic pathways encountered in healthy post–prandial subjects are shown in Figure 3.3 and the changes induced by early and late

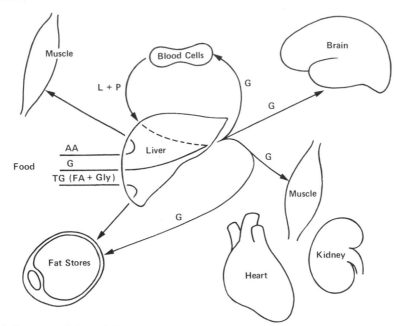

Fig. 3.3 Post–prandial metabolic pathways. AA — amino acids, FA — fatty acids, G — glucose, Gly — glycerol, K — ketones, L — lactate, P — pyruvate, TG — triglycerides

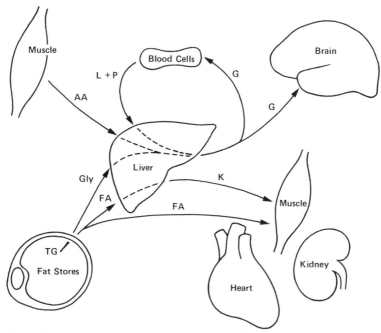

Fig. 3.4 Metabolic pathways in early starvation (for key see Fig. 3.3)

starvation are shown in Figures 3.4. and 3.5. Cahill (1970) has suggested that in early starvation approximately 75 g of protein and 160 g of fatty acids are mobilised each day. Gluconogenseis from the protein produces 180 g of glucose of which 144 g are oxidised completely to water and carbon dioxide by the brain

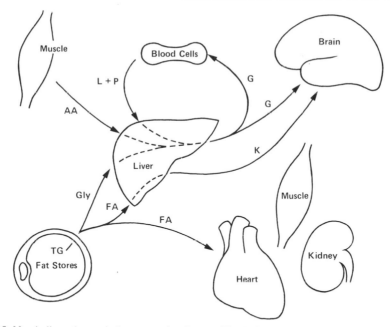

Fig. 3.5 Metabolic pathways in late starvation (key see Fig. 3.3)

and 36 g are oxidised incompletely by glycolytic tissues to lactate and pyruvate from which glucose is resynthesised in the liver by the Cori cycle. In prolonged starvation, Cahill has estimated that as a consequence of ketone utilisation, the daily cerebral glucose requirement is reduced to 44 g. The total daily glucose requirement for the brain and glycolytic tissues is 80 g which is produced mainly by gluconeogenesis in both the liver and kidney of 20 g of protein. Thus protein breakdown is reduced from 75 g/d in early starvation to 20 g/d in late starvation. The increase in the quantity of fat that is burnt from 160 g/d in early starvation to 180 g/d in late starvation is less than might be expected as total energy requirement is reduced in prolonged starvation.

INJURY

The changes in metabolism that follow starvation appear to be purposeful and beneficial with the prime objective being conservation of body tissue and, in particular, body protein. This is achieved mainly by reducing gluconeogenic requirements. As Hunter originally suggested, the changes in metabolism that follow injury may also be purposeful and represent a teleological response designed to mobilise the tissues for defence and repair. However the response to injury is more extensive than the response to starvation; it is governed by changes in a greater number of hormones, it imposes a greater burden upon the tissues of the body (particularly upon the protein reserves as gluconeogenesis is not reduced) and it is not abolished by the simple restoration of nutritional intake. These changes, although more pronounced after certain insults such as burns and sepsis and first described after bony injury (Cuthbertson 1930), may be recognised after traumatic events of any kind.

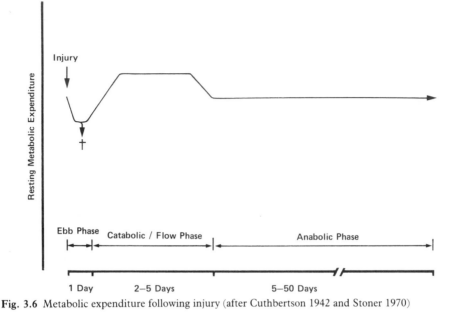

Fig. 3.6 Metabolic expenditure following injury (after Cuthbertson 1942 and Stoner 1970)

The changes in metabolic expenditure that follow injury are shown in Figure 3.6 which is based upon descriptions by Cuthbertson (1942) and Stoner (1970). These changes have been studied extensively after a variety of injuries in man and in experimental animals. Although there are minor differences in response between different species, the broad sequence of events observed is remarkably constant throughout the animal kingdom. After injury, there is a depression of metabolic function with a reduction in oxygen consumption, heat production and body temperature. This period, which lasts for a few hours after injury of moderate severity, was called the 'ebb phase' by Cuthbertson, and in the experimental animal it is associated with impaired function in the tricarboxylic acid cycle (Threlfall 1970). It appears to be a critical phase, for, if the injury inflicted is severe, the metabolic depression increases and the animal dies as a consequence of what Stoner has termed necrobiosis. In man this 'ebb phase' appears to correspond with shock (see Ch. 5). After elective operations, a few patients in the recovery room may be observed to be exhibiting the features of the ebb phase, but by the time they return to the ward this should have abated. If the injury has not been too severe, metabolic function recovers and eventually heat production exceeds that found before injury. Cuthbertson called this the 'flow phase' but it is usually referred to by surgeons as the 'catabolic phase' of injury. Eventually, catabolism diminishes and with increasing appetite and ambulation the patient enters the anabolic phase that is typical of normal convalescence. The use of the term 'catabolic phase' has been criticised by O'Keefe and his colleagues (1974) who emphasise that in particular the negative nitrogen balance that occurs during this period may be a reflection of decreased synthesis rather than increased breakdown of protein. However, the term has much to commend its use; it describes overall changes in metabolism of protein, fat and carbohydrate occurring at a particular stage following injury that is easily recognised by clinicians. Nevertheless the objection to its use is understandable as therapy designed to prevent or diminish breakdown of protein may differ from that designed to promote synthesis. These semantic difficulties could be overcome if the terms catabolism and anabolism were adopted to describe the nett result of synthesis and breakdown. There is evidence to suggest that during the catabolic phase of injury, alterations occur in both synthesis and breakdown of protein, but breakdown exceeds synthesis.

If the patient does not succumb to the initial injury, this ideal sequence of events does not always follow. The development of sepsis increases energy demands (Kinney et al 1970) and the occurrence of myocardial infarction, pulmonary embolism or bronchopneumonia may cause hypoxia, a potent stimulus to tissue catabolism. The loss of lean body mass in these patients may be fatal and of such cases Moore and his colleagues (1963) have observed 'the most destructive processes seen in the study of body composition are those that combine severe injury with invasive sepsis. The body cell mass quickly melts away into a hypotonic ocean of extracellular fluid'. Fortunately, the majority of patients do not suffer severe injury or such complications and there is little change in the total energy requirements following elective operations of moderate severity (Tweedle & Johnston 1971). Although this response to injury is reduced in patients who are nutritionally impoverished before injury (Moore & Ball 1952) mortality and morbidity is particularly severe in these patients (Studley 1936, Bistrian et al 1975).

Following injury, the major pathways of metabolism are similar to those shown for early fasting (Fig. 3.4) but there are important quantitative and qualitative differences. There is an overall increase in energy requirements and in particular there is an increase in gluconeogenic requirements. This is hormonal in origin and consequently is not influenced by infusion of energy (Kinney et al 1970). In early fasting approximately 75 g of protein must be broken down to provide glucose each day but in severely injured patients as much as 250 g of protein may be required. These quantitative and qualitative differences between the metabolic pathways during early fasting and injury become even greater when sepsis occurs. The intolerance of injured patients to exogenous glucose was increased by the onset of sepsis and reduced when sepsis resolved (Askanazi et al 1980). This intolerance was accompanied by an increased excretion of noradrenaline in the urine. Some examples of the rate of protein and energy consumption that occur in hospital patients are shown in Table 3.1.

These composite figures have been derived from observations of a wide variety of medical and surgical patients (Coleman & Dubois 1915, Benedict 1915, Dubois 1924, Cuthbertson 1932, Keys et al 1950, Liljedahl et al 1961, Kinney et al 1970, Tweedle & Johnston 1971, Tweedle 1974, Wilmore et al 1974a, Halmagyi & Kinney 1975). These values are typical of the maximum rates observed in the majority of patients. In some patients, the maximum rate may occur for two or three days only, but in others such as those with extensive burns and sepsis, the maximum rate of loss may be sustained for many days or weeks. Considerable variation may occur according to the age, sex, stature, and previous health of the individual and every effort should be made to estimate these losses in severely ill patients.

Although, in general, total energy production is increased when protein loss is

Table 3.1 Protein and energy loss in health, starvation and injury (see text for sources)

| | Protein loss | | Energy loss | |
	g N/d	g/d	MJ/d	kcal/d
Health	11	70	7.5	1800
Early starvation	9	55	6.7	1600
Late starvation	7	45	5.2	1250
Cholecystectomy	12	75	7.5	1800
Pancreatectomy	16	100	8.4	2000
Oesophago–gastrectomy	14	90	8.4	2000
Small bowel fistula (without sepsis)	20	125	8.0	1900
Ulcerative colitis (severe)	30	190	9.0	2150
Peritonitis	18	110	9.0	2150
Typhoid fever	30	190	10.5	2500
Burns				
0–25%	20	125	11.3	2700
25–50%	25	155	13.2	3150
50–75%	30	190	15.1	3600
Respiratory failure and sepsis	18	110	11.7	2800
Renal failure and sepsis	20	125	11.7	2800
Simple fracture	14	90	8.8	2100

increased, such losses are not always proportional. Thus patients with considerable protein loss from the gastro–intestinal tract may show little increase in energy production in the absence of sepsis. In general, measurements of protein loss and energy production have been much lower than values frequently suggested following attempts to reverse these losses by the provision of exogenous substrates; it is very uncommon to observe protein losses greater than 150 g/d and energy production greater than 12.5 MJ/d (3000 kcal/d). Patients who are suffering from renal failure who are not treated by dialysis may appear to have very low losses of protein, but the daily increase in the urea content of the body represents protein loss. In patients treated by dialysis, losses of protein may exceed those shown in Table 3.1.

Endocrine response and intermediary metabolism

The changes observed in intermediary metabolism following injury are associated with corresponding changes in hormonal secretion. Although both components may be influenced by changes in the other, it is apparent that the major difference between the response to starvation and the response to injury is a consequence of alterations in hormonal secretions that show little response to nutritional modification.

Although there is a small increase in the serum concentration of glucagon, changes in intermediary metabolism during starvation are predominantly a consequence of changes in the serum concentration of insulin. Following injury there are widespread changes in many hormones whose metabolic actions are opposed to insulin. One of the earliest observations was the association of an increased output of urinary steroids following operation and the similarity between changes in postoperative metabolism and those associated with Cushing's disease (Albright 1943). However, not every operation produces a change in urinary excretion of cortisol (Espiner 1966) and it has been suggested that cortisol has a permissive, rather than a promotional role (Ingle 1954, Dudley et al 1959). Studies in animals and in man have shown that adrenaline, noradrenaline and their metabolites appear in the urine in increased quantities after injury (Walker et al 1959, Walker 1965). The plasma concentration of glucagon is also markedly elevated following injury (Meguid & Brennan 1974, Wilmore et al 1974b) and after operation (Russell et al 1975). It would appear that the major catabolic hormone that stimulates breakdown of glycogen, protein and triglyceride following injury is noradrenaline. The principle role of glucagon appears to be the stimulation of hepatic uptake of amino acids such as alanine and perhaps other nitrogenous substances with the subsequent production of glucose from the carbon skeletons and urea from the amine groups.

The thyroid hormones, thyroxine and tri–iodothyronine, are often considered to be catabolic hormones. Patients with thyrotoxicosis have raised serum glucose and free fatty acid concentrations and they break down excessive quantities of their lean body mass and fat stores to fuel their increased basal metabolic expenditure. However, lack of thyroid hormones produces the stunted growth of cretinism which can be prevented by the provision of small quantities of thyroxine. The thyroid hormones are only catabolic when released in excessive quantities. Contrary to original theories, secretion of thyroid stimulating hormone is unaltered after operation (Charters et al 1969, Kirby & Johnston 1971) and there is disagreement about whether serum thyroxine and tri–iodothyronine concentrations are increased or decreased (Schwartz & Roberts 1957, Franksson et al 1959, Burr et al 1975, Becker et al 1976).

During the ebb phase of injury there may be a failure of insulin secretion in response to hyperglycaemia (Allison et al 1967, 1968). During the flow phase, abnormally high serum concentrations of insulin are found but there is a coexistent hyperglycaemia (Wright et al 1974) which may be a reflection of the antagonistic effects of cortisol, glucagon and the catecholamines as indicated in Figure 3.7. It is apparent that increased concentrations of these powerful catabolic hor-

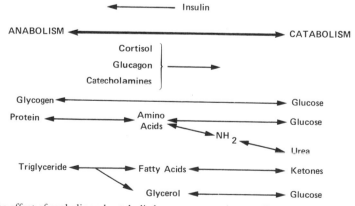

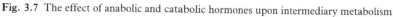

Fig. 3.7 The effect of anabolic and catabolic hormones upon intermediary metabolism

mones may produce hyperglycaemia even in the face of hyperinsulinaemia and treatment of so-called 'traumatic diabetes' requires the use of far greater quantities of insulin than those required for the treatment of diabetes mellitus. Furthermore, these hormonal changes may explain why gluconeogenesis may be inhibited by the infusion of small quantities of glucose before but not after injury (Kinney et al 1970). This important difference in intermediary metabolism explains why the metabolic consequences of injury are far greater and more difficult to counteract than those of simple starvation.

The role of the other anabolic hormones, growth hormone and testosterone, in the metabolic response to injury is uncertain. There have been only a few studies of relatively small numbers of patients over short periods of time (Glick et al 1965, Charters et al 1969, Newsome & Rose 1971, Carstensen et al 1972). It would appear that during oparation plasma growth hormone concentration increases but falls rapidly to normal levels on the day of operation and does not fluctuate during the catabolic or anabolic phases of the response to injury. These findings suggest that it is unlikely that this hormone has any major role in the regulation of metabolism after injury. The secretion of growth hormone appears to be particularly sensitive to the serum glucose concentration and the increased secretion during operation may be in response to the hyperglycaemia that occurs at this time. The observation that postoperative decreases in the urinary excretion of 17–ketosteroids was much greater in males than in females (Tanaka et al 1970) was followed by studies which confirmed that plasma testoterone concentrations fell consistently after operation and normal concentrations were restored by the 4th to 10th day according to the severity of the surgery (Matsumoto et al 1970, Carstensen et al 1972). Although this decrease in the plasma concentration of an anabolic hormone coincides with the catabolic phase of the response to injury, it is difficult to envisage an important role for this hormone after injury or operation in females.

TREATMENT

There is considerable disagreement as to which patients require particular attention to their nutritional requirements. Many surgical patients undergo periods of 5 to 10 days before, during and after operation when oral intake of nutrients is negligible or absent. Most healthy young adults can withstand periods of starvation of this length and the associated metabolic effects of operation without any apparent ill effects, but such starvation may be a fatal insult to a malnourished, elderly patient with cardiac and respiratory impairment undergoing major surgery. There are those who believe that, as the body possesses carbohydrate reserves that will last for only a few hours and subsequent requirements for carbohydrate are met predominantly by gluconeogenesis from protein of the lean body mass, 'no hospital patient should be allowed to starve for more than six hours' (Peaston 1968). A very different view was held by Wilkinson (1955) who observed that 'the basic pattern of chemical behaviour after injury is not readily modified by the administration of calories, protein or water' and Davidson & Passmore (1969) who considered the response to injury to be inevitable and physiological and that there was little justification in attempting to alter it. Most clinicians agree that it is difficult to modify the response to injury but recognise that in certain patients the response may be excessive and contribute to morbidity and mortality.

How can the deleterious effects of the changes in metabolism after injury be modified? In spite of many years of investigation, the initiating factor of this response has not been identified. As Hunter (1791b) observed in his famous treatise, 'I come now to the most difficult part of the subjects; for it is much more easy to describe actions, than to assign motives; and without being able to assign motives, it is impossible to know when or how we may or should check actions or remove them' so also two centuries later did Le Quesne (1961) emphasise 'The whole notion of a compensatory reaction implies that the organ or system in question is attempting to solve or react to the problem with which we think it should be concerned, whereas it may be responding to an entirely different stimulus'.

In spite of these uncertainties it would appear that the alterations in metabolism after injury are a consequence of the predominance of the combined action of the catabolic hormones over the action of anabolic hormones (Fig. 3.7). As the major impetus seems to come from excessive action of catabolic hormones, it may be possible in the future to restrict their action by antagonistic substances but, as yet, attempts to modify the response to injury by hormonal therapy have been restricted to providing exogenous anabolic hormones. Although exogenous growth hormone was without effect upon nitrogen balance after herniorrhaphy (Johnston & Hadden 1963) the degree of traumatic insult imparted by this operation is very small and it is possible that any modification in protein metabolism induced by the therapy may have been correspondingly slight and beyond the sensitivity of the method of study. Other studies have demonstrated that negative nitrogen balance following burns can be reduced by giving exogenous growth hormone, particularly when given with large quantities of protein and non–protein energy (Liljedahl et al 1961, Wilmore et al 1974c).

The development of synthetic compounds with chemical configurations very similar to the natural hormone testosterone was followed by a large number of studies of the effect of these synthetic hormones upon nitrogen balance following operations. Although nitrogen balance following partial gastrectomy was improved by intramuscular injection of synthetic anabolic steroids (Abbott et al 1956, Gilder et al 1957), no improvement was observed following thoracic operations in patients suffering from tuberculosis (Kennedy et al 1959, Webb et al 1960). A significant improvement in nitrogen balance was recorded after inguinal herniorrhaphy and vagotomy and gastro–enterostomy (Johnston & Chenneour 1963) but a significant deterioration in nitrogen balance was observed with the use of the same anabolic steroid in patients receiving large quantities of protein and non–protein energy after abdominal operations (Johnston et al 1966). These conflicting results may reflect many other variables inherent to these studies. In some of these investigations, the control and study groups differed greatly with respect to the sex, age, weight and nutritional intake of the patients studied, the degree of trauma inflicted upon the patient and in the length of the study.

In a study designed to assess the effect of nandralone decanoate in patients receiving both high and low intakes of nutrition after vagotomy and pyloroplasty (Tweedle et al 1973) the nitrogen balance of all the patients receiving the anabolic

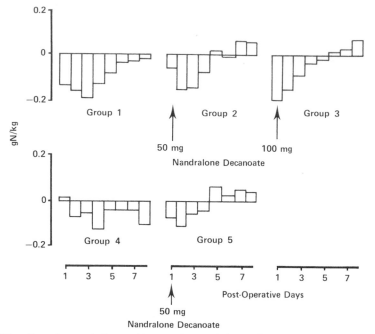

Fig. 3.8 The effect of an anabolic steroid upon nitrogen balance after truncal vagotomy and pyloroplasty

steroid was improved (groups 2, 3 and 5 of Fig. 3.8). The prolonged and rapid effect of this steroid, previously noted in experimental animals (de Visser & Over-beek 1960) was confirmed in man. The greatest improvement in nitrogen balance was produced by a combination of high nutritional intake and the anabolic steroid. Although there was no evidence of any further improvement produced by increasing the dose in patients in group 3, the optimal response may require high-er doses in patients undergoing operations of greater severity. If the urinary nit-rogen is assumed to be solely a product of the breakdown of hydrated protein, the differences between the control group (1) and low–intake groups (2 and 3) repre-sents a saving of 0.8 kg of lean body mass during the eight days of study and the differences between the control group (1) and high intake group (5) represents a saving of 1.4 kg.

Anabolic steroids have been reported to cause cholestatic jaundice and liver damage. Sherlock (1962) has emphasised that all the preparations that have in-duced jaundice or liver damage are active when given orally and all are C17–alkyl substituted testosterones. The anabolic steroid nandralone decanoate used in the study described above does not have this chemical configuration and is inactive when given by mouth. Masculinisation in the female is a further unwanted side effect of some anabolic steroids. The ideal preparation is one with a high anabolic effect and low androgenic effect. The usual method of assessing the relative potency of this unwanted effect is to compare the myotrophic effect of the drug upon the levator ani muscles of the rat with its androgenic effect upon the semi-nal vesicles (Hershberger et al 1953). These and other side effects of treatment with anabolic steroids have usually followed long–term use in debilitating illnesses or abuse by healthy athletes and may have little relevance to their short-term use in promoting protein synthesis after injury.

Nevertheless, anabolic steroids have been used infrequently in the treatment of patients after operation and injury and the mainstay of hormonal therapy has been insulin. Recognising that insulin enhances cellular uptake of amino acids and their incorporation into protein (Manchester 1968, 1970, Pozefsky, et al 1969) and inhibits glycolysis (Ashmore & Weber 1968), Hinton et al (1971) demonstrated that treatment with large quantities of exogenous insulin and glucose reduced protein catabolism after injury and increased urinary excretion of sodium but decreased urinary excretion of potassium. Although these initial studies were performed mainly in patients with burns, the same pattern of response has been observed in patients with other forms of injury and after operation. It should be noted that Hinton and her colleagues wished to study the effect of insulin therapy upon the metabolic response to injury and infused hypertonic solutions of glucose to prevent hypoglycaemia that would be induced by the large doses of insulin. This difference in approach should be compared with standard practice in North America where the unavailability of intravenous fat emulsions for intravenous feeding led to the use of highly concentrated solutions of glucose, insulin being required to prevent hyperglycaemia and hyperosmolarity (Dudrick et al 1970). Although the end result is very similar on both sides of the Atlantic Ocean, the underlying rationale differs, the approach of Hinton et al being based upon hormonal therapy and that of Dudrick et al upon the provision of large quantities of substrate. Because Hinton and her colleagues needed to infuse large quantities of glucose (500 g/d) to prevent hypoglycaemia, it was not possible to be certain that the protein–sparing was induced by the insulin and not by the provision of the large quantity of substrate, but subsequent studies have shown that insulin does have a protein–sparing effect, irrespective of the concomitant infusion of glucose (Woolfson et al 1977).

The quantities of insulin that have been given to counter the adverse hormonal circumstance of the response to injury have shown considerable variation. In most cases it is appropriate to infuse 4 g of glucose with each unit of insulin and to give about 500 g of glucose and 125 units of insulin each day. The patient should have a catheter inserted in the bladder and urine tested each hour. The blood glucose concentration should also be measured at least twice each day. If hyperglycaemia and glucosuria develop, the quantity of insulin should be increased or dangerous hyperosmolarity will occur. In some severely injured patients as much as 600 units each day has failed to prevent the development of hyperglycaemia induced by 500 g of glucose and it is usual to refer to this phenomenon as 'insulin resistance'. Although it is suggested that this post–traumatic resistance to the normal effect of insulin is a consequence of the increased secretions of the catabolic hormones, this remains to be proved. The catecholamines suppress endogenous release of insulin in response to hyperglycaemia (Porte & Robertson 1973) but this mechanism cannot explain the alteration in insulin requirements when both exogenous insulin and glucose are given in large quantities. Frequently, a reduction in insulin requirement is an early sign of improvement in a desperately ill patient. Insulin also promotes cellular uptake of potassium and phosphorus and these elements must be given in addition to glucose or

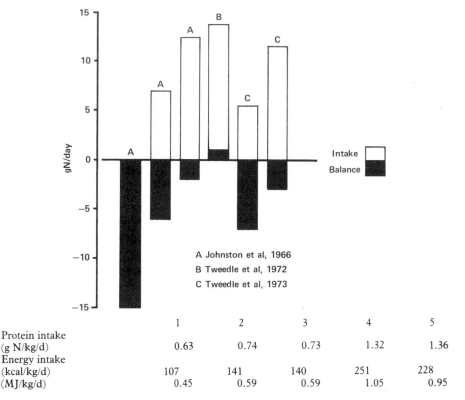

Fig. 3.9 The effect of intravenous nutrition upon nitrogen balance after truncal vagotomy and pyloroplasty

dangerous hypokalaemia and hypophosphataemia may occur. The requirements for insulin, glucose and these elements in a variety of patients are discussed in greater detail in Chapter 8.

Although hormonal changes appear to initiate the metabolic response to injury the deleterious consequences are substrate in nature and it is not surprising that many have attempted to overcome these phenomena by altering the intake of substrate. As described above, the effects of starvation and injury differ in both a qualitative and quantitative manner and the quantities of nutrients that are required to produce a neutral or positive balance after injury are much greater than those required to reverse simple starvation. As these patients frequently have inadequate gastro-intestinal function most patients have been fed intravenously. The requirements differ according to the previous nutritional state of the patient and to the disease or injury from which they are suffering. For some time it was doubted whether it was possible to achieve positive nitrogen balance after operation. It is now apparent that positive balance can be attained if sufficient quantities of protein and non-protein energy are given. It is evident from the results of the three studies depicted in Figure 3.9 that nitrogen balance in the first week following vagotomy and pyloroplasty is determined by nitrogen intake and that the negative balance that usually follows this operation can be reversed by intravenous feeding with 14 g N (87.5 g protein) and 11.3 MJ (2700 kcal) of energy each day (Johnston et al 1966, Tweedle et al 1972, 1973). These quantities are considerably greater than those required to reverse the effects of simple starvation. Nevertheless, the traumatic insult of vagotomy and pyloroplasty is comparatively slight when compared with other elective operations and accidental injuries. As the severity of the traumatic insult increases, the quantity of protein and energy that is required to achieve a positive nitrogen balance increases in an exponential manner. As much as 33 g N (205 g protein) and 14.2 MJ (3400 kcal) of energy are required each day to achieve positive balance following more extensive elective operations such as cardio–oesophagectomy and duodeno–pancreatomy (Loirat et al 1975). When patients develop septic complications following severe injury, it may be impossible to reverse the negative nitrogen balance by increasing intake.

Although the negative nitrogen balance following some injuries may be reversed by increasing intake, it should be noted that this is not due to any decrease in the urinary excretion of nitrogen. The increased excretion following injury remains as a component of the balance, positive balance being achieved by ensuring that intake exceeds output. A small proportion of the infused amino acids is always excreted unutilised (usually less than 5% with modern solutions containing only l–isomers) and a corresponding allowance in intake must be made for this quantity. These features emphasise that in some patients the attainment of positive balance may be an illusory achievement indicating little more than numerical superiority of intake over output with no beneficial effect for the patient.

As discussed above, there can be little doubt that patients who have greatly increased requirements after severe injury and sepsis and in whom ingestion, digestion and absorption of even normal requirements is impossible do require nutritional support. However, there is little evidence that routine support in patients who are undergoing elective operations confers any benefit. Although there was a significant improvement in the weight and the concentration of serum albumin of patients with malignant disease who received intravenous nutrition for 3 days before operations, there was no statistically significant difference in the incidence of major complications when compared with patients who were not fed intravenously (Holter & Fischer 1977). In a similar study in patients undergoing oesophagectomy for carcinoma, intravenous feeding for 5 to 7 days before operation and for 6 to 7 days after operation maintained a positive nitrogen balance before and after operation and wound healing was complete in contrast to that observed in patients who were not fed intravenously (Moghissi et al 1977). It has been known for many years that immune function is impaired in malnourished patients (Cannon 1945) and more recently it has been demonstrated that immune competence can be restored by nutritional repletion (Law et al 1973, Haffejee et al 1978). The incidence of wound infection was reduced in patients fed intravenously for 7–10 days before operations for gastric and oesophageal cancer when compared with controls but there was no change in immunocompetence (Heatley et al 1979). As emphasised elsewhere (Brit. med. J. 1979), both premature enthusiasm and precipitate condemnation must be avoided. The role of peri–operative nutritional repletion remains to be established and many more studies are required with particular emphasis placed upon clinical rather than biochemical responses.

4

Hydrogen ion regulation

Hydrogen ion regulation is disturbed during the course of many illnesses and recognition and treatment of such a disturbance can make a major contribution to the patient's recovery. The term 'hydrogen ion regulation' is used in preference to 'acid–base balance' because the former term emphasises that it is variation in the quantity of free hydrogen ions which causes the disturbances. Although hydrogen ions (H^+) do not exist free in solution, but as H_3O^+ (hydronium molecules) this slight inaccuracy is of no importance to the understanding of the subject. Hydrogen ion regulation should be considered in the same way as sodium or potassium balance, on the basis of its production, transport and elimination.

HYDROGEN ION REGULATION IN HEALTH

Definitions

An acid is a substance which donates hydrogen ions.

A base is a substance which accepts hydrogen ions.

A strong acid is well dissociated and has many hydrogen ions available for donation.

A strong base is well dissociated and will readily accept hydrogen ions.

The degree of dissociation of a substance is affected by the acidity of the solution. A substance which is an acid when in a solution of low acidity may act as a base at a higher acidity; e.g. HCO_3^- is a base at physiological pH but is an acid ($H^+ + CO_3^-$) at a higher pH.

pH is the term which is used to express the acidity or alkalinity of a substance. It is $\dfrac{1}{\text{Log }[H^+]}$, the negative logarithm of the hydrogen ion concentration. Hydrogen ion concentration can be measured directly, and the result given in nanomoles of hydrogen ion per kilogram of water but most clinical laboratories deduce the quantity of hydrogen ion by comparison of the unknown solution with buffer solutions of known pH and express the result in pH units.

A buffer is a mixture of a weak acid and its salt of a strong base in an association which minimises the effects of addition or removal of hydrogen ion from the medium. The most important physiological buffer is the combination of carbonic acid and bicarbonate i.e.

$$H^+ + HCO_3^- \rightleftharpoons H_2CO_3$$

The addition of hydrogen ion to the left-hand side of the equation increases the amount of carbonic acid present, but since this is poorly dissociated and in equilibrium with sodium, the pH of the medium is not changed significantly. The equation moves in the opposite direction if hydrogen ions are removed from the medium.

At body temperature chemical neutrality exists at pH 6.8. Blood is moderately alkaline and the normal pH range is between 7.36–7.44, which is equivalent to 49–36 nmol hydrogen ion per kg body water. The range of viability is usually said to be from pH 6.8–7.7, equivalent to 160–20 nmol hydrogen ion per kg body water.

The intracellular pH cannot be measured easily and since it varies between tissues, no mean intracellular pH value can be given. It depends upon cellular metabolic activity, the supply of oxygen and nutrient material and the efficient removal of metabolic waste products. Hydrogen ions do not readily cross cell membranes so the extracellular and intracellular pH may differ considerably. This will be referred to later.

Hydrogen ion production
Under normal circumstances the body is more concerned to excrete than to retain hydrogen ions. They are produced from respiratory and non-respiratory sources but the relative amounts which are produced are very different.

13 000 mmol hydrogen ion (13 000 $\times$ 10^6 nmol) are produced in each 24-hour period from carbon dioxide

1000 mmol hydrogen ion (1000 $\times$ 10^6 nmol) are produced in each 24-hour period from ingested food and from non-respiratory and organic acids.

These two sources are by convention called 'respiratory' and 'metabolic' respectively but since both are the result of metabolic activities it is more accurate to call them 'respiratory' and 'non-respiratory' sources.

Hydrogen ion homeostasis
Homeostasis is maintained by three processes:
1. Pulmonary excretion
2. Renal excretion
3. Buffers

Pulmonary excretion
Carbon dioxide is produced by cellular metabolic activity. It is not an acid but in solution and in the presence of the enzyme carbonic anhydrase it is converted to carbonic acid,

$$\text{i.e. } CO_2 + H_2O \rightleftharpoons H_2CO_3 \rightleftharpoons H^+ + HCO_3^-$$

Carbonic anhydrase is present inside red blood cells, in the kidneys and the lungs. It increases the speed of what would otherwise be a very slow chemical reaction. Carbonic acid is relatively poorly dissociated at physiological pH, that is, it is a weak acid. It is transported to the lungs where the carbon dioxide is excreted and the equation moves to the left. Thus hydrogen ions and carbon dioxide are in equilibrium and the loss of one carbon dioxide molecule is equivalent to the loss of one hydrogen ion.

To emphasise the importance of this process, it can be demonstrated that if the excretion of gaseous carbon dioxide was totally prevented for five minutes (without allowing the patient to die from hypoxia) the pH would fall by approximately 0.2 pH units. In contrast, if the urinary excretion of hydrogen ion was arrested for one hour, the effect on pH would not be noticeable.

Renal excretion

There are three systems in the kidney by which hydrogen ion excretion is regulated.

The renal tubular cells contain the enzyme glutaminase. This controls the breakdown of the amino acid glutamine, which is present in extracellular fluid, to ammonia (NH_3). Ammonia is also produced from the breakdown of glycine, alanine, leucine and aspartic acid by the action of oxidases. At physiological pH, ammonia behaves as a base and accepts hydrogen ion to become ammonium ion (NH_4^+) which is excreted into the tubular urine in exchange for sodium ions. In this way it both facilitates the excretion of hydrogen ions and the conservation of sodium.

The second system involves the addition of hydrogen ion to monohydrogen phosphate (HPO_4^{2-}) which is excreted as dihydrogen phosphate ($H_2PO_4^-$).

Either carbonic acid or bicarbonate ions can be excreted in the urine as required.

These mechanisms are activated or inhibited according to the amount of hydrogen ion or base which must be excreted. If the extracellular fluid becomes alkaline, the production of ammonia is reduced, monohydrogen phosphate (HPO_4^{2-}) and bicarbonate are excreted and hydrogen ions are retained. The excretion of base is equivalent to the retention of acid; i.e. the excretion or loss of one bicarbonate molecule is accompanied by the retention of one hydrogen ion, and vice versa.

Renal excretion of hydrogen ions ceases at a urinary pH of 4.5.

Buffers

Buffers were defined earlier. Their function is to permit hydrogen ions to be produced and transported to their point of elimination with minimal alteration in the extracellular pH. The most important buffers are:

$$H_2CO_3 \ + \ HCO_3^- \ + \ \text{Cation}$$
$$HHb \ + \ Hb^- \ + \ \text{Cation}$$
$$H_2PO_4 \ + \ HPO_4^{2-} \ + \ \text{Cation}$$

The bicarbonate–carbonic acid buffer is quantitatively the most important. Because carbonic acid is partially dissociated in the extracellular fluid it has itself to be buffered by haemoglobin and the plasma proteins. This reduces the change in pH which would be produced by the transport of carbonic acid from the tissues to the lungs, where it is excreted as carbon dioxide.

Reduced haemoglobin is a better buffer than is oxyhaemoglobin. The removal of oxygen by the tissues increases the ability of haemoglobin to buffer the hydrogen ions produced therein. The plasma proteins are also buffers but, weight for weight, have only one third of the buffering capacity of haemoglobin. As they are present in less than half its amount their total buffering capacity is only one sixth that of haemoglobin. The phosphate buffer is of minor importance in the extracellular fluid but of major importance in the kidneys, as described above.

The pH of buffer pair depends upon the law of mass action, which can be written as:

$$pH = pK + Log \frac{[Base]}{[Acid]}$$

For the carbonic acid–bicarbonate buffer this becomes the Henderson–Hasselbalch equation:

$$e.g. \ pH = pK + Log \frac{[HCO_3^-]}{[H_2CO_3]}$$

The constant K is the dissociation constant of the acid and pK is its negative logarithm, which for carbonic acid is 6.1. The ratio of base to acid in this buffer pair is normally 20, the logarithm of which is 1.3

$$i.e. \ pH = 6.1 + 1.3$$
$$= 7.4$$

The Henderson–Hasselbalch equation can also be written as follows:

$$pH = 6.1 + Log \frac{[HCO_3^-]}{PaCO_2 \ (kPa) \times 0.23}$$

This modification is possible because there is a constant relationship between carbon dioxide tension and carbonic acid. $PaCO_2$ is in kilopascals and the factor 0.23 is the solubility coefficient for carbon dioxide. When $PaCO_2$ is measured in mmHg, the solubility factor is 0.03. The various forms of the equation are useful because if any two of the variables are known it is easy to calculate the third. There are many graphical ways of doing this which eliminate the mathematics. These include the Singer Hastings and the Siggaard–Andersen nomograms. The latter (Fig. 4.1) is one of the more comprehensive versions which shows most of the acute and chronic hydrogen ion disturbances which can occur and it will be referred to again. However the version devised by Nunn (Fig. 4.2) is easier for the beginner to understand and it will be used extensively in the next section. For completeness it should be realised that there are some objections to the use of the Henderson–Hasselbalch equation, which include the fact that the constant K is not absolutely constant.

CLINICAL SYNDROMES OF HYDROGEN ION IMBALANCE

Definitions

Acidaemia: Accumulation of hydrogen ion or loss of base causing a reduction of pH to below 7.35

Acidosis: A change which would result in acidaemia in the absence of compensatory processes

SIGGAARD-ANDERSEN ACID-BASE CHART

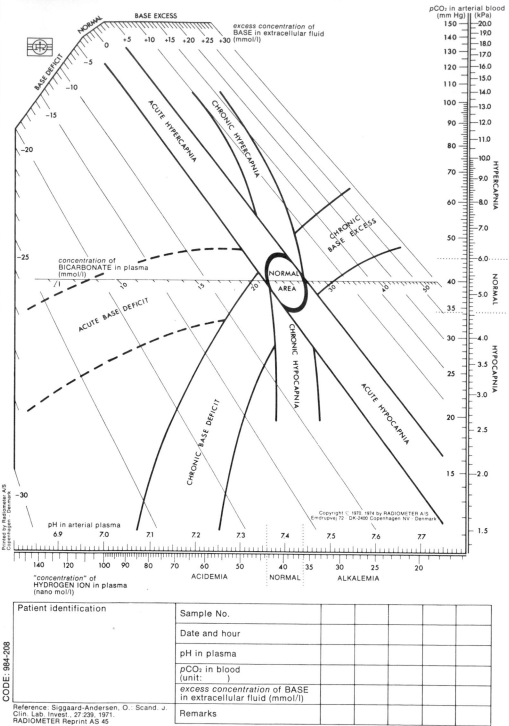

Fig. 4.1 The Siggaard-Andersen acid-base chart. This chart is used in association with the Astrup technique in which pH and Log $PaCO_2$ are plotted against each other for two known gases and a buffer line obtained. The 'actual $PaCO_2$' is then obtained from the 'actual pH' and the point where this falls on the buffer line permits the rest of the data to be obtained. (see text). Reproduced with permission from Radiometer A/S and Professor Siggaard-Andersen

Alkalaemia: Loss of hydrogen ion or accumulation of base causing an elevation of pH above 7.45

Alkalosis: A change which would produce alkalaemia in the absence of compensatory processes

The body's response to a disturbance of hydrogen ion regulation is to attempt to produce its physiological opposite i.e. the natural correction for a non–respiratory acidosis would be a respiratory alkalosis. The degree of correction is some indication of the duration of the disturbance and of the body's homeostatic abilities. It will be remembered that respiratory disturbances alter the hydrogen ion balance much more rapidly than do non–respiratory disturbances. The clinician usually attempts to correct the cause of the disturbance rather than to neutralize it, although in the first instance it may be necessary to apply 'first aid' measures, some of which are described in a later section.

The four simple disturbances of hydrogen ion regulation are described below and shown graphically in Figure 4.2. In addition there are mixed disturbances and others which do not fit easily into this basic classification, some of which will be described at the end of this section.

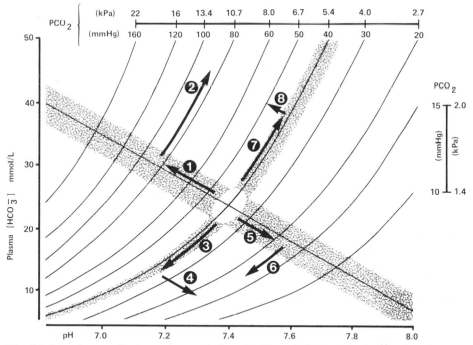

Fig. 4.2 Disturbances of hydrogen ion regulation (after Nunn, J.F. (1960) In *Clinical Physiology*, ed. Campbell E.J.M., Dickinson C.J. & Slater J.D.H.)

1. Respiratory acidaemia
2. Respiratory acidaemia with renal compensation
3. Non-respiratory acidaemia
4. Non-respiratory acidaemia with respiratory compensation
5. Respiratory alkalaemia
6. Respiratory alkalaemia with renal compensation
7. Non-respiratory alkalaemia
8. Non-respiratory alkalaemia with respiratory compensation.
   See text for further details

Respiratory acidaemia

This abnormality is due to carbon dioxide retention, exemplified by arrow 1 on Figure 4.2. As a result the pH falls and there is an immediate rise in plasma bicarbonate. If the disturbance is of short duration no compensation occurs and the pH falls below the normal range. If it is of longer duration renal compensation will be noticeable and the bicarbonate level will rise still further (arrow 2). An acid urine will be produced. The degree of compensation is an index of the duration of the disturbance and a fully compensated respiratory acidaemia (respiratory acidosis), in which the pH has been corrected to within the normal range, must have been present for many hours.

Respiratory acidaemia is synonymous with ventilatory failure (hypoventilation). It may be due to acute or chronic respiratory disease such as bronchitis or emphysema; it may result from central respiratory depression due to drugs, coma or head injuries; it may follow interruption of neuromuscular function by poliomyelitis, polyneuritis and curare–like drugs; it is often seen after surgery or trauma involving the chest wall, abdomen or diaphragm. A more comprehensive list is given in Table 4.1.

Table 4.1 Causes of respiratory acidaemia

Acute or chronic bronchitis, emphysema, status asthmaticus, pulmonary fibrosis, pleural effusion
Pneumothorax, pneumoperitoneum
Drugs — opiates, anaesthetics, sedatives, anxiolytics, curariform agents
Coma, head injury, cerebral tumours, cerebral vascular accidents
Polyneuritis, poliomyelitis, polymyositis, myopathy, myasthenia gravis
Chest or abdominal injury or surgery
Septicaemia

The treatment of respiratory acidaemia is aimed at the underlying cause. This may involve the use of antibiotics, physiotherapy, bronchoscopy and assisted ventilation. Occasionally stimulant drugs or antidotes may be used but the place of respiratory stimulants is very limited and few true drug antidotes exist. Respiratory acidaemia due to opiate drugs can be readily reversed with naloxone (Narcan) but in most other instances of drug–induced respiratory depression it is advisable to assist the patients respiration with a mechanical ventilator until the effects wear off. Central respiratory depression due to a head injury may be an indication for cerebral decompression. Although carbon dioxide is normally a respiratory stimulant, it may ultimately cause respiratory depression and when respiratory acidaemia (carbon dioxide retention) and hypoxaemia coexist, respiratory depression becomes self–perpetuating.

Non-respiratory acidaemia

This condition results either from accumulation of non-gaseous acids or from loss of base. This is shown by arrow 3 in Figure 4.2. The plasma bicarbonate and pH fall. If spontaneous compensation is possible the patient will hyperventilate because acidaemia causes respiratory stimulation. Hyperventilation increases the excretion of carbon dioxide (arrow 4) and the pH rises and the bicarbonate level falls.

Non–respiratory acidaemia may be due to uncompensated diabetes with the accumulation of lactic, aceto–acetic and hydroxybutyric acids. Another common cause is loss of bicarbonate from the gut which may be the result of upper intestinal fistulae or severe diarrhoea. Renal failure, either acute or chronic, is usually accompanied by hydrogen ion retention. Non–respiratory acidaemia frequently follows hypoxia and ischaemia and may be seen acutely during and after cardiac arrest. Lactic acidosis (acidaemia) is of particular interest and is described in greater detail later, but in addition to its association with diabetes, hypoxia and ischaemia, it may result from septicaemia because of anaerobic glycogen metabolism. These and other causes are listed in Table 4.2.

Table 4.2 Causes of non-respiratory acidaemia

Diabetes (uncontrolled)
Renal failure
Intestinal fistula, pancreatic fistulae
Hypoxia, ischaemia, septicaemia
Lactic acid accumulation
Salicylate poisoning (N.B. also produces respiratory alkalaemia)

The treatment of non–respiratory acidaemia depends upon its cause but it may also be necessary to apply biochemical correction by the administration of intravenous sodium bicarbonate solutions, as described below.

Respiratory alkalaemia
Respiratory alkalaemia is caused by the loss of carbon dioxide from the body through hyperventilation. This is not necessarily synonymous with tachypnoea nor with deep breathing and may be difficult to diagnose at the bedside. If the patient is producing more than the usual volume of carbon dioxide he has to ventilate his lungs with a greater than normal minute volume in order to maintain his arterial carbon dioxide tension at the normal level. Pyrexia, thyrotoxicosis, catabolic and anabolic processes increase the production of carbon dioxide. Many respiratory diseases cause an increase in physiological dead space and necessitate deeper breathing to maintain the carbon dioxide tension within the normal range but although the patient may appear to be breathing hard he is not necessarily hyperventilating. The diagnosis of hyperventilation can only be made with certainty if the arterial carbon dioxide tension is found to be below the normal range (hypocapnia).

Respiratory alkalaemia is demonstrated in Figure 4.2 by arrow 5. Because the $PaCO_2$ falls the plasma bicarbonate also falls and the pH rises.

The correction for a respiratory alkalaemia is a non–respiratory acidaemia (arrow 6). The kidneys excrete bicarbonate and monohydrogen phosphate and retain hydrogen ion.

Hyperventilation (hypocapnia) causes vasoconstriction which reduces the blood flow through the brain, skin and voluntary muscles and may cause hypoxaemia in these tissues. As a result lactic acid accumulates because of anaerobic glycogen metabolism. Lactic acid may also be formed in the overactive respiratory muscles if the patient is breathing spontaneously, although not during mechanical ventilation. These processes help to correct the alkalaemia.

The causes of hyperventilation include pain, anxiety, hysteria, hypoxia and re-

Table 4.3 Causes of respiratory alkalaemia

Pain, anxiety, hysteria
Hypoxia due to: bronchopneumonia
pneumothorax
pulmonary oedema
pulmonary thrombo–embolism
Adult respiratory distress syndrome
Cerebral vascular accidents
Artificial ventilation
Hepatic failure
Salicylate poisoning (also causes non–respiratory acidaemia)
Non–respiratory acidaemia

spiratory diseases such as bronchopneumonia, asthma or thrombo–embolism (Table 4.3). Hyperventilation may be the only obvious sign of a pneumothorax. In the operating room or intensive therapy unit it may be the consequence of accidental or deliberate overventilation with a mechanical ventilator (IPPV). It has been shown that 'inappropriate' hyperventilation, that is, hyperventilation which has no obvious cause, can be one of the early signs of post–traumatic respiratory insufficiency (adult respiratory distress syndrome, 'shock lung', described in Ch. 7).

The treatment of respiratory alkalaemia depends upon the underlying cause. Hyperventilation which is caused by pain or anxiety must be treated with the appropriate analgesic or anxiolytic drug, but before using any drug which may depress respiration it is important to establish that the patient is not coincidentally hypoxic. All analgesic, sedative and anxiolytic drugs cause respiratory depression and are contra–indicated in most respiratory diseases. If hyperventilation is a symptom of a non–respiratory acidaemia such as that caused by salicylate poisoning, diabetic keto–acidosis or renal failure, the appropriate treatment must be given. If it is due to a cerebral disorder it may be necessary to artificially depress the respiratory centre with drugs so that the patient does not suffer its side effects or become exhausted. This is a potentially dangerous form of treatment which must be performed only if the medical attendant is fully aware of its hazards. During IPPV a moderate level of hyperventilation is often desirable because it raises the patient's pain threshold and depresses his respiratory centre and intrathoracic receptors and thereby reduces his inclination to breathe against the ventilator.

Non-respiratory alkalaemia

This is caused by excessive loss of hydrogen ion or retention of base and is represented by arrow 7 in Figure 4.2. The pH and plasma bicarbonate are both increased. The spontaneous compensation should be to produce a respiratory acidaemia (arrow 8) but this rarely happens to any appreciable extent. Although acidaemia is an effective respiratory stimulant, alkalaemia is not a true respiratory depressant.

Non–respiratory alkalaemia may result from a number of causes, some of which are listed in Table 4.4. Vomiting of acid gastric juice due to pyloric stenosis or other upper gastro–intestinal disorders is an important cause of this con-

Table 4.4 Causes of non-respiratory alkalaemia

Vomiting, nasogastric aspiration
'Antacid' or bicarbonate therapy
Large volume blood transfusion
Hypokalaemia

dition. A less obvious cause is continuous drainage of gastric secretions through a nasogastric tube. It may also follow the administration of sodium bicarbonate or other bases (including 'antacids') intravenously or by mouth.

The transfusion of large volumes of blood may cause a transient acidaemia because stored blood has a low pH and contains citrate (citric acid) anticoagulant. If the blood is warmed during infusion this effect is reduced and within a short time of the transfusion the citrate is metabolised to bicarbonate and a non–respiratory alkalaemia produced. If the patient's liver function is grossly depressed, citrate may accumulate and the pH be lowered.

The treatment of non–respiratory alkalaemia depends upon its cause and severity. In most cases it can be left to the kidneys to correct by excreting basic ions (bicarbonate, phosphate) and retaining hydrogen ion. If treatment is necessary an infusion of normal saline will provide chloride ions and encourage the excretion of bicarbonate ions. When the pH is greater than 7.55 and when renal compensation cannot be expected, hydrogen ions can be given in the form of ammonium chloride or arginine hydrochloride which are metabolised and release hydrochloric acid. Rarely, dilute hydrochloric acid is infused. The details of treatment with arginine hydrochloride are given later.

Hypokalaemic alkalosis
It has been realised for many years that there is an inverse relationship between hydrogen and potassium ions. There are two ways in which this may manifest itself. Patients who become hypokalaemic frequently excrete an acid urine because hydrogen ions are exchanged for potassium ions in the renal tubules. The second explanation is slightly more debateable. Most of the body's potassium is stored inside cells and when the extracellular concentration of potassium falls, potassium diffuses from the intracellular compartment into the plasma. To maintain ionic equilibrium hydrogen ions move in the reverse direction and the pH rises. This explanation is not entirely satisfactory because most cell membranes are almost impermeable to hydrogen ions but the permeability characteristics of cell membranes are not uniform and the explanation given is probably correct.

Mixed disturbances
In clinical medicine mixed hydrogen ion disturbances are common. In severely ill patients a mixture of a non–respiratory with a respiratory acidosis is the usual combination due to cardiorespiratory failure and renal impairment but any mixed disturbance may be encountered and its interpretation may be difficult unless the sequence of clinical events is carefully evaluated. This point cannot be over–emphasised; the interpretation of the results of hydrogen ion analysis must be carried out at the patient's bedside after all of the symptoms have been considered in chronological order.

Lactic acidosis

The normal level of lactic acid in the serum, measured as lactate, is 0.4–1.3 mmol/l. This figure is often exceeded during exercise, particularly when an oxygen debt is incurred, through the anaerobic metabolism of glycogen. After the exercise period, the lactate is either metabolised via carbon dioxide and water, or reconverted to glucose. Most of the lactate in the body is produced in the liver, kidneys, skin and voluntary muscles; it is metabolised and excreted by the liver, kidneys and lungs.

In severe dehydration and in shock of all kinds (cardiogenic, haemorrhagic, septicaemic), inadequate tissue perfusion and hypoxia increase anaerobic glycolysis and large amounts of lactic acid are produced. The serum lactate level may exceed 9 mmol/l. This depresses myocardial contractility, decreases the responsiveness of the cardiovascular system to catecholamines and may also cause coma. Acidaemia stimulates the respiratory centre and causes hyperventilation, which may be the only obvious sign of the disturbance. Abdominal pain, nausea and vomiting may complete the picture.

An acceptable definition of lactic acidosis is a condition where there are clinical signs of acidaemia with a blood lactate which is greater than 5 mmol/l and a pH of less than 7.25. The correct term would be 'lactic acidaemia' but familiarity makes 'lactic acidosis' more usual. The serum lactate level is not routinely measured but the presence of lactic acidosis may be inferred from the clinical signs together with a low pH and an anion gap which is greater than 20 mmol/l.

The type of lactic acidosis described above and which is associated with shock or cellular ischaemia has been known for many years (Type A) but it has recently been recognised that a more insidious form exists (Type B). This is caused by certain drugs or poisons, by metabolic disorders such as diabetes, liver disease or renal disease or is occasionally associated with malignant conditions such as leukaemia and with certain rare hereditary metabolic disorders (Table 4.5).

Table 4.5 Causes of lactic acidosis

Type A	Type B _(No primary circulatory or hypoxic insult)_		
Hypotension	Phenformin	Diabetes	Glycogen storage disease Type I
Poor tissue perfusion	Metformin	Liver failure	
	Sorbitol	Renal failure	Hepatic fructose diphosphatase deficiency
Hypoxaemia			
	Ethanol	Infection	Methylmalonic aciduria
Shock: Cardiogenic			
Haemorrhagic	Fructose	Leukaemia	
Hypovolaemic			Leigh's
Septicaemic	Methanol	Reticuloses	encephalomyopathy
	Salicylates	Pancreatitis	

The commonest causes of Type B lactic acidosis are diabetic keto–acidosis and the use of the oral hypoglycaemic drug phenformin. Less frequently metformin may be involved. Lactic acidosis is not a feature of stable diabetes but occurs when fat is metabolised in default of carbohydrate.

Phenformin and metformin probably cause acidosis by interfering with glu-coneogenesis. Sorbitol, ethanol and fructose are used as intravenous energy sources and are rapidly converted to lactate by the liver. The rate of lactate clearance is reduced in liver disease and the use of these substances may be contraindicated therein. This aspect of lactate metabolism is discussed elsewhere.

Acute or acute on chronic ethanol poisoning may cause lactic acidosis because they potentiate the conversion of pyruvate to lactate through the action of alcohol dehydrogenase.

There is a correlation between the level of blood lactate and mortality rate. Although actual figures vary quite widely and the underlying cause may be more important than the serum lactate levels, when the level exceeds 15 mmol/l survival is unlikely. In lactic acidosis associated with septicaemic shock the mortality rate ranges between 75 and 100%. In that due to phenformin the mortality is approximately 50%. Since alternative oral hypoglycaemic agents are available the continued use of this potentially lethal drug is questionable.

The treatment of lactic acidosis is described later but it is vital to include the treatment of the underlying condition. Cardiovascular and respiratory failure are potentially reversible with the appropriate treatment. If the patient is in renal failure dialysis will efficiently, if temporarily, reverse the abnormality.

Interpretation of hydrogen ion and carbon dioxide concentrations

pH measurements are made with a hydrogen ion–sensitive glass electrode calibrated against buffer solutions of known pH. Carbon dioxide tension is measured in one of two ways; in the first the glass electrode is separated from the fluid to be analysed by a carbon dioxide–permeable membrane and a bicarbonate solution. This is the Severinghaus electrode. The pH of bicarbonate solutions which are equilibrated with carbon dioxide bears a linear relationship with the log of PCO_2. The second method is based upon the Astrup technique which depends upon the validity of two assumptions; the first is that when arterial blood is equilibrated with CO_2 in a tonometer, it behaves in the same way as it does in the body; i.e. that the in vitro and in vivo CO_2 dissociation curves are identical. The second assumption is that the relationship between pH and log $PaCO_2$ is linear over a clinically useful range. Neither of these assumptions is strictly correct but the effects of the inaccuracies are unimportant in practice.

Log $PaCO_2$ and pH form the co–ordinates of the Siggaard–Andersen acid base chart (Fig. 4.1). This is a graphical form of the Henderson–Hasselbalch equation ($pH = pK + Log \frac{[Base]}{[Acid]}$). The chart contains other data which include the 'plasma hydrogen-carbonate' (the standard bicarbonate) and the base excess. When the sample of blood is taken, its 'actual pH' is measured and noted. Two aliquots of the blood are then placed in tonometers and exposed to two mixtures of carbon dioxide in oxygen (usually 3% CO_2 and 8% CO_2). After equilibration the pH of the two blood samples is measured. Knowing the $PaCO_2$ of the gas mixtures two points can be marked on the Siggaard–Andersen chart and a straight line drawn between them. The 'actual pH' point is then marked on this line and the $PaCO_2$ and other values derived. These calculations are usually performed automatically by the analyser and the results displayed digitally or printed.

The analyses are made upon arterial or arterialised blood which must be collected into heparinised syringes or capillary tubes, free from gas bubbles. The sample must be placed in ice to retard white cell metabolism, which would affect the pH reading, and the analyses must be made without delay.

Results. The results are usually presented in the following sequence:

	Range
Actual pH	7.36–7.44
Actual $PaCO_2$	4.55–6.0 kPa (34–45 mmHg)
Base excess	–2 to +2 mmol/litre
Standard bicarbonate	24 mmol/litre

The PaO_2 is also usually given.

The 'actual' pH is the balance between the respiratory and non–respiratory components of the Henderson–Hasselbalch equation.

The 'actual' $PaCO_2$ is an indication of the patient's alveolar ventilation ($\dot{V}_A$). The alveolar ventilation is the volume of the air breathed which actually reaches the alveoli and takes part in gas exchange. It is the expired minute volume ventilation ($\dot{V}_E$) minus the dead space ($\dot{V}_D$) i.e. $\dot{V}_A = \dot{V}_E - (f \times \dot{V}_D)$ where f is the ventilatory frequency. If it can be assumed that the patient's dead space volume is remaining constant, then the $PaCO_2$ is inversely related to the minute volume ventilation.

There is an approximately inverse relationship between the $PaCO_2$ and the alveolar ventilation. If the $PaCO_2$ is half the normal value this implies that the alveolar ventilation is twice what it needs to be and vice versa. It does not indicate the reason for the disturbance nor whether it is primary or secondary (compensatory).

The 'base excess' is a measurement of the bicarbonate buffer in the extracellular fluid. It is a non-respiratory factor. If it is positive it means that there is an excess of bicarbonate in the extracellular fluid and if negative (usually called a 'base deficit') there is too little.

Two other results are also frequently given by the laboratory, namely the standard bicarbonate and the total buffer base.

The standard bicarbonate value is defined as the bicarbonate content of arterial blood at a $PaCO_2$ of 5.5 kPa (41 mmHg) and pH 7.40 and at 37°C. The $PaCO_2$ is specified to eliminate the effects of variation in the respiratory component from the calculation. It is of little additional value to the base excess and should be similar to the venous bicarbonate level.

The total buffer base represents the buffering power of whole blood and includes haemoglobin, plasma proteins and minor buffers such as phosphate. Its significance and value are frequently debated and its clinical importance small. As an example, chronic loss of red cells in anaemia reduces the buffering capacity of haemoglobin but since this is accompanied by an increase in total bicarbonate content as the haematocrit falls, any change is hardly significant. Acute blood loss has so many other consequences that the relative importance of a minor reduction in buffering power is not great.

CLINICAL FEATURES OF HYDROGEN ION IMBALANCE

The clinical evidence of a hydrogen ion disturbance may be obvious or its presence may be inferred from the underlying disease. For example patients who have renal disease, unstable diabetes or acute on chronic bronchitis may be expected to have an acidosis or acidaemia but the clinical symptoms are not always obvious. The main symptoms and signs of acidaemia have been mentioned earlier; they include hyperventilation but severe acidaemia may also cause cardiovascular failure and oliguria. Patients with respiratory acidaemia cannot hyperventilate, by definition. The signs of carbon dioxide retention include warm, red or purplish skin, a bounding pulse and, sometimes, hypertension. Pre–terminally these patients may develop peripheral circulatory failure.

The signs of alkalaemia are less clear–cut. Tetany, with or without epileptiform convulsions, is the most obvious, and usually the skin is pale and cold. The patient may be confused or restless.

Hydrogen ion abnormalities exert most of their ill effects upon cell membranes and intracellular processes. The only feature that can be demonstrated easily is their effect upon the oxyhaemoglobin dissociation curve. Acidaemia shifts the curve to the right, which makes haemoglobin release its oxygen more readily and alkalaemia has the reverse effect. This can be demonstrated at the bedside with a device which measures $P50$ — the partial pressure of oxygen at which haemoglobin is 50% saturated.

The essential measurement of hydrogen ion disturbance, the arterial pH, base excess, lactate etc. have been discussed at some length already. In addition to these measurements it is helpful to test routinely the pH of other secretions, particularly when abnormal losses are occurring. The obvious example of this is gastric secretion when the patient is either vomiting or undergoing continuous nasogastric aspiration. A surprising number of patients have achlorhydria and loss of secretions here would not have the same effect.

Whenever external losses are occurring, whether from the stomach, pancreatic or biliary drains, fistulae, ileostomies or the large bowel, their volume and pH should be measured. It goes without saying that routine urinalysis in sick patients should always include measurement of its pH.

CORRECTION OF NON–RESPIRATORY DISTURBANCES

The measurement of base excess permits corrections of the non–respiratory component of hydrogen ion balance to be made. The extracellular fluid volume is approximately one third of the patient's body weight (kg). Sodium bicarbonate solution is usually available in two strengths; 8.4% which contains 1 mmol bicarbonate per ml of solution and 2.54% which contains approximately 0.3 mmol bicarbonate per ml of solution. The correction is therefore made as follows:

Base deficit (mmol/litre) × 0.3 body weight (kg) = ml molar sodium bicarbonate

e.g. A patient who has a body weight of 60 kg has an extracellular volume of 20 litres. If his base deficit is 10 mmol/litre he requires 10 × 20 = 200 ml of 8.4% sodium bicarbonate or 600 ml of 2.54% sodium bicarbonate.

In severe lactic acidosis there is some evidence that rapid correction of the hydrogen ion abnormality is vital and in some cases up to 2500 mmol of sodium bicarbonate have been given in 24 hours. In less severe acidaemic states it is probably safer to administer not more than 500 mmol sodium bicarbonate in a 24–hour period although up to 200 mmol bicarbonate may be given in 2 hours if care is taken.

In any severe disturbance of hydrogen ion regulation patient monitoring must be of a very high order. This includes individual care in an intensive therapy unit, rigid attention to fluid balance and frequent blood gas and hydrogen ion analyses. The latter may need to be repeated at hourly intervals until the patient's clinical and biochemical status are satisfactory.

If the patient has a base excess it is corrected with arginine hydrochloride as follows:

$$\text{Base excess (mmol/litre)} \times 0.3 \text{ body weight (kg)} = \text{ml molar arginine hydrochloride}$$

Molar arginine hydrochloride contains 20 g/100 ml. Unless the base excess is greater than +5 or the base deficit greater than –5 it should not require correction, provided that the renal function is adequate.

Lactic acidosis is corrected by the administration of sodium bicarbonate which may be required in this condition because lactic acid is being produced continuously and not being metabolised. Many authorities state that the rapid correction of acidaemia is the most important step in its treatment, but it must be remembered that for every mmol of bicarbonate administered the patient receives one mmol of sodium. This may cause hypervolaemia and pulmonary oedema.

The correction of acidaemia involves general resuscitative measures which include the use of blood volume expanders.

It is impossible to state the optimum rate at which bicarbonate solutions should be infused to correct a non–respiratory acidaemia. There are at least two reasons for this. The problem of sodium and water overload is mentioned above. In addition, hydrogen ion disturbances involve both the intracellular and extracellular compartments. It is relatively easy to correct extracellular disturbances but the hydrogen ion status of the intracellular space is unknown at such a time. Too–rapid correction could cause acute ionic disequilibrium with unforeseeable results. Bicarbonate does not pass quickly across the blood–brain barrier and a patient whose extracellular base deficit has been corrected may continue to hyperventilate for 24–36 hours until the pH of the cerebrospinal fluid returns to normal. In most instances the base deficit or base excess need only be partially corrected. For example, if the base deficit is –10 mmol/l, half of the calculated amount is given and the estimation repeated.

5

Shock

There are few topics that will provoke more heated arguments among specialists in every field of medicine than the subject of shock. After a few months on the wards, the junior doctor will have little difficulty in recognising the shocked patient. After many years of experience, his chief may find great difficulty in defining shock and perhaps after a few decades he will decide that the wisest policy is not to attempt a precise definition. Shock is most easily understood if it is considered at a cellular level. The cell depends upon the extracellular fluid to supply it with nutrients and to remove from it the waste products of metabolism. This concept of an internal environment that was of constant composition was enunciated by the great physiologist, Claude Bernard (1949):

'Qu'est – ce que ce milieu intérieur? C'est le sang, non pas à la vérité le sang tout entier, mais la partie fluide du sang, le plasma sanguin, ensemble de tous liquides interstitiels, source et confluent de tous les échanges élémentaires'.

A French surgeon, Le Drau (1743) was probably the first to use the word shock in his treatise on gunshot wounds and the early writings on the topic naturally emphasised the circulation and the role of hypovolaemia (Hunter 1791, O'Shaughnessy 1831, Crile 1899, Blalock 1939). The recognition that shock due to inadequate peripheral circulation might occur in patients who were normovolaemic directed attention to the pumping function of the heart. Then it became apparent that shocked patients might have an adequate blood pressure and peripheral circulation and the importance of adequate oxygenation was recognised. The development of sophisticated techniques to aid the circulation, respiratory exchange, hepatic detoxification and renal excretion has certainly reduced the mortality of shock, but many patients still succumb to this syndrome because of the profound effects of generalised infection. Thus the cell may exist in an internal environment that initially is not grossly disturbed but it and ultimately the organism may die as a consequence of bacterial toxins.

It is apparent that shock may occur as a consequence of many varieties of insult, either physical or chemical, and many patients are shocked because of a combination of these aetiological factors. Although the initial effect may be confined to one aspect of the circulation, ultimately the effects are apparent within the three components of the circulation, the heart, the vessels and the blood itself. It is beyond the scope of this book to provide a complete description of the aetiology, pathology and treatment of the many forms of shock. More extensive accounts may be found in the reference list. This account will be confined to a brief description of the major causes of the different types of shock, the signs and symptoms associated with each variety and the methods of treatment, with particular emphasis upon the role of intravenous infusion.

Classification

There have been many classifications of shock published in the medical literature indicating the failure to produce a universally acceptable classification. The classification shown in Table 5.1 and discussed in greater detail below has been derived to enable the doctor to approach the shocked patient in a logical and systematic manner to ensure rapid diagnosis and treatment which are essential to a successful outcome. However, rapid diagnosis is not always possible in shocked patients. Nevertheless, this scheme does encourage a complete assessment of the patient so that in the initial stages an empirical approach may be taken which may be life–saving.

Table 5.1 The causes of shock

Neurogenic shock
Hypovolaemic shock
  Blood loss
  Plasma loss
  Water and electrolyte loss
Cardiogenic shock
Pulmonary shock
Septic shock
Acute adrenal insufficiency
Anaphylaxis

NEUROGENIC SHOCK

This form of shock is commonly encountered in everyday life and its cause is essentially emotional with stimulation of the medullary centres. It develops rapidly due to fright or severe pain such as a broken bone or a blow to the testes. There is a peripheral vasodilatation associated with bradycardia (hence its alternative title of vasovagal shock). The patient may lose consciousness (fainting). The blood pressure may be very low but the feature that distinguishes it from hypovolaemic shock is the slow pulse rate. The treatment required is to lie the patient down until the cardiovascular system recovers. Many texts ignore this form of shock or are dismissive about its importance. Nevertheless, the columns of the more sensational newspapers are a testimony to the number of people who may die from this form of shock.

HYPOVOLAEMIC SHOCK

Hypovolaemic shock (or oligaemic shock as it is sometimes called) is the commonest form of shock in surgical practice. The fluid lost may be blood, plasma or water. The appreciation of the massive quantities of fluid that may be lost externally or internally as a consequence of disease, injury or operation has resulted in rapid and effective treatment and death from this form of shock is now far less common in hospital practice. It is unfortunate that many of the major advances have occurred due to man's inhumanity in various wars (Howard & Brown 1970).

Blood loss

In Great Britain, haemorrhagic shock is most commonly due to loss of blood in the gastro–intestinal tract. The relative frequency of the causes of severe gastro–intestinal haemorrhage in general hospital practice are shown in Table 5.2. Severe and sudden haemorrhage may also occur due to ruptured ectopic pregnancy and placenta praevia. Although massive blood loss may occur due to musculo-skeletal injuries, it is not usually as rapid as the above examples. Fortunately, ex-sanguination from gunshot and knife wounds is a rare event but fatal haemor-rhage from rupture of an aortic aneurysm may occur before surgical intervention can be undertaken.

Table 5.2 The site of gastro–intestinal haemorrhage (after Shepherd 1975)

Peptic ulceration	80%
Mucosal erosions	10%
Portal hypertension	5%
Other sites	5%
Hiatus hernia	
Neoplasms	
Diverticula	

The effect of haemorrhage depends both upon the rate of loss and the volume. Previously healthy individuals can usually withstand a loss of 10 to 15% of their blood volume (about 500–750 ml in a 70 kg male) without any marked change in their pulse rate or blood pressure. Initially there is vasoconstriction with a re-duced blood volume and no alteration in the packed cell volume. During the next 24 hours, the blood volume is gradually restored by diffusion of interstitial fluid into the intravascular compartment. This mechanism has been called transcapil-lary refilling by Moore (1959). The haemoglobin concentration and the packed cell volume fall as a consequence of the haemodilution. During the next month, there is a gradual restoration of red blood cell volume by haemopoiesis. The only therapy required in such cases is the prescribing of oral iron to aid the haemo-poiesis.

The loss of 15 to 25% of blood volume (about 750–1250 ml in a 70 kg male) is associated with tachycardia, hypotension and oliguria but many of the patients are not shocked. The systolic blood pressure is usually between 80 and 100 mmHg and the pulse rate is about 100 per minute with a reduced pressure. The reduced blood pressure and vasoconstriction produces a fall in glomerular filtration rate which is coupled with renal tubular retention of sodium and water due to secretion of aldosterone and antidiuretic hormone respectively. These four factors account for the oliguria which aids restoration of blood volume. Although such patients may not present the typical appearance of shock they are teetering on the verge and any further minor insult may cause the development of rapidly fatal shock; restoration of circulating blood volume by immediate intravenous in-fusion is essential.

A fit young male may not be shocked by the loss of 30% of his blood volume

(1500 ml in a 70 kg male) but the majority of patients in hospital practice will exhibit the fully developed picture of haemorrhagic shock. The skin is cold and pale and the patient may be sweating due to release of catecholamines. The mucous membranes may be pale or cyanotic due to inadequate oxygenation. The pulse rate may be in excess of 120 beats per minute. The systolic blood pressure is usually below 70 mmHg and the diastolic blood pressure in often unrecordable. The central venous pressure recorded at the level of the right atrium is usually negative and catheterisation of the urinary bladder may demonstrate anuria. In the early stages the patient is often alert and extremely anxious but if the condition progresses he lapses into spells of semi–consciousness and becomes uncooperative, often trying to remove his infusion cannula! Eventually his air hunger gives way to irregular respiration and death occurs. Immediate and effective treatment of patients presenting with this clinical picture can produce a remarkable transformation in two or three hours; a delay of 30 min in instituting such treatment can be fatal.

Treatment
If it is immediately feasible the source of haemorrhage should be controlled and if infusion apparatus is not immediately available, the legs should be elevated and may be bound with compression bandages to increase the venous return to the heart. Oxygen may be given by mask or by nasal tubes. However, the major aim of therapy is the rapid restoration of circulating blood volume. It has been suggested that intra–arterial infusion produces a more rapid restoration than intravenous infusion but very few clinicians use the intra–arterial route. The veins are collapsed and it may be necessary to perform a 'cut–down' at the wrist, elbow, ankle or groin or to insert a cannula into the subclavian or jugular veins in the neck. In the moribund, serious consideration should be given to infusion at more than one site.

When an adequate infusion system has been established there are three major questions to be answered.:
1. Which solution should be infused?
2. What quantity should be infused?
3. How rapidly should it be infused?

Which solution? There is an old surgical maxim that the ideal replacement solution has the composition of the solution that has been lost. 'Thus blood should be given to the patient with haemorrhagic shock, plasma to the burned patient and electrolyte solutions in severe vomiting' (MacFarlane & Thomas 1977). However this apparently logical approach may not be the best available in haemorrhagic shock.

Although the infusion of whole blood increases the oxygen–carrying capacity of the blood by increasing the content of haemoglobin, there is a concomitant increase in viscosity so that there is a decrease in peripheral blood flow. The effective oxygen–carrying capacity depends on both of these factors and, surprisingly, the maximum effective oxygen–carrying capacity of the blood appears to be achieved with a packed cell volume of 30% (Hint 1968). Thus, the homeostatic response of transcapillary refilling may improve tissue oxygenation and it has been suggested that intentional haemodilution should be an initial step in the treatment of haemorrhagic shock if the packed cell volume is above 35% (Lillehei & Dietzmann 1974, Messmer 1975). Such haemodilution can be achieved most successfully with a colloidal solution. Plasma or plasma protein fraction can be used but high or low molecular weight dextran solutions may be particularly useful in this respect as they withdraw additional water from the interstitial space, 500 ml of dextran retaining an additional 750 ml of water. There is a further possible benefit in the use of dextran solutions: studies in animals and man have indicated that as well as loss of blood in haemorrhagic shock there occur changes in the distribution of blood both within the macrocirculation and the microcirculation. In the macrocirculation blood flow in the coronary, pulmonary and cerebral circulations is maintained at the expense of reduced circulation in the splanchnic, dermal and renal circulation. In the microcirculation there is pooling of blood in the capillaries with rouleaux formation producing a stagnant anoxia. It has been suggested that dextran solutions, particularly those of low molecular weight, may have specific rheological properties, reducing the tendency for rouleaux formation by inducing electromagnetic changes on the surface of the red cells (Susuki & Shoemaker 1964) and thereby improving tissue oxygenation (Gruber 1969.)

Isotopic studies suggested that there was a contraction of extracellular fluid volume after injury with a reduction of the 'functional' extracellular fluid volume in the immediate postoperative period, probably due to internal redistribution of the interstitial fluid (Shires et al 1961). Subsequent studies suggested that this reduction in 'functional' extracellular fluid volume was particularly severe in haemorrhagic shock and that the extent was out of proportion to the loss of blood (Shires & Carrico 1966). As a consequence of these studies and the observation that many battle casualties appeared to require greater quantities of intravenous fluids than might be expected from conventional assessment, a number of resuscitation teams have infused battle and civilian casualties with vast quantities of crystalloidal solutions. In many cases the quantities infused were probably far greater than those envisaged by Shires and his colleagues. Although there may have been other contributary factors, there is little doubt that overenthusiastic infusion of crystalloidal solutions has been a major factor in the high incidence of pulmonary insufficiency observed in these casualties.

In Great Britain, there has been far less support for the concept of intentional haemodilution in the treatment of haemorrhagic shock and, as emphasised above, in the initial stages of a rapidly fatal haemorrhage the packed cell volume may be unaltered. In most cases the sensible approach is to obtain a sample of blood sufficient for baseline haematological assessment and for cross–matching and to ensure that a satisfactory infusion system has been established, infusing crystalloidal or colloidal solutions until the blood has been cross–matched in the usual fashion. In the interim, the quantity of blood required can be assessed. However, in a few cases it is apparent that infusion of blood is needed urgently or the patient will die from hypoxia. In such cases the doctor should not hesitate to infuse group O Rhesus negative blood of low antibody titre held specifically in reserve by blood banks for this purpose. Haematologists are naturally concerned that such blood should only be used in dire emergency and usually question whether the situation justifies its use, but if the doctor is convinced of its urgent need, he should not be deterred.

Blood substitutes

It is apparent from Table 5.7 that if a solution could be manufactured which possessed the major features of an ideal plasma substitute and which would also transport oxygen and carbon dioxide, then that solution would make an ideal blood substitute. Encouraging results have been obtained with the use of fluorocarbon emulsions and solutions of stroma–free haemoglobin as blood substitutes (Geyer 1973, Rush 1974). However the fluorocarbon emulsions may be toxic to the body tissues, stroma–free haemoglobin has a half–life of only two hours and there is no convincing evidence yet that either solution will maintain adequate tissue oxygenation in humans inspiring normal concentrations of oxygen.

What quantity? Unfortunately, there is no ideal method of determining the quantity of replacement fluid required and previous experience is of great value. There are few examples in clinical practice where urgent and effective treatment has greater rewards and the junior doctor should not hesitate to seek the advice and assistance of his senior colleagues. Although the patient and other observers should be questioned about the extent of the blood loss, they are usually very unreliable witnesses and give a grossly exaggerated opinion as to the extent of the blood loss. It is not uncommon to listen to patients and to their relatives describing in vivid detail the massive volumes that have been lost and yet subsequent measurements of the patient's haemoglobin and packed cell volume show no change over a period of days, indicating the trivial quantities that have been lost. However, doctors often err in the opposite direction and underestimate the quantity that has been lost. This, as many anaesthetists will testify, is particularly likely when surgeons estimate the amount of blood lost during operation. In the operating theatre, the swabs should be weighed in all major cases and the volume in the suction bottle should be measured, although evaporation from the swabs invariably produces an underestimation of the total blood loss.

The blood lost from injuries can vary considerably and there have been many attempts to produce an index upon which a rapid but approximate estimate can be based. Perhaps the most simple and useful is to measure the wound size in units of an adult open hand or closed fist, each unit indicating a loss of 500 ml (Grant & Reeve 1941). But it should be remembered that some tissues are particularly vascular and occasionally patients have been seen who have lost 1500 ml of blood from simple scalp lacerations. Certainly, studies of battle and civilian injuries have shown that blood loss from external and internal wounds is usually underestimated, often by considerable amounts (Prentice et al 1954, Clarke et al 1961.) Underestimation of blood lost is particularly likely in patients with concealed haemorrhage.

The commonest cause of concealed haemorrhage is that due to closed fractures, particularly of the long bone. Not only is blood lost from the fracture, but also from the lacerated soft tissues surrounding the fracture. Typical quantities of blood lost from fractures are shown in Table 5.3. It is not uncommon for inexperienced doctors to request only one litre of blood for patients with multiple

Table 5.3 Typical blood loss associated with closed fractures

Pelvis (major fracture)	3 l
(minor fracture)	1 l
Femur	0.5–1.5 l
Tibia plus fibula	0.5–1.0 l
Humerus	0.5–1.0 l
Radius plus ulna	0.5 l

fractures whose ultimate blood loss may be in excess of five litres. Sometimes the soft tissue damaged may be far greater than might be expected from the bony injury. In particular, large quantities of blood may be lost in the retroperitoneal tissue following blunt injury to the back and the only apparent bone injury may be fractures of a few transverse processes of the lumbar vertebrae. The loss of the psoas shadow on the plain film of the abdomen may be useful in such cases and occasionally there may be an increase in the serum amylase concentration due to involvement of the pancreas. Ultimately, this retroperitoneal extravasation becomes apparent with discolouration spreading forwards round the flanks. Intraperitoneal loss due to blunt injury was often undiagnosed in the past, but the more frequent use of diagnostic peritoneal lavage using a catheter has resulted in more accurate qualitative and quantitive assessment than obtained with needle aspiration in the four quadrants of the abdomen. In 304 patients undergoing diagnostic peritoneal lavage for suspected intraperitoneal haemorrhage (Root et al 1965), a false positive diagnosis was made in only three (1%) and a false negative diagnosis in nine (3%). Suspected blood loss in the upper and lower parts of the intestinal tract can now be confirmed easily by fibre–optic endoscopy. It is surprising how frequently blood loss into the pleural cavity is overlooked, as needle aspiration allows easy and accurate confirmation.

The colour of the skin and mucous membranes should be observed and the so–called 'vital signs' (pulse, respiratory rate and blood pressure) recorded. How ever, these indices do not reflect blood volumes, but more accurately reflect the body's ability to compensate for the blood loss. Although it is now apparent that transcapillary refilling in response to haemorrhage is a rapid phenomenon occurring in a few hours, the haemoglobin concentration and the packed cell volume are poor indicators of the volume of blood lost in the early stages and later the picture may be confused because of the use of plasma expanders.

A logical method of calculating the blood lost would be from measurement of actual total blood volume and calculations of expected blood volume according to equations derived by Moore et al (1963):

Males $2.84 \, l/m^2$ (approximately 7% body weight)
Females $2.47 \, l/m^2$ (approximately 6% body weight)

Blood volume can now be measured accurately by dilution techniques using radio–isotopes. The plasma volume can be measured using radio-iodinated human serum albumin (RISA) and a commercial instrument, the volumetron, can be used for this purpose. The total blood volume can then be calculated by use of the packed cell volume or, more accurately, the red blood cell volume can be measured by the re – injection of the patient's own red cells which have been labelled with ^{51}Cr. The red blood cell volume can also be calculated using the volume-tron. The calculation of total blood volume by these techniques may be valuable in many patients (for example, in confirming the pre-operative expansion of the blood volume after adrenergic blockade in a patient with a phaeochromocytoma) and the concept of repeated estimations to monitor therapy in patients with haemorrhagic shock is extremely attractive (Friedman et al 1966). Unfortunately, the technique depends upon thorough mixing of the isotopes within the circulation and, as discussed above, there is an alteration in the macrocirculation and microcirculation in haemorrhagic shock which precludes such mixing. Consequently, measurement of blood volume by these techniques has not proved to be as useful as initial expectations (Prout 1968).

The urinary output is a simple and excellent indication of the state of the circulation in shock. In a normotensive individual, urine formation becomes impaired if the systolic blood pressure falls below 90 mmHg. Although a patient may have lost 1500 ml, if his urine output is in excess of 25 ml per hour it is unlikely that he will exhibit any gross circulatory failure (normal output is approximately 50 ml per hour). Shocked patients should have a urinary catheter inserted and urinary output recorded at least hourly. The restoration of adequate urine formation in a previously anuric or oliguric patient is a welcome indication of the adequacy of volume replacement. The routine measurement of central venous pressure in the assessment and treatment of patients with haemorrhagic shock was a major advance. Although central venous pressure is dependent upon blood volume, other factors discussed below also influence this measurement and it soon became apparent that changes in central venous pressure did not parallel changes in blood volume (Conn 1967).

How rapidly?   If the patient is pale, cold and sweating and has a rapid thready pulse, the quantity of blood loss is likely to be at least one litre. Unless there is a previous history or evidence of cardiac failure, there is little to be gained from slow infusion and one litre of colloidal solution should be infused during the next hour. During this time the vital signs should be recorded every 15 min, the electrodes for cardiographic recording attached to the chest and urinary and central venous catheters inserted. The response to this initial therapy will usually give some indication of the severity of the problem. The rate of further infusion should be gained by this response and in particular by changes in central venous pressure.

Central venous pressure
The central venous pressure is the pressure recorded in the great veins of the chest or the right atrium. Central venous pressure is dependent upon:
1. Intrathoracic pressure
2. Venous return to the heart
3. The function of the right side of the heart

Thus, central venous pressure is elevated in patients with increased expiratory resistance which may be due to disease or caused by intermittent positive pressure ventilation (IPPV), particularly if positive end – expiratory pressure (PEEP) is applied. If these respiratory phenomena can be excluded, then central venous pressure reflects the ability of the right side of the heart to cope with the venous return. Thus, central venous pressure will rise if there is obstruction to the out-flow from the right ventricle (e.g. left ventricular failure, pulmonary embolism and pulmonary artery stenosis) or if there is an abnormally high venous return to the heart beyond the capability of the pumping mechanism of the right side of the heart (e.g. over-transfusion).

This simple, valuable and inexpensive technique can be used in any patient where there is a risk of over-transfusion. A wide bore intravenous catheter of at least 1 mm internal diameter should be used to ensure accurate recording. The catheter should be introduced by percutaneous puncture, but occasionally a cut-down is required. The ideal point of insertion is in the antecubital fossa (see Ch. 9) and the catheter should then be threaded proximally into the superior vena cava. The position of the tip of the catheter should be confirmed by radiological examination. If it is impossible to insert the catheter into an antecubital vein, then it may be inserted into the external jugular vein or the subclavian vein, but air embolism has occurred with the use of the external jugular vein and pneumothorax and haemothorax with the use of the subclavian vein (by either the

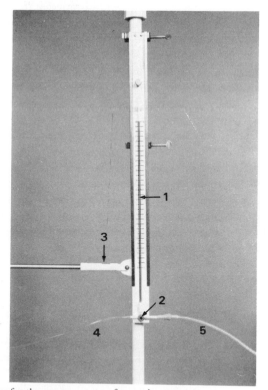

Fig. 5.1 A manometer for the measurement of central venous pressure

1. Manometer
2. Two-way stop-cock
3. Spirit level to calibrate the manometer (see text)
4. Infusion tubing connected to intravenous catheter
5. Infusion tubing connected to intravenous infusion set

supraclavicular or infraclavicular routes). The manometer should be assembled as shown in Figure 5.1 and having filled the system the infusion line should be connected to the catheter. By adjustment of the three–way tap, the recording limb of the manometer can be connected to the central vein and disconnected from the infusion bottle. Fluctuations in the height of the column should then be noted due to respiration and the column of fluid should fall until the central venous pressure is recorded. If fluctuation is not observed then this may indicate that the tip of the catheter has impinged on the wall of the vein and by judicious manipulation it is often possible to resite the catheter tip within the lumen of the vein. The central venous pressure apparatus should not be used for routine infusion. It is possible to record central venous pressure at regular intervals throughout the day and to infuse only 200 ml of fluid through this system. However, it can be used as a convenient alternative infusion system for electrolyte solutions and on occasion for the infusion of dextran. Plasma, blood or intravenous nutrients should never be infused through this system.

Central venous pressure has been recorded from the level of the clavicle and from the mid–cardiac point. It is apparent that different values will be obtained according to the choice of zero level. However, in practice these differences in recording techniques are not of any great significance, as an individual measurement of central venous pressure is not of particular relevance. It is the change of central venous pressure in response to the rapid infusion of fluid over a short period that is of significance. If the infusion of 200 ml of fluid over a 5–minute period produces an increase in central venous pressure of 5 cm, then the right side of the heart is unlikely to be able to cope with further large–scale infusion. This may indicate a normal or increased blood volume and adequate heart function, but in some cases it may indicate inadequate blood volume and inadequate heart function. In the latter patients heart function may improve following the use of cardiac stimulants and blood volume then restored according to the central venous pressure. Although central venous pressure is determined by the three major factors discussed above and isolated measurements are less significant than changes in pressure, the pressure recorded at the mid – thoracic point has a normal range of 5–15 cm of water and the common therapeutic implications of differing ranges of central venous pressure are shown in Table 5.4.

Table 5.4

Central venous pressure (cm water)	Probable clinical state	Treatment
0–5	Hypovolaemia	Fluid replacement
6–10	Hypovolaemia or normovolaemia	Assess response to trial of fluid replacement
10–15	Normovolaemia or hypervolaemia	Replace fluid as it is lost
15	Hypervolaemia or heart failure	Restrict intravenous infusion Consider the use of diuretics and cardiac stimulants

Pulmonary artery wedge pressure

As discussed in detail above, central venous pressure indicates the ability of the right side of the heart to cope with the venous return. In some situations this is a reflection of the function of the left side of the heart. Usually it is fairly obvious whether the main problem is right or left ventricular failure, but in some circumstances such distinction can only be made by measuring the function of the left side of the heart. It is now possible to insert a catheter into an antecubital vein and to thread it onwards under the influence of natural blood flow, so that eventually the catheter tip passes into the pulmonary artery (Zohnan & Williams 1959). This technique has recently been modified with the commercial development of the Swan – Ganz catheter (Swan & Ganz 1975) which has an inflatable balloon at its tip (Fig. 5.2). The balloon can then be inflated and wedged in a radicle of the pulmonary artery. With the exception of the comparatively few patients who suffer from pulmonary vascular disease, pulmonary wedge pressure is a reliable index of left ventricular end – diastolic pressure which is a very sensitive indicator of left ventricular function. In some cases left ventricular end – diastolic pressure may increase without significant increases in right atrial pressure (i.e. central venous pressure) with the subsequent development of pulmonary oedema. Further modifications of this technique with triple lumen catheters have allowed simultaneous measurements of right atrial pressure, pulmonary wedge pressure and the sampling of mixed venous blood from the pulmonary artery. The most recent advance has been the development of a catheter containing a thermistor at the catheter tip which allows measurement of cardiac output by a thermodilution

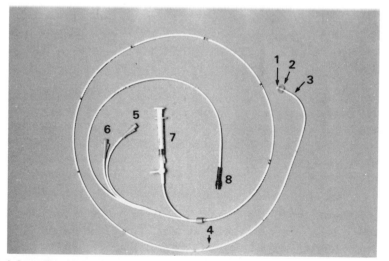

Fig. 5.2 A Swan-Ganz catheter

1. Orifice for measurement of pulmonary arterial wedge pressure
2. Inflated balloon (0.8–1.5 ml)
3. Thermistor (inside catheter)
4. Orifice for infusion of ice-cold saline (and measurement of right atrial pressure)
5. Luer connection for (1)
6. Luer connection for (4)
7. Syringe for inflation of (2)
8. Electrical connections for (3)

technique following the infusion of ice – cold saline through the lumen used for the measurement of right atrial pressure. These techniques are commonly used in shocked patients in North America, but have been introduced only recently in Great Britain. Cardiac catheterisation in any form is not without hazard and the precise role of these techniques remains to be evaluated. However, it would appear that their judicious use will allow the bedside attainment of valuable information which was previously unobtainable in severely shocked patients.

Plasma loss

It is often forgotten that intracoelomic exudation involves the internal or third space loss of protein – rich fluid. Thus peritonitis from any cause (but particularly that due to pancreatitis) and carcinomatosis peritonei may produce a fall in circulating plasma volume. A similar third space loss of protein–rich fluid can occur into crushed limbs. However, the commonest cause of plasma loss occurs in burns or scalds and the quantities involved may be very large. The burn injury increases capillary permeability so that plasma is lost as an interstitial inflammatory oedema in spite of the increased lymphatic flow. The plasma can be seen collecting in subcutaneous blisters or exuding from the raw surface if the skin has been lost. This dramatic and visual loss usually forms but a small percentage of the total loss, for as much as eight litres of protein–rich inflammatory oedema may accumulate in the interstitial spaces. It has long been known that the volume of replacement fluid required is proportional to the magnitude of the burn and this has recently been confirmed in a study of 1027 patients (Davies 1975a, b). There have been many systems devised for quantifying the extent of the burn injury and one of the simplest and most useful is shown in Table 5.5. This 'rule of nines' refers to the extent of third degree burns (full–thickness burns). Second degree burns should be included in the summation as one half of their extent.

Table 5.5 The estimation of the area of burns in adults*

Head and neck	9%
Trunk — front	18%
back	18%
Upper limbs (9% each)	18%
Lower limbs (18% each)	36%
Perineum	1%

* see Chapter 11 for estimation in children

The requirement for large quantities of sodium in the effective treatment of burns was shown in one of the earliest studies of the metabolic consequences of injury (Davidson 1926) and many clinicians still believe that large quantities of crystalloidal solutions are the only requirement for effective treatment (Baxter & Shires 1968, Monafo 1970). In this form of treatment Ringer's lactate solution is usually infused at the rate of 4 ml/kg body weight per % burn during the first 24 hours and at a reduced rate during the subsequent days as determined by the response to therapy. However, most doctors believe that these ionic solutions have little effect in restoring plasma volume and advise concomitant infusion of large quantities of colloidal solutions such as plasma, albumin or dextran (Haynes et al 1955, Wilkinson 1958, Moore 1970, Davies et al 1977a, b). The type of regimen

Table 5.6 Fluid requirement in patients with burns (first day)

1. Colloid solution (plasma, albumin or dextran)
   0.5 ml/kg body weight per % burn

2. Electrolyte solution (0.9% saline or Ringer's lactate soln.)
   1.5 ml/kg body weight per % burn

3. Water (5% glucose soln.)
   2000 ml

Example: An 80 kg patient with 30% burns requires
1. Colloid solution	80 × 30 × 0.5	= 1200 ml
2. Electrolyte solution	80 × 30 × 1.5	= 3600 ml
3. 5% glucose solution		= 2000 ml
	Total	= 6800 ml

used in such therapy is shown in Table 5.6. The colloid and electrolyte content is reduced by half during the second day of treatment, but it should be noted that this regimen is modified according to the patient's response. As in other types of shock, the urine output is considered to be a vital index of the response to treatment and a urine flow of 30–50 ml/h is an indication that fluid replacement is keeping pace with fluid loss. If the urine flow falls below 20 ml/h, the quantity of isotonic dextrose should be increased and the quantity of electrolyte solution should be decreased. It has been suggested that oliguria should be treated by the infusion of hypertonic solutions and mannitol but Wilkinson (1958) has emphasised that oliguria is a normal response during the early phase of injury and renal failure occurs in less than 2% of patients with burns (Cason 1966). A fall in arterial blood presure or central venous pressure may be indicative of an inadequate colloid replacement. Many patients with severe burns require a tracheostomy with a subsequent increase of approximately one litre in their daily requirement of isotonic dextrose. When the definitive treatment of the burns by exposure, dressing or grafting is begun, the electrolyte requirements are greatly reduced. Anaemia is produced by the burn injury and by subsequent haemolysis (Davies & Topley 1956). The extent of the anaemia should be documented by daily estimations of the packed cell volume which should be maintained at 35%. In severe cases this may require the additional infusion of 500 ml of whole blood each day. Patients with burns covering more than 80% of the body surface have been successfully treated using this type of regimen. These requirements can be reduced by nursing patients in a warm (30–34°C) and dry (18–24% relative humidity) atmosphere (Barr et al 1968). If possible, patients with extensive burns should be treated in specialised units which are usually supervised by plastic surgeons.

The energy and protein requirements of patients with burns are greatly increased due to increased evaporative and non–evaporative heat loss and increased protein catabolism (Davies 1970). The increase in energy and protein requirements is proportional to the extent of the burn and patients with full–thickness burns extending to 50–75% of the body surface area may require 15 MJ/d (3600 kcal/d) of non–protein energy and 30 g Nd (190 g protein per day). In many of the patients normal feeding is impossible as the face is involved in the thermal injury and anorexia and nausea are frequent complaints. Consequently, the large nutritional requirements must be given enterally by tube feeding or parenterally. Initially, post–traumatic ileus may necessitate the use of intravenous feeding. However, the risk of infective complications associated with intravenous feeding is particularly high in patients with thermal injuries and tube feeding should replace intravenous feeding as soon as it is feasible. If possible, the central catheter should be inserted into the superior vena cava through healthy skin. The nutrient requirements for enteral and parenteral feeding are discussed in greater detail in Chapters 8 and 10. Although nutritional support is an essential component of the successful treatment of patients with major burns it is important to recognise that the initial fluid requirement is determined by the need to resuscitate the patient from his shocked state. The infusion of nutrient fluids should not be considered until the patient is haemodynamically stable (which is usually achieved about the second day after injury).

Plasma substitutes

At this point it is convenient to consider the solutions that may be used as alternatives to plasma. It is preferable to use the term plasma substitute for such solutions and to retain the term plasma expander for solutions such as dextran, which, as a consequence of its considerable oncotic properties, will withdraw water from the interstitial space and thereby expand the plasma volume even further than the volume infused. The properties that would be possessed by the ideal plasma substitute are shown in Table 5.7 and some of the advantages and disadvantages of plasma substitutes now available are shown in Table 5.8. It is apparent that the plasma substitutes available at present are far from ideal and a considerable amount of time and money is being spent in this field. It should be noted that the different features of each substitute may be used with advantage in different clinical conditions. If a hypoalbuminaemic patient is suffering from congestive heart failure and oedema that is resistant to diuretic therapy, the main requirement is to increase the oncotic pressure of the plasma to mobilise the peripheral oedema. In order to avoid placing undue stress upon a failing heart, it is preferable to achieve this by the infusion of as small a quantity of fluid as possible. The oncotic effect of 50 ml of 20% salt–poor albumin, 200 ml of 5% albumin or 200 ml of plasma protein fraction is equivalent to one unit of plasma. If the patient is suffering from hypovolaemic shock and the clinician wishes to infuse a plasma substitute that will be excreted in a relatively shory time when

Table 5.7 The features of an ideal plasma substitute

Maintains oncotic pressure
Compatible with blood
Similar rheological properties to blood
No interference with blood typing or cross–matching
Beneficial effect upon haemostasis
Will act as a hydrogen ion buffer
Remains in the circulation for the required period of time
Non–toxic and non–pyrogenic
No antigenicity
No risk of transmitting hepatitis
Freely available
Inexpensive
Withstands storage

Table 5.8 The advantages and disadvantages of plasma and its substitutes

	Half-life	Hepatitis risk	Hypersensitivity reactions	Effect on coagulation	Interference with blood typing	Availability	Cost
Plasma (fresh frozen)	Days	Present	Rare	Improvement	None	Sometimes scarce	Expensive
Albumin	Days	None	Rare	None	None	Sometimes scarce	Very expensive
Plasma protein fraction	Days	None	Rare	None	None	Sometimes scarce	Expensive
Dextran 40	5 h	None	<0.1%	Impairment	Yes	Freely available	Inexpensive
Dextran 70	8 h	None	<0.1%	Impairment	Yes	Freely available	Inexpensive
Hydroxyethyl starch	8 h	None	Rare	Slight impairment	None	Freely available	Inexpensive
Gelatin	<5 h	None	Rare	None	None	Freely available	Inexpensive

blood will be available, a low molecular weight dextran or gelatin solution would be a sensible choice.

Albumin. The major indication for the infusion of plasma or its substitutes is the need to infuse a substance that will remain in the intravascular compartment and maintain oncotic pressure. The most effective component of the plasma proteins in the maintenance of oncotic pressure is albumin which has a . lower molecular weight than the globulins. A major advantage in comparison with plasma is its freedom from the risk of transmitting hepatitis. Concentrated solutions with low sodium content are particularly beneficial in the treatment of patients with hypoalbuminaemia and oedema due to secondary aldosteronism. Unfortunately, solutions of albumin are in scarce supply and are extremely expensive.

Dextrans. Dextrans are polysaccharides of glucose and they have been used in clinical practice for many years. The molecular weight can be adjusted during production and dextran can be dissolved in isotonic solutions of glucose or saline so that the solution may be given different properties. The two solutions in common use have molecular weights of 40 000 (Dextran 40, low molecular weight dextran, LMWD) and 70 000 (Dextran 70, high molecular weight dextran, HMWD). Occasionally, solutions are used that have a molecular weight of 120 000. The major portion of dextran 40 is excreted by the kidneys and the major portion of dextran 70 is oxidised to water and carbon dioxide. Consequently, the half–life of dextran 40 in the circulation is five hours or less and there is very little remaining after 24 hours but the half–life of dextran 70 is eight hours and it requires 48 hours for complete removal from the circulation. This persistence in the circulation of dextran 70 may be an advantage or disadvantage according to circumstance. Thus, the persistence in the bloodstream of small quantities of dextran 70 may be used for prophylactic antithrombotic effect but, if the quantity infused is too great, the plasma volume may be increased so much that congestive failure occurs, particularly in the elderly.

The rheological properties of dextran 40 in improving blood flow in the microcirculation following haemorrhagic shock have been discussed above. It is also used in the treatment of incipient gangrene in patients suffering from peripheral vascular disease but it is uncertain whether any benefit is due to any specific rheological property or whether it reflects the effects of haemodilution. One gram of dextran retains 20–25 ml of water in the circulation (Appel 1971) so that infusion of 500 ml of a 10% solution of dextran 40 increase the plasma volume by 1000–1250 ml, the extra water being withdrawn from the interstitial fluid. The osmotic pressure of a 10% solution of dextran 40 is 2400 mmHg (320 kPa) and of a 6% solution of dextran 70 is 800 mmHg (106 kPa). This effect should be born in mind when dextran solutions are infused in patients with cardiac failure. Dextrans exert an antithrombotic effect and are used prophylactically to prevent deep venous thrombosis (Jansen 1972). Unfortunately dextran interferes with typing and cross–matching of blood and it is important to withdraw sufficient blood for the purpose of cross–matching before beginning the infusion of dextran. Hypersensitivity reactions, usually mild, with nausea, headache, flushing, and pain in the lumbar region but occasionally amounting to anaphylactic shock, occur in less than 0.1% of infusions (Michelson 1968).

Hydroxyethyl starch. Although the incidence of hypersensitivity reactions due to dextran is very low, a plasma substitute with less antigenicity would be beneficial. Hydroxyethyl starch (HES) like the dextrans is a polysaccharide of glucose. Although reactions to these starches can occur, they are extremely rare (Geyer 1970) and they do not interfere with typing and cross – matching of blood. When infused as a 6% solution, it has a half–life in the circulation of about 8 hours but it persists in small amounts in the circulation for up to 60 days (Schier et al 1974). Unfortunately, the ultimate fate of hydroxyethyl starch is uncertain but its high molecular weight (130 000–450 000 according to the method of preparation) and its similarity to glycogen would suggest that it is oxidised in a similar manner to other starches. Clinical evaluation of hydroxyethyl starch is being undertaken in many countries and in some its use is increasing at the expense of dextran.

Gelatin. One of the first substances to be tried as a plasma substitute was gelatin, but the solutions proved difficult to produce and sterilise and hypersensitivity was a common problem (Hogan 1915). These problems have now been overcome although anaphylaxis following infusion of modern solutions of gelatin has been recorded (Lemd 1973). A variety of commercial preparations are available with molecular weights of 20 000–45 000. The half–life of these preparations in the circulation is less than 5 hours, the major pathway of excretion being by the kidneys. Gelatin does not interfere with the typing and cross–matching of blood and has no effect on haemostasis. Because of this and the lower incidence of hypersensitivity reactions, solutions of gelatin are being used with increasing frequency as an alternative to dextran when a plasma substitute is required.

Water and electrolyte loss
Deficiency of water and electrolytes has been discussed in detail in Chapter 2. It is unusual in Great Britain to witness shock due to loss of water and electrolytes alone. Occasionally patients are seen in a shocked state following large losses of fluid by vomiting and diarrhoea induced by dysenteric organisms. Most patients with dysentery and those with large 'third space' loss into the bowel lumen and peritoneal cavity receive appropriate intravenous therapy before they become shocked, but there are areas in the world where, due to geographical or social difficulties, such therapy may be delayed. The loss of water and sodium from the dermis and into the interstitial space following thermal injury and the quantities required for treatment has been discussed above.

As emphasised in Chapter 2, the major requirement is for isotonic saline. Although a variety of solutions have been manufactured that resemble more closely the composition of extracellular fluid such as Ringer's and Hartmann's solutions, the use of these solutions is usually an unnecessary refinement as adequate renal function will correct any acid–base deficit. The lactate content of Hartmann's solution provides an additional 28 mmol of base in each litre which should be compared with the 13 000 mmol of carbon dioxide excreted by the lungs and the 4500 mmol of bicarbonate reabsorbed by the kidney each day. In acidotic patients, the amounts of carbon dioxide and of bicarbonate excreted may be much greater. Nevertheless, potassium additives may be required, particularly in dysenteric patients. A method of calculating the quantity of isotonic saline required is described in Chapter 2 but in practice it is usually sufficient to be guided by the response of the central venous pressure and urine output.

Table 5.9 Causes of cardiogenic shock

Myocardial damage	Severe, acute valve lesions[†]
Myocardial infarction	Ruptured aortic valve cusp
Viral myocarditis	Mitral regurgitation
Arrhythmias[*]	Ruptured sinus of Valsalva
Tachycardia	Cardiac tamponade
Atrial fibrillation	Dissecting aortic aneurysm
Atrial flutter	
Atrial tachycardia	
Ventricular tachycardia	
Brachycardia	
Heart block	

[*] Arrhythmias will rarely lead to cardiogenic shock unless there is co–existent heart disease
[†] These may be spontaneous or secondary to infective endocarditis

CARDIOGENIC SHOCK

Cardiogenic shock may be produced by the conditions shown in Table 5.9. A detailed description of the treatment is beyond the scope of this book. Cardiogenic shock has been reported in up to 10% of patients with myocardial infarction. It is usually associated with the destruction of at least 30% of the left ventricular myocardium (Page et al 1971). Even in favourable cases the long–term prognosis is still poor. However, most other causes of cardiogenic shock, although less common, can be completely and rapidly reversed with appropriate treatment. Consequently it is imperative to make an accurate diagnosis as soon as possible before irreparable damage occurs. If cardiogenic shock is suspected the advice of a cardiologist should be sought and if possible the patient transferred to a coronary care unit for assessment. The role of digitalisation in the treatment of septic shock is discussed later in this chapter.

PULMONARY SHOCK

Although monographs written about shock usually discuss the many varied insults that the lungs may suffer due to shock and emphasise the importance of adequate ventilation and gaseous exchange in shocked patients, many ignore the possibility that the primary insult may occur in the lungs. Patients with severe pulmonary pathology may exhibit the classical features of the shocked state with tachypnoea, tachycardia, reduced cardiac output and arterial blood pressure and abnormal gas tensions in the arterial blood. The causes of pulmonary shock are shown in Table 5.10.

Table 5.10 The causes of pulmonary shock

Pulmonary embolism
Pulmonary atelectasis
Pneumothorax
Haemothorax
Fat embolism
Shock lung

Patients occasionally become shocked following the development of pulmonary atelectasis. Bronchial obstruction producing pulmonary atelectasis may be caused by a plug of mucus (particularly after operation in patients with chronic chest disease), foreign bodies, tumour, or enlarged hilar nodes. In addition to tachypnoea, cyanosis and tachycardia, the trachea is usually deviated to the affected side and there are signs of atelectasis on that side. A chest X–ray will confirm the diagnosis and bronchoscopy should be performed to establish and possibly remove the cause. Severe respiratory insufficiency and shock may occur due to rapidly progressive haemothorax or pneumothorax, particularly if the latter is of the tension variety. The trachea is deviated to the opposite side and on the affected side, breath sounds are absent with a stony dull note on percussion in haemothorax and a tympanitic note in pneumothorax. A chest X–ray will confirm the diagnosis and a chest drain should be inserted. Thoracotomy may ultimately be required to treat the underlying pathology.

Although emboli of fat are frequently found in the lungs at post mortem in patients dying after severe injury, the clinical syndrome of fat embolism with its characteristically severe arterial hypoxaemia is far less common (Sevitt 1962). There is considerable disagreement as to whether the fat originates from bone marrow or is produced by coalescence of plasma lipids and as to whether disturbed cerebral function and death are due to cerebral emboli or to cerebral anoxia as a consequence of the pulmonary emboli. Most clinicians believe that the fat does originate from the bone marrow and that arterial hypoxaemia due to the pulmonary lesion is the major cause of altered cerebral function and death (Watson 1970, Prys–Roberts et al 1970). The syndrome usually develops within the first two days of injury and the cerebral manifestations are frequently the first sign noted by the clinician. As well as altered consciousness ranging from irritability and hallucination to frank coma, the patient is febrile and may also exhibit spasticity of the limbs and sometimes decerebrate rigidity. Petechial haemorrhages in the skin over the shoulders, chest and in the axilla usually occur about the second day. In addition to tachypnoea, tachycardia, and arterial hypotension the patient is usually cyanosed and has a reduced arterial oxygen tension. The diagnosis is confirmed by demonstrating fat globules in the urine or sputum. Most patients require intermittent positive pressure ventilation with high concentrations of oxygen in the inspired gases to correct the hypoxaemia (further details of this form of therapy are given under septic shock in this chapter and under post–traumatic pulmonary insufficiency in Chapter 7). Heparin is usually given to stimulate lipase activity (Cobb et al 1959). This clears the plasma of the excessive quantities of fat but there is no clear evidence that it has any effect upon survival. Pulmonary atelectasis, pneumothorax, haemothorax and fat embolism are uncommon causes of pulmonary shock, the majority of cases being due to pulmonary embolism.

Pulmonary embolism

Large venous emboli may block both pulmonary arteries but it is apparent that even a small pulmonary embolus that is indetectable clinically or radiologically may produce severe shock and the patient may die. In patients with large emboli, the reduced right ventricular output (and consequently reduced left ventricular output and reduced arterial oxygen tension) reflect the obstruction in the pulmonary arteries and the occurrence of the shocked state is not unexpected. The observation of severe shock due to small pulmonary emboli is more difficult to explain. It is usually assumed that the emboli release or provoke the release from local tissue of substances such as histamine or 5 – hydroxytryptamine which have profound effects upon the cardiovascular system. Nevertheless, proof of such proposed phenomena is lacking. The most consistent feature of pulmonary embolism is tachypnoea which is responsible for a reduction in arterial carbon dioxide tension. If pulmonary embolism is suspected and the arterial carbon dioxide is normal or raised, the diagnosis is unlikely to be correct. In such cases, myocardial infarction or the development of shock lung (see later in this chapter under septic shock) should be considered. Classically, the patient complains of severe chest pain, becomes breathless and very anxious. The pain is usually pleuritic in nature when a small infarct produces peripheral infarction, but may be retrosternal and crushing in nature with massive emboli that impact in the pulmonary trunk. Haemoptysis may occur following pulmonary infarction. In addition to the tachypnoea, the patient is often cyanosed and has a tachycardia with reduced cardiac output and arterial blood pressure. The central venous pressure is usually raised. Respiratory movement may be impaired and rhales and a pleural rub may be heard over the appropriate area of the chest. Although wedge–shaped infarcts, pleural effusion and decreased vascularity may be noted on the chest X–ray, in the majority of patients this investigation is of little help in early diagnosis. Pulmonary angiography is the most accurate method of diagnosing pulmonary emboli but this technique is not available in every hospital (Williams et al 1963). Combined ventilation and perfusion scanning using radio–isotopes may be helpful (Lavender 1979) when preservation of ventilation with deficient perfusion is pathognomonic of vascular occlusion. The classical electrocardiographic changes of right ventricular strain with large S waves in lead I and large Q waves and inverted T waves in lead III are seen rarely and usually indicate a massive embolus in one or both pulmonary arteries.

Treatment
The treatment of pulmonary embolism is highly controversial and a detailed discussion is beyond the scope of this book. In Great Britain the majority of patients are treated with anticoagulants in the belief that this will prevent the further development of thrombosis in the calf, thigh or pelvic veins from which the clot originated and hopefully will prevent the addition of thrombus to the embolus in the pulmonary vasculature. In other countries various forms of venous ligation or division are popular to prevent further dissemination up the inferior vena cava (Moretz et al 1959, De Weese & Hunter 1963). These operations are not popular in Great Britain because of a high mortality, the development of large collateral veins which may transmit pulmonary emboli within weeks of operation and the high incidence of pain, oedema, phlebitis, and ulceration that can occur in the lower extremities. Dissolution of the pulmonary embolus by various thrombolytic agents such as urokinase is an attractive concept but unfortunately systemic complications due to bleeding severely limit its use (Soutter et al 1972). Further evaluation of the infusion of these thrombolytic agents through a catheter introduced into the pulmonary artery is required. In patients who survive long enough after

massive pulmonary embolism, emergency pulmonary embolectomy may be indicated.

SEPTIC SHOCK

The onset of septic shock may be mistaken for the onset of many other forms of shock discussed in this chapter and organisms may be found in the bloodstream of patients with these other varieties of shock. Nevertheless, the recogition of organisms within the bloodstream of shocked patients should not be ignored. The diagnosis of septic shock is frequently made retrospectively when it is apparent that the initial diagnosis was incorrect and there are many patients who bear the scars of laparotomy and thoracotomy as testimony to the difficulty that experienced clinicians may have in establishing the diagnosis. A major factor in this difficulty is the knowledge that less than half of the patients who are ultimately shown to be suffering from septic shock have detectable organisms in their bloodstreams during the first 24 hours (Ledingham & McArdle 1978). In these cases it is assumed that the shock state is due to the liberation of toxins into the bloodstream by the bacteria. The presence of circulating endotoxin can be indicated by the Limulus Lysate gelation method but the sensitivity of the test may make the clinical significance of a positive result uncertain (Fossard et al 1974).

The source of the sepsis may arise within any organ of the body, but the gastro-intestinal tract is by far the commonest site of origin (Ledingham et al 1980). The source determines the organisms involved and influences the prognosis, mortality being as high as 84% in faecal peritonitis (Neely et al 1971). Two thirds of patients suffering from septic shock have Gram–negative septicaemia. This difference in the incidence of Gram – positive and Gram – negative organisms found in patients suffering from septic shock reflects the difference in the ability of these bacteria to produce a shock state when liberated into the bloodstream. Only 10% of patients suffering from staphyloccal septicaemia become shocked, but 50% of the patients with aerobic Gram–negative bacilli and 30% with Bacteroides in their bloodstream develop shock (Lancet 1963). It has been suggested that the clinical features of Gram–negative and Gram–positive shock differ as they are produced by different mechanisms (Kwaan & Weil 1969). Patients suffering from Gram–negative shock have been observed to undergo an initial period of increased tissue perfusion with dilatation of the capillary bed and increased cardiac output. The classical features of hypodynamic shock ultimately occur many hours after this hyperdymanic phase. Although this sequence may be observed occasionally, it occurs in a very small minority of patients and consequently it is usually impossible to distinguish clinically between patients with Gram–positive or Gram–negative septicaemia.

The diagnosis of septic shock depends predominantly upon the demonstration of organisms within the bloodstream and the exclusion of other causes of the shock state. Blood should be taken under sterile conditions and cultured in suitable media under aerobic and anaerobic conditions. It is often useful to ask the bacteriologist to examine the blood immediately under a microscope using Gram's stain, as the identification of Gram–positive or Gram–negative bacteria may be a valuable indication as to the initial choice of antibiotics. Blood samples should be taken immediately and during the peak of any episode of pyrexia and repeated at least daily until the organism is isolated. Thereafter, it is probably sufficient to repeat the cultures every 48 hours. As well as sending blood to the laboratory for culture, bacterial swabs from body orifices and any fluid or pus that my be obtained by direct or indirect means should also be sent. In many institutions, additional information may be rapidly obtained by the expert examination of samples using gas – liquid chromatography. The advice of an experienced bacteriologist is invaluable and is best obtained by discussion at the bedside when the bacteriologist has seen the patient rather than by less informative communication by telephone. Although septic shock is usually bacterial in origin, it may be produced by fungi. Septicaemia due to *Candida albicans* usually occurs in desperately ill patients who have been given broad–spectrum antibiotics. Although many very ill patients may grow Candida from swabs taken from natural orifices during the course of their illness and recover, invasion of the bloodstream is usually fatal.

Although diagnosis ultimately depends upon the demonstration of septicaemia in a shocked patient with no other obvious cause for the shocked state, there may be one or two associated phenomena that may suggest the correct diagnosis. Obviously the known existence of a septic focus and the potential for developing sepsis in certain types of disease should increase the clinician's awareness that septicaemia may be present. Patients suffering from Gram–negative septicaemia usually have a severe thrombocytopenia but this is unusual in patients with Gram–positive septicaemia. If the thrombocytopenia persists in spite of treatment, the prognosis is poor. Rarely, thrombocytopenia due to intravascular coagulation may occur in patients with septic shock and this possibility should be excluded by measurement of the fibrin degradation products and fibrinogen content of the blood. Haemolysis may occur in both Gram–positive or Gram–negative septicaemia but is more common and severe in the former. In many patients there is an initial leucopenia which is followed by a prominent leucocytosis, but the initial leucopenia is frequently missed. As with thrombocytopenia, persisting leucopenia has a grave prognosis. Patients suffering from septic shock are usually hypoxic, hypocapnoeic and have a moderate degree of metabolic acidosis, but these features may be found in patients suffering from other forms of shock. Similarly, the other biochemical changes such as hyponatraemia and mild icterus which are frequently observed are not peculiar to septic shock. The kidneys appear to be particularly sensitive to the development of septic shock and, although it is usually evident to the doctor only after some hours have elapsed, an early feature of septic shock is a dramatic fall in the sodium content of the urine. This inability to excrete any excessive intravenous infusion of sodium salts contributes to the dilution of all the compartments of the body fluid that occurs in patients with septic shock. The development of shock lung is almost always indicative of septicaemia but in the majority of patients, this complication occurs after the shock state has become established and septicaemia has usually been diagnosed. Shock lung (or post–traumatic pulmonary insufficiency as it is better named) is discussed in detail in Chapter 7. In many of the patients a supraventricular tachycardia gives way to atrial fibrillation. Persistent heart block or atrial flutter is a grave sign, particularly in patients with no previous evidence of cardiac disease.

Treatment

Although the ultimate aim must be to eradicate the source of infection, the immediate requirement is to restore the *milieu intérieur* to as near normality as possible by providing the cell with adequate oxygen and substrate and removing waste products. This may require support and therapy for the heart, lungs, and kidneys as well as providing necessary fluid. When this has been achieved attention can be directed to effective treatment of the septic focus. In the meantime, antibiotics should be given to limit the extent of the sepsis. It is unusual in surgical practice for the initial septic focus to be eradicated by antibiotics alone.

Fluid requirement.   Although extracorporeal loss may not be obvious in septic shock, absolute hypovolaemia is a common feature of septic shock due to the increased insensible loss produced by fever, the loss of protein into the interstitial fluid through damaged capillary endothelium and frequently due to 'third space loss' into the gastro-intestinal tract. In addition, the required blood volume may be greater than normal if there is vasodilation. The urgent requirement is for colloid and the solution used will depend upon availability and the patient's clinical state. Although it has been shown in experiments with animals that haemodilution improves oxygen availability (discussed in detail under haemorrhagic shock above), patients with septic shock are usually anaemic and if whole blood is immediately available then it should be infused without delay. If blood is not available, a plasma expander is required. Although albumin with a low sodium content is the most ideal, it is very expensive and not always available. Plasma, plasma protein fraction (PPF), gelatin or dextran 70 are the fluids most frequently used. Crystalloid solutions may be infused after 1–1.5 litres of colloid solution have been given according to requirements estimated from fluid balance calculations and measurements of serum electrolyte concentration, packed cell volume and plasma osmolality. Post–traumatic pulmonary insufficiency is a common sequel of septic shock (see Chapter 7) and infusion of excessive quantities of crystalloid solutions may be an important factor in its development. As many of these patients have inadequate gastro–intestinal function, intravenous feeding is frequently necessary in spite of persisting bacteraemia but nutrient requirements may be ignored for two or three days until the patient is haemodynamically stable.

Cardiovascular function.   It is advisable to prescribe digitalis at an early stage in elderly patients to improve myocardial function and lessen the risk of developing atrial fibrillation (Ledingham et al 1980). Rapid digitalisation is necessary and the dose required should be determined by expert appraisal of the electrocardiographic changes. Measurement of the digoxin concentration in the blood should be made over the ensuing days to determine maintenance requirements. Isoprenaline has also been given as an alternative inotropic drug to digitalis but dopamine is now used more frequently as it also dilates the mesenteric and renal vessels in addition to its effect on the heart. It should be given via a separate infusion set using a volumetric pump. The rate of infusion is adjusted according to the haemodynamic response as indicated by the difference between the core and peripheral temperature, urine output, blood pressure, central venous pressure and cardiac rate. Cardiac output, right atrial pressure, pulmonary artery pressure and pulmonary wedge pressure are being measured in these patients with increasing frequency by the use of Swan–Ganz catheters (Swan & Ganz 1975) as described under hypovolaemic shock. Many other drugs which affect the heart and blood vessels have been used in septic shock and it is likely that many more will be developed. As most of these drugs produce very undesirable effects if used injudiciously, they should not be used by the inexperienced. Although they may have profound effects upon the cardiovascular system there is no evidence that they have influenced the dreadful mortality of patients with septic shock.

Respiratory function.   Severe hypoxaemia is a common finding in patients with septic shock, many of whom ultimately develop post–traumatic pulmonary insufficiency. Although this hypoxaemia may be due in part to decreased cardiac output and intrapulmonary shunting of blood, the major factor in its production is the decrease in pulmonary gas exchange due to the increase in lung water. This interstitial oedema is sometimes apparent before the fluid retention discussed above is particularly advanced. Subsequent pulmonary infection is usually inevitable. The aetiology and treatment of post – traumatic pulmonary insufficiency is discussed in detail in Chapter 7.

An increase in inspired oxygen concentration combined with intermittent positive pressure ventilation (IPPV) is necessary in most patients to correct severe hypoxaemia. It has been shown that when this therapy is begun soon after the development of the shock state, further deterioration of pulmonary gas exchange is reduced or prevented (Milligan et al 1974) and perhaps the elective use of IPPV should be considered in patients with satisfactory arterial oxygen tension. IPPV also relieves the patient of the energy demands of breathing which may be considerable in these patients (Bursztein et al 1978). The use of positive end–expiratory pressure (PEEP) may improve the pulmonary gas exchange by reducing alveolar collapse. However, excessive PEEP may reduce venous return to the heart and increase pulmonary capillary resistance (Powers et al 1973). The subsequent fall in cardiac output may outweigh any benefit in pulmonary gas exchange and PEEP should not be used in excess of 10–15 cm of water. The oxygen tension of the inspired gases should be determined by measurement of the arterial oxygen tension. The lowest inspired oxygen tension that will produce satisfactory arterial oxygen tension should be used (Benatar et al 1973). Recently, attempts have been made to remove water from the lungs by combining the infusion of albumin with diuretics or dialysis (Bone 1978).

Renal function.   Although it is not always evident at the bedside, deterioration in renal function is an early feature of septic shock. Initially the volume of urine formed each hour may not alter, particularly if there has been little fall in systolic blood pressure, but the ability of the kidneys to concentrate urine is impaired. The treatment of renal failure is discussed in detail in Chapter 7. Furosemide and ethacrynic acid usually have little effect upon renal function in patients who are shocked. If renal failure is not established, renal function may be protected by maintaining renal perfusion using dopamine and maintaining diuresis with infusion of 200 ml of 20% mannitol solution. If renal failure becomes established, it is important to restrict fluid intake immediately and to begin dialysis early so that fluid overload is avoided, as this has a particularly deleterious effect on pulmonary function. The development of renal failure is a grave prognostic sign in patients with septic shock.

Antibiotics.   A wide variety of antibiotics have been used in the treatment of septic shock and, as the identity of the invading organism is often unknown, it is usual to prescribe combinations of antibiotics that will cover a wide spectrum of organisms until the results of bacteriological investigations are available. *E. coli*, Bacteroides, Klebsiella, enterococci and Proteus are the common bacteria that are found in patients who develop septic shock following gastro–intestinal surgery. A combination of gentamycin, ampicillin and metronidazole is particularly useful in such patients. Gentamycin is excreted by the kidney and in patients with adequate renal function 80 mg should be given three times a day by intramuscular injection. The aim should be to achieve a peak serum concentration of 5–8 μg/ml one hour after injection and the dosage should be modified accordingly. The drug is ototoxic at serum concentrations greater than 10 μg/ml and this is most likely to occur in patients with impaired renal function. Gentamycin is inactive against enterococci and anaerobic organisms. Ampicillin is a very effective drug in the treatment of enterococci and is excreted in the bile as well as the urine. It can be given intravenously in doses of 500 mg every 6 hours. Anaerobic bacteria are commonly incriminated in septic shock following colonic surgery and metronidazole is highly effective against these organisms. It is given by intravenous infusion of 400 mg every 8 hours.

Many patients with septic shock ultimately become colonised with *Candida albicans*, particularly if they have been treated with mixtures of broad–spectrum antibiotics for lengthy periods of time. The fungus can be grown from the skin creases and body orifices of many patients in intensive care units but only rarely is it cultured from the bloodstream. Its presence in the skin and body orifices can be ignored, the organism disappearing with the patient's recovery. However, invasion of the bloodstream is a very grave event and recovery is uncommon although treatment with amphotericin B or 5–fluorocytosine is occasionally effective. If invasion of the bloodstream is suspected but cannot be proved by culture, an opthalmologist may be able to identify the colonies in the retina.

The above account provides a broad outline of antibiotic therapy in septic shock. There are many alternative combinations of antibiotics favoured by different clinicians which may be just as effective. In general, it is important to start antibiotic therapy as soon as the diagnosis is suspected and to give adequate quantities of antibiotics that will be effective against a broad spectrum of pathogens. Expert advice from an experienced bacteriologist should be obtained as soon as possible.

Surgical intervention.   Although the septic foci of a few patients will respond to antibiotic therapy and those of a few other patients may discharge spontaneously to the body surface, a large number of patients suffering from septic shock require further surgery. It is wise to regard antibiotic therapy as a prophylactic manoeuvre to abate the septic process until resuscitation of the patient has enabled definitive treatment of the sepsis to be performed. It has recently been suggested that resuscitation and appropriate surgical intervention may be more important to a successful outcome than optimal antibiotic selection (Young et al 1977). However, demonstration of the necessity for further surgery and its timing may present the surgeon with considerable problems. Frequently it is quite obvious that the patient has a septic focus but it may be impossible to identify the site with any degree of confidence in spite of sophisticated methods of investigation. Although ultrasonic investigations may accurately locate collections of fluid that may not be revealed by routine radiological examination, adequate investigation by this technique may be impossible due to interference by drains, drainage bags, tension sutures and previous incisions. Isotopic imaging of abscesses with gallium is available in a few institutions but the isotope is usually available on only one day of the week, the patient must be transported to the counting room and accurate results require further scanning one week later. If the surgeon is convinced that there is a septic focus within the abdomen he should not hesitate in performing a laparotomy after discussion with his anaesthetic colleagues about the optimal timing for operation. Such operations should be performed by experienced surgeons and the anaesthetic given by an experienced anaesthetist. The use of epidural anaesthesia may reduce the toxic effects of general anaesthetic agents upon the lungs and liver. If no abnormality is found on laparotomy, the majority of patients suffer no ill efects (Ledingham & McArdle 1978).

The surgery should be directed towards drainage of abscesses and exteriorisation of leaking anastomoses and the surgeon should remember that he is operating to eradicate sepsis and save life rather than to perform a technically brilliant but time–consuming operation. It is advisable to insert a large number of tube drains to which suction can be applied and which may also be used for irrigation. In some patients it is obvious that in spite of the surgical intervention pus, blood or bowel content will continue to collect in one area within the abnormal cavity. A sump drain should be inserted into this area to obviate the chance of the tube drain becoming blocked. In many of these patients it is often useful to insert a tube into the jejunum through which the patient may subsequently be fed, thereby avoiding the need for intravenous feeding in a septic patient. Some patients who have gastric and colonic stasis due to intraperitoneal sepsis may be able to absorp nutrients that are infused directly into the jejunum.

Corticosteroids. The role of corticosteroids in septic shock remains highly controversial. It has been shown that the mortality of septic shock induced in experimental animals may be reduced if steroids are given at the same time as the endotoxin. This protection is believed to be due to stabilisation of cellular and subcellular membranes, particularly those of the lysosomes whose enzymes may effect oxygen utilisation by the mitochondria if released into the cell. There is little evidence to suggest that corticosteroids have any effect in septic shock in man. One controlled trial did suggest that steroids reduced mortality due to septic shock (Schummer 1976). However, many patients who have suffered septic shock die many weeks later from organ failure. Nevertheless many clinicians give 50–150 mg/kg of hydrocortisone by intravenous injection when septic shock has been diagnosed.

ACUTE ADRENAL INSUFFICIENCY

Acute adrenal insufficiency may occur as a classical Addisonian crisis due to destruction of the adrenal glands by disease or following bilateral adrenalectomy. Unexpected stress may require a greater level of cortisol than is being provided by routine replacement therapy. If any patient who is receiving steroid therapy is to undergo operation it is necessary to determine before the operation whether his adrenals can respond to pituitary stimulation by performing an ACTH stimulation test. If there is any doubt, it is advisable to give increased quantities of steroids parenterally immediately before, during and after operation. If such a patient becomes shocked, he should be given 500 mg of hydrocortisone intravenously before time is spent seeking another cause for the shock state. In the past, many patients suffering from septicaemic shock (particularly of pneumococcal origin) were thought to have acute adrenal insufficiency and were given large doses of steroids. It is now considered that acute adrenal failure occurs very infrequently in septicaemia.

ANAPHYLAXIS

Anaphylactic shock is produced by the liberation of vaso–active substances due to antigen–antibody interaction in the body. Histamine is probably the most important mediator and the concentration in the blood correlates with the degree of hypotension (Fisher 1977). The blood pools in the capillary beds and there is considerable dyspnoea due to laryngeal oedema and bronchiolar constriction. It usually occurs following treatment with drugs, horse serum and other foreign proteins, particularly when given parenterally. Although the event may be forgotten, the patient has usually been given the agent previously. Anaphylaxis is uncommon, occuring in 0.06% of patients in hospital (Boston Collaborative Drug Surveillance Program 1973) but atopic patients have a greater susceptibility. The most effective therapy is to inject 500 μg adrenaline intramuscularly every 15 minutes until the patient can breathe easily and is normotensive. Adrenaline is an alpha and beta receptor agonist producing arteriolar constriction and bronchodilation respectively. It is advisable to inject 10 mg chlorpheniramine intramuscularly which has a prolonged H_1 antagonistic effect and should prevent relapse. Emergency tracheostomy and intravenous infusion are rarely required.

6

Nutritional requirements in gastro–intestinal disease

The nutritional consequences of disease in the liver and the pancreas are discussed in Chapter 7. The nutritional deficits and requirements associated with other common disease processes of the gastro–intestinal tract are considered in this chapter.

A rigid approach to treatment is not to be encouraged and may be dangerous. Each patient has different requirements influenced by age, sex, previous nutritional state, the severity of the pathological process and the presence of co–existent disease. Patients who have been vomiting because of pyloric obstruction for a period of five days are likely to have a fluid deficit of at least 3 litres and to be hypokalaemic. In an otherwise healthy young adult with duodenal ulceration, the infusion of 2 litres of isotonic saline solution, 1 litre of isotonic glucose solution and appropriate quantities of potassium chloride over a period of 12 h will produce a rapid improvement in the clinical picture. Such infusion in a marasmic 70–year–old patient with a carcinoma of the gastric antrum who has co–existent heart disease and poor renal function may end in the death of the patient due to congestive heart failure or cardiac arrhythmia. Doctors should be trained to treat patients and not pathological processes.

The commonest cause of abnormality in the quantity or quality of the body fluids is the loss of the gastro–intestinal secretion. As emphasised in Chapter 2 the loss of fluid may be external due to vomiting, aspiration, fistulae or diarrhoea, interstitial into the bowel wall, or internal translocation into the bowel lumen or peritoneal cavity. The usual quantity and content of the gastro–intestinal secretions are shown in Table 6.1 but these may be altered by disease. If there is obstruction in the lower gastro–intestinal tract, initially some reabsorption of fluid may occur in the small bowel so that the condition progresses slowly and some compensation by transfer of fluid from the intracellular fluid to the extracellular

Table 6.1 The volume and electrolyte content of the daily intestinal secretions

| Secretion | Volume | Concentration (mmol/l) | | | |
		Na^+	K^+	Cl^-	HCO_3^-
Saliva	1500	15	30	10	30
Gastric	2000	50	15	120	–
Small bowel	3000	140	10	100	30
Bile	600	140	5	100	35
Pancreatic	700	140	5	70	100

fluid may occur. If the obstruction is in the upper bowel, copious vomiting (or aspiration) is an early feature and the patient's condition deteriorates rapidly. The content of the fluid lost also depends upon the site of the lesion. The major sites of absorption of some important nutrients from the gastro–intestinal tract are shown in Table 6.2.

Table 6.2 The major sites of intestinal absorption in health

Site	Substances	Comments
Duodenum Proximal jejunum	Water Water–soluble vitamins and drugs Electrolytes Sugars	These substances may be absorbed efficiently in the distal jejunum and ileum but it is unusual for the transport systems in the proximal small intestine to become saturated
Distal jejunum Proximal ileum	Proteins Fats Fat–soluble vitamins	Abnormalities of assimilation are more commonly due to defects in digestion rather than absorption
Distal ileum	Bile salts Cholesterol Vitamin B_{12}	Disease or resection of the ileum produces abnormalities of absorption of these substances which cannot be overcome by absorption elsewhere in the intestine

OESOPHAGEAL OBSTRUCTION

The oesophagus may be obstructed by benign or malignant disease with progressive difficulty in swallowing solids and then fluids. A carcinoma of the gastric cardia may present in a similar manner. Ultimately the patient may be unable to swallow his saliva. Although oesophageal obstruction may develop rapidly, in the majority of patients its progress is slow and malnutrition is a common feature. Surgical correction is usually required and many surgeons suggest that, if feasible, surgery should be delayed for 2 or 3 weeks to allow some nutritional repletion of the patient to be achieved (Moghissi et al 1977). In the past, this nutritional repletion has been achieved by intravenous feeding but fine–bore nasogastric feeding tubes can now be passed through oesophageal strictures using the biopsy channel of a flexible endoscope and nasogastric feeding is being used more frequently in these patients. Modern naso–enteral feeding tubes do not irritate the oesophagus and do not interfere with the healing of the anastomosis. Only non–viscous, low–residue commercial tube feeds will flow through these narrow bore tubes (see Ch. 10 for additional details).

After operation, although digestion and absorption in the stomach and small bowel is unaffected for more than two days, the onset of normal fluid and solid intake is usually delayed for some days until the integrity of the oesophageal anastomosis is assured. If at operation the surgeon advances a fine bore nasogastric tube into the duodenum or jejunum, intestinal feeding can be begun when bowel sounds are heard, the patient being able to tolerate the fine–bore tube for many days. If required, an additional tube of greater diameter can be brought out through a pharyngostomy (Fig. 6.1) to allow suction drainage at the anastomosis and from the stomach. Although the incidence of complications following gastrostomy or jejunostomy is low, haemorrhage, volvulus, perigastric and subphrenic

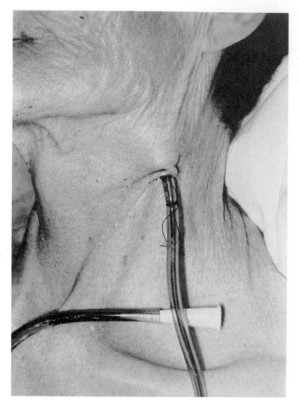

Fig. 6.1 Pharyngostomy

abscess, intestinal obstruction and failure of spontaneous closure may occur and gastrostomy or jejunostomy should only be performed if the above methods have failed.

PYLORIC OBSTRUCTION

Pyloric obstruction may be organic (e.g. carcinoma of the gastric antrum or duodenal ulcer) or functional (e.g. postoperative stasis). Gastric juice is mainly hydrochloric acid with some sodium and potassium chloride. In established pyloric obstruction the kidneys conserve sodium so effectively that sodium disappears completely from the urine. This conservation of sodium is so well developed that in spite of the patient suffering metabolic alkalosis with an increase in the extracellular concentration of bicarbonate, hydrogen ions are exchanged for sodium ions in the renal tubule so that the patient excretes an acidic urine (Gamble & Ross 1925, Le Quesne 1961). There may be a compensatory respiratory acidosis (see Ch. 4). In some patients in whom the ability to secrete acid has been reduced by gastritis or neoplastic infiltration, the gastric juice may be mainly mucus and the alkalosis correspondingly less severe. Potassium loss is usually not severe in the initial stages until, like hydrogen, potassium ions are exchanged for sodium ions in the renal tubules. In such cases the hypokalaemia may be severe and associated with abnormal myocardial contraction and the appearance of J waves on the electrocardiograph. The major clinical features are those of saline deficit with thirst, sunken eyes and ultimately circulatory collapse (see Ch. 2) and the major therapeutic requirement is for intravenous infusion of saline. When the extracellular fluid volume has been restored to normal, renal function is sufficient to correct the metabolic alkalosis and potassium can be conserved. It is advisable to include potassium chloride in the infusion even in patients without evidence of hypokalaemia. As discussed in Chapter 2, the serum concentration of potassium may be normal in patients who have lost large quantities of intracellular potassium. When the extracellular fluid volume is re-expanded with saline alone there may be a rapid decrease in the serum concentration of potassium. If the patient is very anaemic due to loss of blood from the tumour or peptic ulceration (a feature that may not be apparent in the initial stages due to haemoconcentration), it is advisable to replace some of the lost fluids as whole blood.

HIGH INTESTINAL OBSTRUCTION

Obstruction in the third or fourth part of the duodenum or high in the jejunum results in the vomiting or aspiration of gastric, biliary, duodenal, pancreatic and upper jejunal secretions. The same secretions may be lost from duodenal and jejunal fistulae. It is apparent from Table 6.1 that large volumes of fluid may be lost in this manner and treatment must be prompt and effective or the patient may succumb in the early stages from circulatory collapse. If it is impossible or inappropriate to restore normal continuity of the bowel by early operation, then it is essential to collect all the aspirate and exudate and record the volume and to analyse the electrolyte content. As with all gastro–intestinal secretions, the predominant constituent of these high intestinal juices is sodium chloride but they also contain larger quantities of potassium and bicarbonate than gastric juice. The bicarbonate concentration of pancreatic juice is particularly high after stimulation with secretin. After obstruction in the small bowel, the ability to absorb electrolytes and water is lost in the bowel above the obstruction (Shields 1965). Initially, the loss of water and electrolytes into the bowel occurs at the normal rate, but as the condition of the bowel deteriorates the rate of loss increases.

Patients with high intestinal obstruction require urgent surgical correction of the abnormality after adequate resuscitation. The patient cannot be restored to normal until the obstruction has been relieved and operation should not be delayed because of some minor abnormality of homeostasis. Every hour that is lost means an increase in the oedema in the bowel, a greater risk of interference with the blood supply and consequently an increased risk of leakage from any suture line. The surgeon must constantly assess the relative risks of operating too early on a patient who has been inadequately resuscitated and too late upon a patient whose fluid and electrolyte losses have been completely restored.

HIGH INTESTINAL FISTULAE

The mortality associated with high intestinal fistulae may be as high as 60% (Edmunds et al 1960). Much of the morbidity and mortality is due to the corro-

Table 6.3 Gastro–cutaneous fistulae

Diagnosis	Operation(s)	Site	Result	Days
Carcinoma of splenic flexure	Left hemicolectomy and splenectomy	greater curvature	closed	8
Recurrent duodenal ulceration	Polya gastrectomy	suture line	closed	9
Duodenal ulcer	Truncal vagotomy and antrectomy	suture line	closed	10
Recurrent duodenal ulceration	Bilroth II partial gastrectomy	suture line	closed	10
Carcinoma of stomach	Polya partial gastrectomy	suture line	death from respiratory failure	18
Carcinoma of stomach	Oesophago–gastrectomy	suture line	closed	11

Table 6.3 (*cont.*) Duodeno–cutaneous fistulae

Diagnosis	Operation(s)	Site	Result	Days
Carcinoma of stomach	Polya partial gastrectomy	afferent loop	death from malignant dissemination	49
Carcinoma of stomach	Polya partial gastrectomy	afferent loop	closed	21
Cholelithiasis	Cholecystectomy	duodenum	death from pulmonary embolism	3
Chronic pancreatitis	1. Total pancreatectomy 2. Repeat choledocho-jejunostomy	choledochojejunostomy	closed	50
Cholelithiasis, choledochal stenosis, acute pancreatitis	1. Cholecystectomy, exploration of CBD, duodenotomy and sphincteroplasty 2. Drainage of pancreatic abscess	sphincteroplasty	closed	42
Cholelithiasis	Cholecystectomy, exploration of CBD and duodenotomy	duodenotomy	closed	24
Cholelithiasis and choledochal stenosis	1. Cholecystectomy, exploration of CBD, duodenotomy and sphincteroplasty 2. Resuture of duodenotomy	duodenotomy	closed	33

sive action of the biliary and pancreatic secretions. It is often safer to delay operation in patients with intestinal fistulae as re-operation is often followed by a recurrence of the fistulae as the sutures 'cut out' of the oedematous, friable tissue. In the past, a consequence of this delay in surgical correction was the development of painful 'autodigestion' of the skin around the fistula and deliberate starvation to reduce the volume of intestinal secretions. In spite of the use of pastes based upon aluminium, zinc and karaya, the problems of skin excoriation were considerable. To a great extent this problem has been surmounted by the use of sheets of Stomadhesive® in which a small hole can be cut to allow the passage of the fistulous discharge whilst protecting the surrounding skin. Discharge from a cutaneous fistula can be reduced to a minimum by a combination of intraluminal aspiration by a tube passed through the nose and intravenous feeding. The details of 13 consecutive patients with gastric or duodenal fistula who were treated by this method are shown in Table 6.3. Three patients died from causes which were not directly related to their fistulae (but which might not have occurred if fistulae had not developed). The remaining fistulae healed without the need for surgical interference in 8–50 days (Tweedle 1980a). This morbidity and mortality is considerably less than previously reported by Edmunds and his colleagues (1960).

Although many fistulae of the small bowel will heal if enteral nutrition is provided in the form of low residue diets (Bury et al 1971), their use inevitably induces gastro-intestinal secretion and it is preferable to provide intravenous nutrition for patients with high intestinal fistulae.

LOW INTESTINAL OBSTRUCTION

Obstruction in the ileum is usually less dramatic then obstruction in the jejunum because until the later stages there is a greater capacity for intestinal absorption. In the upper small bowel secretion exceeds absorption, but in the lower small bowel absorption greatly exceeds secretion. The major requirement is for saline. The loss of potassium and bicarbonate ions is much less than in high intestinal obstruction and metabolic acidosis is uncommon. If the patient is very anaemic due to blood loss from a tumour or Crohn's disease, it is advisable to replace some of the lost fluid with whole blood.

STRANGULATION

If the bowel becomes obstructed due to entrapment in a hernial orifice or due to volvulus, the blood supply may be impaired at an early stage or, more commonly, at a later stage as the fluid content of the bowel wall and lumen increases. Initially it is the low-pressure venous drainage that is occluded and because the high-pressure arterial supply is unaffected, fluid continues to flow into the affected segment but not out of it and the rate of fluid loss into the bowel is dramatically increased. As the state of the loop of bowel deteriorates, bleeding may occur into bowel wall and lumen and even into the mesentery and the patient's condition deteriorates. Ultimately the arterial supply is affected and unless this is restored within minutes, the bowel will not be viable at operation and resection is inevitable. If surgical relief is delayed too long then the bowel may perforate with the development of peritonitis. In patients with strangulated bowel it is imperative that laparotomy should be performed as soon as possible. The circulating blood volume should be restored to normal by the rapid infusion of isotonic saline and 500 ml of colloid with frequent monitoring of the central venous pressure and urine output. In this manner, the majority of patients can be prepared for anaesthesia and operation within two hours of admission to hospital.

SHORT BOWEL SYNDROME

Massive resection of small bowel must be performed on occasion as a consequence of extensive gangrene due to mesenteric vascular disease or mid-gut volvulus. A similar clinical state may arise following repeated resections of the small bowel for regional enteritis. This condition is usually called 'the short bowel syndrome'. The effects of resection depend upon the quantity and quality of small bowel remaining and the relative lengths of jejunum and ileum (Pullan 1959, Wright & Tilson 1971). Resection of either the entire jejunum or the entire ileum may not produce any visible nutritional deficit although iron deficiency anaemia is common with the former and vitamin B_{12} deficiency is inevitable with the latter. In any patient, nutritional problems are fewer if the ileocaecal valve and the large bowel can be preserved, presumably due to the effects upon intestinal transit. A similar effect may be produced surgically by interposing a reversed segment of small bowel (Venables et al 1966). Patients may show little or no long–term nutritional effects following resection of 80% of the small bowel if the ileocaecal valve is preserved. This remarkable result is a consequence of the adaptation that occurs over a period of months. The successful recovery from massive resection of the small bowel can be subdivided conveniently into three stages (Pullan 1959):

First stage
Initially there is a profuse, watery diarrhoea and as much as 10 litres may be lost daily from the bowel. This is due mainly to a reduction in the absorptive area and the irritative effect of gastric hyperacidity. The major requirement is for fluid and electrolyte replacement. This stage usually lasts for 2 to 4 weeks.

Second stage
Over a period of weeks there is considerable villous proliferation so that ultimately the mucosal surface area of the small bowel may approach that before resection. Absorption of fluid and electrolytes may revert to normal. However, during the first and second stages the absorption of substrate will be extremely poor. If the patient has been saved from dehydration during the first stage, he must now be saved from starvation. Absorption of all substrates may be increased by reducing transit time with codeine phosphate syrup and by reducing the bulk of the intestinal contents using low–residue diets (see Ch. 10). If the ileum has been resected, the normal enterohepatic circulation of bile salts is interrupted and the bile salt level is reduced. As a consequence, fat digestion and absorption may be affected and steatorrhoea is common in patients. Medium–chain triglycerides (6–12 carbon atoms in length) are water–soluble and, it was believed, would be easi-

ly absorbed into the portal vein without requiring bile salts. Although their use has proved beneficial in some patients, others have been unable to absorb them and diarrhoea has followed their use. Bile salts are potent cathartics and their addition to the diet has produced more problems than benefit.

Third stage
If the patient be saved from starvation, then there is usually a slow improvement in absorption of substrate. This stage of adaptation may take up to six years. However, even when complete adaptation has occurred, it is unusual for the patient to be able to digest and absorb the type of diet that he consumed before his resection, and it is very rare to observe obesity in these patients. Most patients must restrict their daily intake of fat to 50 g and they must eat 'little and often'. During this stage, various specific deficiencies of nutrients such as vitamin B_{12} may become apparent.

In patients with the short bowel syndrome, the aim of treatment is to avoid death due to dehydration and starvation until sufficient adaptation has occurred in the bowel to allow the digestion and absorption of sufficient nourishment to maintain life. In a few patients, resection has been so extensive that insufficient bowel has been left to be compatible with life even after adaptation is complete. In these patients, life can be maintained only by intravenous feeding.

The distal ileum is the site of absorption of bile salts and loss of normal function due to disease or excision of the ileum interferes with the enterohepatic circulation of bile acids producing a decrease in the total bile salt pool and a change in the lithogenic index of the bile (Heaton & Read 1969, Dowling et al 1972). In these patients the incidence of cholelithiasis may be as high as 34% (Heaton & Read 1969). The logical approach to prophylaxis and treatment would be to give bile salts orally but unfortunately, as discussed above, these salts frequently induce severe diarrhoea. The distal ileum is also the site of absorption of vitamin B_{12} and unless these patients receive regular intramuscular injections of this vitamin they will develop megaloblastic anaemia and other cellular dysplasias.

ILEOSTOMY

Similar but less severe nutritional problems may be encountered after the formation of an ileostomy. The majority of patients who have an ileostomy do not suffer from any metabolic consequences. Following a variable period of ileus, the ileostomy usually begins to function about 36 hours after operation and during

Table 6.4 The daily volume and content of ileostomy effluent from six healthy patients

	Mean	S.D.
Volume (ml)	531	260
Sodium (mmol/l)	121	23
Potassium (mmol/l)	8.7	3.3
Calcium (mmol/l)	15.9	6.1
Magnesium (mmol/l)	7.4	2.9
Nitrogen (g/l)	1.1	0.7
Osmolarity (mosmol/l)	352	69

the first week the daily volume of effluent may be as great as two litres. However, the volume usually decreases after the first week and the effluent becomes more solid. The daily volume and content of the effluent of six patients with ileostomies that had been fashioned for longer than six months and who had no evidence of residual disease in the small bowel is shown in Table 6.4. It is apparent that the daily loss of nitrogen and minerals is very similar to normal loss in the faeces but loss of water is much greater (usually about 100 ml in faeces).

There may be specific nutritional deficiencies in patients who have undergone resection of the terminal ileum in additon to colectomy (usually patients who have been suffering from regional enteritis). In these patients, transit time from mouth to stoma may be reduced with an increase in the loss of water, sodium and potassium when compared with patients who had not undergone significant ileal resection (Nuguid et al 1961, Hill et al 1975a). Although the patient may enjoy excellent health, there may be a reduction in renal excretion of water and sodium because of this increased ileal loss (Clarke et al 1967) and a failure to restore the chronic pre–operative deficits in total body water and total body sodium produced by the inflammatory bowel disease for which the operation was performed (Hill et al 1975b). Excessive losses of water and of minerals may be most effectively reduced by treatment with codeine phosphate and to a lesser extent by Lomotil® (a proprietary tablet containing 2.5 mg diphenoxylate and 0.025 mg atropine) but the use of the hydrophilic colloid Isogel® (a proprietary mixture of cellulose and mucilage) increases the loss of water and of minerals (Newton 1978) although the consistency of the effluent may be increased. As might be expected from the consequences of ileal resection, an increased incidence of cholelithiasis occurs in patients with ileostomies (Hill et al 1975c), the incidence being greater in those who have more than 10 cm of ileum resected than in those who have less than 10 cm resected.

INFLAMMATORY BOWEL DISEASE

Profuse, watery diarrhoea is the major feature of acute infections of the gastro–intestinal tract due to Shigella, Salmonella or *Vibrio cholerae* and the major requirement is for rapid intravenous infusion of isotonic saline. In severe cases, the loss of mucus and blood may necessitate the infusion of small quantities of plasma protein fraction or whole blood.

Inflammation of the bowel due to amoebiasis, tuberculosis, actinomycosis regional enteritis or ulcerative colitis may present as an acute diarrhoeal illness but usually the clinical picture is of a more chronic wasting disease. The patients are usually malnourished and anaemic due to loss of protein and blood from the gastro–intestinal tract and these losses may be increased due to the development of fistulae. The involvement of the small bowel, particularly in regional enteritis, may severely affect absorption adding to the patients's malnourishment. Although specific treatment with appropriate antibiotics may rid the patient of amoebae, tubercle bacilli and actinomycoses and the inflammatory process may 'burn itself out' or respond to steroid therapy in patients with regional enteritis or ulcerative colitis, many of these patients require difficult and extensive surgical procedures with a correspondingly high rate of morbidity and mortality.

Defective absorption and the presence of fistulae frequently militate against the effective use of the gastro–intestinal tract for nutritional repletion and the intravenous route is required. In these patients, intravenous feeding is used to replenish a malnourished patient but recently the use of intravenous feeding to promote healing or remission in patients with regional enteritis or ulcerative colitis has evoked great interest. In the initial study (Truelove & Jewell 1974) no less than 36 of 49 patients with severe attacks of ulcerative colitis became symptom–free within five days of starting intravenous feeding and stopping oral intake except for small quantities of water. Patients who did not respond underwent urgent operation. Two–thirds of the patients who went into remission remained symptom–free during the period of review, which averaged 3 years. The authors of this report were so impressed with the results which were collected over 5 years that they suggested that this method of treatment should be adopted to select those patients who require surgery. Subsequently, this group has been successful in obtaining remission of symptoms by intravenous feeding in six patients with membranous colitis (Goodman & Truelove 1976).

The concept of providing large quantities of intravenous nutrients and ensuring total bowel rest in malnourished patients with inflammatory bowel disease is attractive and there have been further enthusiastic reports of this form of therapy in patients with regional enteritis and ulcerative colitis (MacFadyen & Dudrick 1976, Reilly et al 1976). In both of these studies, the response rate was higher in patients with regional enteritis than in those with ulcerative colitis.

It is not surprising that in the absence of distal obstruction, enterocutaneous fistulae will heal, particularly if the bowel is empty. Nor is it surprising that stenoses due mainly to mucosal and submucosal inflammation will improve or disappear. However, regional enteritis affects all layers of the bowel wall and fibrosis in the muscle coat will not respond to this therapy. Both regional enteritis and ulcerative colitis may undergo spontaneous remission and many of these patients have also been treated with steroids or salazopyrine or both. None of these studies contained a control group and consequently it is impossible to be certain that intravenous feeding will produce an improved rate of remission when compared with other methods of treatment. Furthermore, only the passage of time will tell whether an improved rate of remission will hold any long–term benefit with a lower incidence of surgical intervention and a decreased morbidity and mortality. However, regardless of any possible role in producing remission of the disease process, the need for nutritional repletion in patients who are malnourished as a consequence of the disease process is quite apparent.

Patients with non–specific inflammatory disease of the large bowel (diverticular disease) may present with haemorrhage, paracolic abscesses, fistulae or with large bowel obstruction. Fluid replacement in the treatment of haemorrhage is discussed in detail in Chapter 5.

The problems that may be encountered during intravenous infusion in the presence of sepsis are discussed in Chapter 9. Fistulae of the small bowel have been discussed above. The treatment of fistulae of the large bowel is usually less difficult, particularly in the absence of sepsis. In effect, the patient has a colostomy which in the absence of distal stenosis and the eradication of local disease will heal spontaneously. The rate of healing will be increased if the quantity of the fistulous discharge (faeces) is reduced to a minimum by use of a low residue diet (either natural as advised by a dietitian, or commercial). There is rarely any need to feed such patients by vein.

LARGE BOWEL OBSTRUCTION

In the absence of chronic inflammatory disease, secretion in the large bowel is minimal and consequently the onset and course of obstruction is usually gradual and undramatic. However, the large bowel has a comparatively poorly developed facility for absorption of water and electrolytes and although abdominal distension rather than vomiting is the major feature, the condition may have been present for one or two weeks and the loss of fluid into the lumen of the bowel may be considerable. Obstruction is usually due to tumour or inflammation and in most cases resuscitation can be undertaken over many hours, but in some patients the ileocaecal valve is competent and dangerous dilation of the caecum may be observed on the X–ray with no evidence of dilation of the small bowel. In these cases resuscitation must be rapid to allow urgent laparotomy to be undertaken before rupture occurs. Patients with neoplastic and inflammatory disease of the large bowel are frequently anaemic and hypoproteinaemic and the use of small quantities of whole blood or other forms of colloid may be indicated in the restoration of the extracellular fluid volume.

The bacterial content of the large bowel is particularly inimical and if the blood supply is impaired there is a grave danger of perforation and release of colonic bacteria into the peritoneal cavity with the subsequent development of rapidly fatal septicaemia. Obstruction due to volvulus or adhesions usually follows the more benign pattern described above. However, in the later stages there is a danger of strangulation occurring. If this is suspected, resuscitation must be rapid to allow urgent laparotomy (see above under strangulation of the small bowel). A similar but more rapid and dangerous picture may emerge following mesenteric occlusion which carries a high mortality.

VILLOUS ADENOMA OF THE LARGE BOWEL

This uncommon tumour occurs most frequently in the rectum and secretes mucus that is rich in potassium (Eisenberg et al 1964). In the majority of patients the losses are not severe, but occasionally up to 3 litres a day may be lost and the patient may present with muscle weakness, hypokalaemia and hyponatreamia. Large quantities of oral and intravenous potassium chloride may be required to prepare these patients for surgery. Although these tumours account for less than 3% of all tumours of the large bowel and only occasionally produce such severe losses, the possibility should always be considered, particularly when a tumour of the large bowel is observed to be bulky, friable and velvety with a broad base.

7

Organ failure

The importance of considering the nutritional requirements of the individual and avoiding a narrow approach that is restricted to the nutritional consequences of specific diseases was stressed in the last chapter. However, the function of many organs is particularly susceptible to metabolic changes induced by disease elsewhere in the body and, in turn, altered function within these organs may have profound effects upon metabolism in general. Unfortunately, as techniques of resuscitation improve, it is increasingly common to observe patients in the intensive care unit surviving an initial insult that in previous years would have been fatal, only to succumb, sometimes weeks later, from inadequate function of an individual organ. This is particularly likely to occur in patients who suffer septic complications following gastro–intestinal surgery (see under septic shock in Ch. 5).

CARDIAC FAILURE

Cardiogenic shock has been considered in Chapter 5. This narrative will be restricted to the nutritional requirements of patients with congestive cardiac failure and cardiac cachexia.

Congestive cardiac failure

Total body sodium and total body water are increased in patients suffering from congestive cardiac failure. The sodium retention emanates from an increase in the secretion of aldosterone (Goldberger 1957) and this effect is particularly pronounced in patients undergoing cardiac surgery when secretion of aldosterone is further stimulated as part of the metabolic response to injury (Wilson et al 1954). A corresponding quantity of water is retained by the kidneys to maintain normal tonicity of the body fluids, but ultimately the reduction in the *vis a tergo* of the failing left ventricle severely reduces glomerular filtration rate and the rate of fluid retention increases. Failure of the right ventricle produces an increase in central venous pressure and a corresponding increase in the hydostatic pressure in the venules disturbs the normal equilibrium in the capillary bed (see Ch. 1) and the patient develops peripheral oedema. The liver may be affected by the hypoxia that is a consequence of the reduced cardiac output and of congestion resulting from the increased central venous pressure and a reduction in the synthesis of albumin contributes to the cardiac oedema. The generalised tissue hypoxia produces a metabolic acidosis and, if the patient develops pulmonary oedema due to left ventricular failure, the additional insult of a respiratory acidosis is of grave prognosis.

Patients in congestive cardiac failure should not be given infusions of saline and those receiving an oral intake should receive a diet that contains low quantities of this mineral. However, when diuretics are prescribed, such dietary refinement is unnecessary and the only restriction that is required is to ensure that no salt is added at table. Infusion should be restricted to one litre of isotonic glucose solution each day. The slow infusion of 'packed cells' in anaemic patients or salt-free albumin in hypoalbuminaemic patients may have a dramatic effect in initiating a diuresis by the mobilisation of water from the periphery. The use of diuretics such as furosemide and ethacrynic acid may produce hypokalaemia which must be corrected to prevent the development of cardiac arrhythmias. Hypokalaemia also reduces the contractility of the heart.

Cardiac cachexia

Patients suffering from congestive heart failure are frequently malnourished, particularly those with rheumatic disease of the heart valves. The cause of their commonly observed poor appetite is unknown but the inadequate intake of protein is reinforced by the defective hepatic function discussed above and hypoalbuminaemia is an obvious feature of their inanition. A recent survey of the results of replacement of the aortic valve in 411 patients revealed that there was a very significant difference ($P < 0.001$) in the operative mortality rate between two groups of patients divided at the lower limit of the normal range for serum albumin concentration (3.5 g/100 ml) in that hospital (Griepp 1977). The hypoxia that afflicts the liver also affects metabolism at a cellular level throughout the body as may be indicated by defective cerebration. In addition drug intoxication, the nephrotic syndrome and, less commonly, protein–losing gastro–enteropathy and malabsorption of fat may contribute to the cachexia (Pittman & Cohen 1964). Malnourished patients undergoing open-heart surgery required artificial ventilation for longer periods of time, took longer to regain ambulation and suffered more complications such as pneumonia and renal failure after operation than a similar group of patients who had no evidence of malnutrition before cardiac surgery. However, in a randomised trial, the postoperative provision of 5 g/d of nitrogen and 4.18 MJ/d (1000 kcal/d) of energy by intravenous infusion in addition to oral intake was not associated with any improvement in ventilation, ambulation or length of postoperative stay in hospital, but there was a significant increase in the cost of treatment (Abel et al 1976). As the oral intake of these patients was negligible it is apparent that their postoperative intake of substrate was insufficient, even for sedentary requirements. Unfortunately, the provision of adequate protein and energy substrate by intravenous infusion is extremely difficult in these patients as any overloading of the circulation, however slight, may have disastrous consequences (Moghissi 1979).

RENAL FAILURE

Comprehensive accounts of the treatment of acute and chronic renal failure may be found in many general textbooks of medicine and in monographs. This brief discussion emphasises certain important features relating to the nutritional requirements of patients with acute renal failure.

Water and mineral requirements
The term oliguria is commonly used when the daily output of urine is less than 500 ml. Oliguria and anuria can arise due to a deficit of water alone or a combined deficit of water and sodium. However, the most common cause of oliguria is hypovolaemia (this is sometimes referred to as prerenal failure) but anuria usually indicates renal damage, reversible or otherwise. In a classical description, Bull et al (1950) divided the clinical course of 'acute tubular necrosis' into four stages:

Stage of onset
The patient is usually suffering from severe shock with a reduction in renal blood flow.

Stage of anuria or oliguria
As a consequence of the reduction in renal blood flow, glomerular filtration rate and urine output are drastically reduced. The ability to concentrate the urine is impaired as indicated by its low osmolarity and concentrations of urea and electrolytes. The plasma concentrations of urea and potassium rise and if uncorrected the patient may die from cardiac arrest as a consequence of hyperkalaemia. The inability to excrete H^+ produces a metabolic acidosis and the patient may hyperventilate to excrete carbon dioxide. It may take up to three weeks before the kidneys recover.

Early diuretic phase
Glomerular function recovers at an earlier stage than tubular function and the glomerular filtrate is excreted with little tubular modification. During this stage large quantities of dilute urine may be passed and the patient may die from dehydration.

Late diuretic phase
As tubular function recovers the urine becomes more concentrated and the extent of the diuresis diminishes until renal function is restored to normal.

It is important to establish as early as possible whether oliguria is due to hypovolaemia or renal failure. The most informative investigation is to measure the solute concentrations in the urine as shown in Table 7.1. The patient with renal failure is unable to concentrate his urine to any great extent. The specific gravity is low although the concentration of urea may be higher in the urine than in the plasma, the urine may have the same osmolarity as the plasma. This contrasts with the urine of a patient with hypovolaemia which will be highly concentrated. The specific gravity will exceed 1.020 and frequently exceed 1.030. The osmolarity will always be greater than 400 mosmol/l and usually greater than 100 mosmol/l. The urine/plasma osmolar ratio will exceed 1.5 and the urea ratio will exceed 10. It is advisable to catherise the patient to monitor progress and it should

Table 7.1 Urinary concentration in hypovolaemia and renal failure

	Hypovolaemia	Renal failure
Specific gravity	> 1.020	< 1.010
Osmolarity (mosmol/l)	> 400	< 400
$\dfrac{\text{Urinary osmolarity}}{\text{Plasma osmolarity}}$	> 1.5	< 1.1
$\dfrac{\text{Urinary urea concentration}}{\text{Plasma urea concentration}}$	> 10	< 5

not be forgotten that in cases of sudden onset, the urine in the bladder at the time of catheterisation may have been there for two or three hours and be unrepresentative of the patient's condition.

In addition to these measurements, the central venous pressure will be low in hypovolaemia and normal or raised in patients with renal failure (see Ch. 5). If the patient is suffering from cardiogenic shock, the urine will be concentrated as in hypovolaemia but the central venous pressure will be increased. If the patient is oliguric and dehydration is suspected, the response to infusion of 500 ml isotonic glucose should be observed. If this water load is combined with the infusion of 100 ml of 20% solution of mannitol and there is no response, acute tubular necrosis should be suspected and no attempt should be made to force a diuresis by infusion of further quantities of fluid. In the past many patients died from pulmonary oedema or cardiac failure due to mistaken attempts to force a diuresis. In patients with established renal failure, daily intake should restricted to adequate requirements for insensible loss (see Ch. 2) plus the previous day's losses from the gastro–intestinal tract and any urine passed. The most useful method for assessing the fluid balance of patients over a period of days is accurate weighing. If the patient is not receiving adequate substrate intake he will lose about 200–400 g/d due to starvation. The major fluid requirement is for isotonic glucose (although intravenous feeding may be used in conjunction with dialysis — see below). The electrolyte requirement is very low and should be adjusted according to the concentrations in the serum.

Substrate requirements

In spite of recent advances, including peritoneal dialysis and haemodialysis, the mortality of acute renal failure remains high with survival rates of 30–40% being observed after surgery or injury (Berne & Barbour 1971, London & Burton 1972). The most obvious biochemical abnormality of patients suffering from renal failure is retention of nitrogenous end–products of protein metabolism (urea, creatinine and uric acid). Until recently, it was customary to attempt to reduce the production of nitrogenous waste with a diet containing a low content of protein (or none at all) and a high content of carbohydrate to ensure that there was no requirement for gluconeogenesis from protein (Borst 1948, Bull et al 1949). However, the patient's muscle mass usually wasted at an alarming rate and catabolism of protein was found to occur at rates in excess of 100 g/d despite the high intake of carbohydrate (Cameron et al 1967, Lee et al 1967).

Urea can be used as a source of nitrogen in the synthesis of non–essential amino acids (Rose & Dekker 1956) and this mechanism was used beneficially in the treatment of patients with chronic renal failure by Giordano (1963) and Giovannetti & Maggiore (1964). Positive nitrogen balance was achieved in uraemic patients who received the minimum daily requirements of each essential amino acid and a high non–protein energy intake. This oral diet is frequently referred to as a 'Giordano–Giovannetti' diet and the use of a similar type of intravenous diet in the treatment of acute and chronic renal failure has been studied in many centres.

In early, uncontrolled studies it was observed that the use of these intravenous diets was associated with a decrease in uraemia, hyperkalaemia, hyperphosphataemia, hypermagnesaemia, hypocalcaemia and acidosis that are the biochemical consequences of acute renal failure (Dudrick et al 1970, Abel et al 1973a) and chronic renal failure (Bergstrom et al 1972). However, the improvement may have been a consequence of spontaneous improvement in renal function that was unrelated to the use of these diets. Nevertheless, in a prospective double–blind study, 21 of 28 patients receiving an intravenous 'renal failure fluid' recovered from acute renal failure compared with only 11 of 25 patients who received glucose alone (Abel et al 1973b). Statistically significant differences were also observed between the two groups in the rate of change in the concentrations of urea and creatinine in the blood. However, in this study 61% of the patients receiving the 'renal failure fluid' were dialysed but only 44% of the patients receiving glucose alone were dialysed, a factor that may have influenced these results. As the patients receiving glucose alone did so for a mean period of 13.5 days, it is possible that survival was related to the general effects of the nutritional therapy, rather than to any effect upon renal function.

There is evidence to suggest that patients suffering from renal failure have difficulty in synthesising histidine (Bergstrom et al 1972). Man's ability to synthesise non–essential aminoacids is discussed in greater detail in Chapter 8. A major contribution to the treatment of patients with renal failure was the demonstration that regular haemodialysis could remove the nitrogenous waste produced by the daily metabolism of 60 g of mixed protein (Silva et al 1964). Many patients with renal failure have been infused with greater quantities of protein (Lee et al 1967, 1968) and malnourished patients with renal failure should not be denied an adequate supply of protein. No advantage has been shown in using solutions containing essential amino acids alone compared with solutions containing a mixture of essential and non–essential amino acids and there may be other as–yet unrecognised disadvantages in addition to those discussed above. As amino acids will cross the membranes of the filters in the artificial kidney, it is wasteful to infuse solutions of amino acids during or immediately before dialysis.

Ureteric transplantation

The ureters may be transplanted into the colon or into an ileal conduit following cystectomy or to relieve ureteric obstruction in patients with inoperable pelvic tumours. Transplantation of the ureters into the bowel frequently produces a metabolic acidosis due to a combination of renal damage and absorption of urinary contents in the bowel. Reflux of urine up the ureters from the colon produces an ascending pyelonephritis and consequently diminishes the ability of the renal tubules to exchange H^+ for Na^+ and K^+ (see Ch. 4). In the colon, the urine acts as an irritant provoking a mucous discharge rich in K^+; NH_4^+ and Cl^- are absorbed. The patient exhibits a hypokalaemic, hyperchloraemic acidosis and should be treated with sodium bicarbonate and appropriate antibiotics for his infection. These features are less pronounced in patients with ileal conduits, but may still be observed. In spite of these complications many patients have survived for 20 years or more following ureterocolic anastomoses and Turner–Warwick (1969) has observed that 'a patient with a metastatic bladder tumour is frequently denied the personal convenience of a cloacal diversion, in spite of the fact that the prognosis of his bladder tumour is far shorter than that of his kidney function following uretero–sigmoidostomy'.

HEPATIC FAILURE

The liver is the most complex organ in the body, synthesising albumin, most of the globulins, fibrinogen, prothrombin and most of the other factors for blood coagulation. It is the major site of amination, deamination and transamination of keto acids and amino acids and is therefore essential for the development and maintenance of the lean body mass. The major site of glycogen storage is in the liver which, under the influence of insulin and glucagon, ensures that sufficient glucose is provided for peripheral tissues and the brain, if necessary by gluconeogenesis from amino acids such as alanine. Triglycerides and cholesterol esters may be synthesised in the liver which may also oxidise free fatty acids released from peripheral fat stores. Fat–soluble vitamins are stored in the liver. The liver is also the major site of detoxification, the kidney being able to excrete urea only after the liver has synthesised this compound from the more toxic ammonia. The end–products of haemoglobin breakdown and many other pigments are excreted in the bile which is also essential for normal digestion of fat. Each step in these complicated biochemical pathways is controlled by a specific enzyme in the liver.

It is evident that failure of this organ has numerous effects on body function and is frequently fatal. Because of the protean consequences of liver failure, treatment is particularly difficult. Heroic methods of treatment involving extracorporeal perfusion through an animal's liver and homotransplantation have been tried in relatively few patients. The majority of patients have been treated by more conservative methods (Sherlock 1969). The nutritional support of patients with acute hepatic failure is discussed below.

Water and mineral requirements
Patients with established hepatic failure are frequently overloaded with water and salt. The fluid retention may be evident as peripheral oedema or as ascites, particularly if there is any degree of portal hypertension. The retention of abnormal quantities of sodium is due to increased concentrations of serum aldosterone which may be a consequence of increase secretion (Lavagh 1962) or decreased breakdown of aldosterone by the liver (Chart et al 1956). Most patients with cirrhosis are hyponatraemic but total body sodium is increased and sodium is not required. On the contrary, intake should be less than 10 mmol/d and treatment

with an aldosterone antagonist, spironolactone, may produce a diuresis and a reduction in the oedema and ascites.

The water overloading is mainly a secondary phenomenon occurring pari passu with the retention of sodium. Water excretion may be impaired in patients with cirrhosis and increased concentrations of antidiuretic hormone have been found in the peripheral blood of cirrhotic patients (Lee & Bisset 1958). As with patients in renal failure, daily intake of water should not exceed appropriate quantities for insensible loss plus the previous day's urinary output. If it proves possible to induce a diuresis, one litre of water will be sufficient. Accurate daily weighing is the most convenient method of measuring the change in total body water.

Substrate requirements

Until recently, hepatic coma was considered to be produced by toxic waste products of protein metabolism and in particular by ammonia. As the liver was unable to convert these toxic products into less toxic substances such as urea, patients with hepatic coma were denied protein. Indeed, cathartics and enemata have been used to purge the gastro–intestinal tract of dietary protein and of blood from oesophageal and gastric varices, thereby preventing the formation of ammonia in the intestines (Brown et al 1971). If lactulose is used, it also induces a change in bacterial flora which may diminish the production of ammonia and other toxic nitrogenous substances (Bircher et al 1966). As this form of therapy does appear to produce improvement in some patients, the role of ammonia or other toxic end–products of protein metabolism in the aetiology of hepatic encephalopathy cannot be dismissed. However, there has been no evidence of a correlation between the severity of the hyperammonaemia and the encephalopathy as should exist if one was cause and the other effect. Furthermore, there is no evidence to suggest that ammonia has any toxic effect upon the brain in the concentrations that have been observed in man and it must be concluded that increased concentrations of ammonia in the blood are only indicative that a change has occurred in the patient's metabolism that may produce hepatic encephalopathy.

In recent years changes in the concentrations of neurotransmitters in the central and in the peripheral nervous system have been extensively investigated and it has been suggested that replacement of the true neurotransmitters dopamine and noradrenaline by false neurotransmitters such as octopamine and phenylethanolamine could produce many of the clinical manifestations of hepatic failure and in particular of hepatic encephalopathy (Fischer & Baldessarini 1971). The aromatic amino acids tyrosine (TYR), phenylalanine (PHE) and tryptophane (TRP) are important precursors in the synthesis of neurotransmitters and they compete with the branched chain amino acids valine (VAL), leucine (LEU) and isoleucine (ILEU) (Orlowski et al 1974). In normal man and dog the molar ratio

$$\frac{VAL + LEU + ILEU}{PHE + TYR}$$

was found to be 3.0–3.5 in the plasma but in patients or dogs with hepatic encephalopathy this ratio was reduced to 1–1.5 (Fischer et al 1975). A hypothesis was then proposed that changes in this molar ratio were responsible for the development of hepatic encephalopathy (Soeters & Fischer 1976). An important contribution to this hypothesis was the observation of an improvement in hepatic encephalopathy apparently induced by restoration of abnormal concentrations of plasma amino acids to normal levels following infusion of an amino acid solution containing large quantities of the branched chain amino acids, small quantities of phenylalanine and tryptophane and no tyrosine (Fischer et al 1976). Unfortunately, in an extensive study of patients with a variety of hepatic diseases, although there was a correlation between the molar ratio and the histological severity of hepatic disease, changes in the ratio appeared to be independent of the presence of hepatic encephalopathy and did not reflect changes in the clinical condition (Morgan et al 1978). Nevertheless, manipulation of plasma amino acid concentrations may prove to be a useful method of therapy in patients with hepatic disease, although it should be emphasised that this therapy is directed at the biochemical consequences of hepatic disease and it is unlikely to influence the progress of the hepatic pathology.

Although it is apparent that it is one or more products of protein metabolism that produces hepatic encephalopathy, patients in hepatic failure, like those in renal failure, do require enough protein for replacement of functional and structural proteins. In particular, the hypoalbuminaemia that is common in these patients is a major factor in the development of oedema and ascites. Diuretics are frequently ineffective in these patients, unless water is mobilised from the extracellular space by an increase in the oncotic pressure following infusion of salt–free albumin. Patients often improve dramatically following infusion of albumin but relapse when the infusions are stopped and there is no improvement in life expectancy (Wilkinson & Sherlock 1962).

POST–TRAUMATIC PULMONARY INSUFFICIENCY

In Chapter 5, it was emphasised that with prompt treatment death from haemorrhagic shock can be prevented in most patients. Such an event is now uncommon in hospital and provided that blood pressure and perfusion are rapidly restored, the tissues are not permanently damaged. Unfortunately, it has become increasingly apparent that many of the severely injured patients, although responding satisfactorily to haemodynamic resuscitation, ultimately die from pulmonary failure. The cause of this progressive deterioration in pulmonary function is obscure and the subject of much controversy. The syndrome has been known by many titles (shock lung, adult respiratory distress syndrome, wet lung, stiff lung, Da Nang lung, septic lung, white lung and congestive atelectasis are among the most common) that tend to reflect current opinions about possible aetiological factors. Post–traumatic pulmonary insufficiency is the most frequently used title. It was the title of an early monograph on the subject (Moore et al 1969).

Aetiology

It is usual to find that the lungs of patients with this syndrome have been subjected to more than one insult. By far the most common combination is that of inadequate perfusion and sepsis. Other common features include direct or indirect pulmonary contusion by blows or shock waves, inhalation, prolonged ventilation (particularly with high tensions of oxygen), massive blood transfusion and excessive intravenous infusion of fluids (particularly of those containing sodium).

Clinical features

Moore and his colleagues (1969) suggested that patients who are developing progressive pulmonary insufficiency after resuscitation from severe injury appear to pass through four distinct phases:

Phase I   Injury and resuscitation
Phase II   Circulatory stabilisation and beginning of respiratory difficulty
Phase III   Progressive pulmonary insufficiency
Phase IV   Terminal hypoxia and hypercarbia

This scheme can be criticised on semantic grounds as pulmonary insufficiency is only evident in phases III and IV. Furthermore, the syndrome can develop at an earlier stage before adequate haemodynamic resuscitation has been achieved, although this is an unusual occurrence. Nevertheless this approach does emphasise the important features and the clinical sequence culminating in respiratory failure that may follow major injury or operation.

The onset of pulmonary insufficiency is usually sudden. The patient has been stable haemodynamically for several hours up to one week after the original injury. The first clinical indication that all is not well is usually an increase in respiratory rate which is frequently overlooked. This is followed by an increase in heart rate but falling systemic blood pressure and frequently a rise in the patient's temperature. In the first few hours clinical and radiological examination of the chest fails to reveal any abnormality. However, even at this stage, the arterial oxygen tension is usually only 60 mmHg (8 kPa) when the patient is breathing room air and if the oxygen content of the inspired air is increased, the rise in arterial oxygen tension is usually lower than would be expected. This increase in alveolar/arterial oxygen gradient is due to perfusion of poorly ventilated segments of the lungs. This wasteful perfusion of poorly ventilated segments is usually referred to as shunting.

Over the next few hours the patient's condition may deteriorate rapidly with increasing alveolar/arterial oxygen gradients that indicate more than half of the output of the right ventricle is being shunted through non–ventilated segments of the lung. The patient may be hypoxic in spite of being ventilated mechanically with 100% oxygen. At this stage, there is evidence of poor air entry and moist sounds on auscultation. The change in the chest X–ray may be dramatic with the typical opaque appearance of florid pulmonary oedema but most patients show an improvement in arterial oxygen tension with an increase in systemic blood pressure and a small decrease in tachycardia. In the majority of patients, infection of the compromised lungs now occurs in spite of the use of prophylactic antibiotics. The organisms are rarely those that are associated with common respiratory infections usually being of the Pseudomonas, Proteus, Klebsiella and Aerobacter strains that are typically found in intensive units. Nevertheless, these infections are usually autogenous. It is not uncommon to successfully clear the patient's bloodstream of one organism for it to be replaced by another. An increasingly frequent sequence of events is the successful eradication of one or more species of bacteria by appropriate antibiotics to be followed by a fatal septicaemia due to *Candida albicans*.

In spite of expert treatment, approximately half of the patients who develop post–traumatic pulmonary insufficiency die and although complete recovery does occur, many of those who do not succumb are left with such permanent fibrotic and degenerative changes in their lungs that they are frequently unable to return to their occupations.

Pathology

The histological picture varies according to the stage of the syndrome (Blaisdell 1974). During the first 18 hours after the development of shock, petechial haemorrhages and engorgement of the capillaries and small veins are the first signs of damage in the lungs. Alveolar congestion and patchy atelectasis is more evident in the lower and middle lobes. Within 24 hours of onset there is intra–alveolar haemorrhage and thrombo–emboli may be observed in small vessels. There is interstitial and alveolar oedema and radiological evidence of pulmonary oedema may now be evident. During the subsequent 48 hours there is a gradual progression with diffuse haemorrhagic consolidation of the lungs so that they may resemble liver at post mortem. Hyaline membranes develop in the alveoli. By the fifth day infection is now the predominant feature with severe confluent bronchopneumonia.

Prophylaxis and treatment

Prophylaxis and treatment of any condition is difficult when the cause is uncertain. The possibility that platelet and other micro–aggregates may have a role in the production of post–traumatic pulmonary insufficiency (Blaisdell et al 1970) and the knowledge that such micro–aggregates that are present in stored blood are small enough to pass through the filters of standard infusion sets (Connell & Swank 1973) has led to the routine use of filters with smaller pore size in patients receiving large quantities of blood. There is little evidence to show that the use of these filters has influenced the incidence of post–traumatic pulmonary insufficiency (see Ch. 9).

One of the earliest changes to be observed during the development of the syndrome is an increase in pulmonary water and there is little doubt that the high incidence of pulmonary insufficiency following injury in the Vietnam War (Proctor et al, Hirsch et al 1971) was associated with the infusion of large quantities of crystalloidal solutions. Some doctors believe that injudicious infusion of saline is evident in every case, but the increase in pulmonary water can occur before overloading with fluid is evident elsewhere in the body (Riordan & Walters 1968). Renal function is impaired in septic shock and although not evident clinically one of the earliest signs of its development is the inability to excrete a saline load. Exceeding the sodium requirements of septic patients may be an important factor in the development of post–traumatic pulmonary insufficiency.

Those clinicians who believe that corticosteroids have a stabilising effect on cellular and subcellular membranes in patients with septic shock give 50–150 mg/kg of hydrocortisone by intravenous injection when septic shock has been diagnosed and may repeat this dose during the first 48 hours (Schummer & Nyhus 1970). Most do so in the particular belief that this therapy reduces the incidence of post–traumatic pulmonary insufficiency in patients with septic shock. The important role of sepsis in the development of post–traumatic pulmonary insufficiency has been discussed above. The incidence of this syndrome would be considerably reduced by a decrease in the incidence of septic complications in hospital patients. Many more surgical procedures are being performed in patients who are given prophylactic antibiotics. If sepsis is recognised prompt and adequate treatment is required. The treatment of septic shock has been discussed in Chapter 5.

Although high concentrations of oxygen may damage the lungs (Morgan 1968) and the extent of the damage appears to be proportional to the oxygen concentration and the time that it is delivered, the syndrome can occur in patients who are not ventilated or inspiring increased concentrations of oxygen. In the majority of patients suffering from respiratory failure, an inspired oxygen concentration of 35 – 45% is usually sufficient to produce an acceptable arterial oxygen concentration and it is doubtful whether the lungs will be damaged by exposure to this concentration for a few days. However, in a few patients with post–traumatic pulmonary insufficiency hypoxaemia may exist in spite of ventilation with 100% oxygen.

As high concentrations of inspired oxygen may be a factor in the development of post–traumatic pulmonary insufficiency, it is important to select as low a concentration as possible that will ensure adequate arterial oxygen tension (Benatar et al 1973) when intermittent positive pressure ventilation is necessary. In a previous healthy adult, the arterial oxygen tension should exceed 70 mmHg (9.3 kPa) and preferably approach 90 mmHg (12 kPa). However, many patients who have suffered from chronic pulmonary diseases do not exhibit clinical signs of anoxia when their arterial tension is 60 mmHg (8 kPa). Anoxia may produce changes in the patient's cerebral state and the nail beds are usually grey or blue. A persistent, unexplained tachycardia may be the only sign. Arterial blood oxygen concentration should be measured at least daily in these patients and the use of arterial catheters allows more frequent estimations to be made. The inspired gases should be humidified with sterile water at 37°C to avoid dehydration. In many patients requiring ventilation, increased arterial oxygen concentration can be achieved at any given inspired oxygen concentration by using positive end–expiratory pressure (PEEP) to reduce alveolar collapse at the end of the expiratory phase. However, positive end–expiratory pressure may reduce venous return and cardiac output (Powers et al 1973). The hydrostatic pressures existing across the capillary walls in the lungs are such that fluid constantly passes from the capillary into the interstitial space, regardless of the oncotic pressure. This fluid is removed by the well–developed lymphatic system which may possibly be imparied by excessive positive end–expiratory pressure which should not be used in excess of 15 mm of water. Notwithstanding any improvement in arterial oxygenation, the use of intermittent positive pressure ventilation reduces the patient's energy requirements by 25–40% (Bursztein et al 1978).

In a few patients in whom adequate arterial oxygenation cannot be obtained by the use of intermittent positive pressure ventilation and in whom adequate pulmonary function might be expected upon recovery, extracorporeal oxygenation may be considered (Hill et al 1972).

PANCREATIC FAILURE

It is apparent from Table 7.2 that the pancreas is essential for the normal assimilation of ingested nutrients. Not only does the pancreas secrete a wide variety of hydrolytic enzymes into the lumen of the gut, it also secretes peptide hormones into the bloodstream, some of which affect secretion elsewhere in the gastro–intestinal tract and others which control the ultimate destination and fate of the products of digestion.

Table 7.2 The secretions of the pancreas

Exocrine	Endocrine
a. Sodium bicarbonate	Insulin
b. Proteolytic enzymes	Glucagon
Chymotrypsinogen	Pancreatic polypeptide
Trypsinogen	
Elastase	Somatostatin
Carboxypeptidases	
Ribonuclease	
Deoxyribonuclease	
c. Lipolytic enzymes	
Lipases	
Esterases	
d. Amylolytic enzymes	
Amylase	

Exocrine failure

In spite of the numerous enzymes secreted by the pancreas, the major portion of the organ must be destroyed thereby reducing stimulated secretion to about 10% of normal before clinical signs such as steatorrhoea and creatorrhoea develop. Following total pancreatectomy, moderate quantities of protein may be hydrolysed by gastric pepsin and the peptidases of the succus entericus, starch by salivary amylase and maltose, lactose and fructose by the disaccharidases of the succus entericus. However, although lipases are found in gastric juice and in the succus entericus, digestion of fat is grossly disturbed by total pancreatectomy and the frequent passage of bulky, pale, foul–smelling and unformed stools is inevitable. These stools are irritant and the subsequent intestinal hurry and malabsorption aggravates the nutritional effects of deficient digestion. Patients suffering from chronic pancreatitis and those who have undergone pancreatic surgery are frequently severely malnourished. There is evidence to suggest that lipolysis is adequate in patients suffering from chronic pancreatitis. However, absorption of fatty acids is interfered with by excessive quantities of lecithin which requires pancreatic phospholipase for its digestion (Shimoda et al 1974).

A variety of extracts of animal pancreas is now available to compensate for deficient exocrine secretion. Each preparation differs in content and in strength and correct dosage should be ensured by reference to the manufacturer's literature. Not every manufacturer states the proteolytic, lipolytic and amylolytic activity of the product. One extract contains pepsin and a few contain ox bile. The extracts may be in the form of tablets, capsules or granules. The extract should be taken immediately before, during or immediately after the meal but they are frequently unpalatable and it may be impossible to persuade the patient to ingest the required quantity. Some patients prefer to sprinkle the contents over their food but it can be unappetising to witness the soup digested before consumption. The optimum pH for most of the pancreatic enzymes is about 7 and this is achieved in the duodenum under natural conditions by the alkaline pancreatic juices neutralising the acidic chyme from the stomach. Ingested extracts may be destroyed by the acid in the stomach and extracts contained in gelatine capsules may be more effective (Taylor et al 1979).

Endocrine failure

In health it is known that the endocrine pancreas secretes the peptide hormones insulin, glucagon, pancreatic polypeptide and somatostatin (growth hormone–release inhibiting hormone). The discovery of the last two hormones is a compatively recent event and it is possible that the pancreas may contain other as yet undiscovered small quantities of other hormones such as gastrin but in health the content of these hormones is trivial when compared with other sites in the gastro–intestinal tract (Polack & Bloom 1979). However, rare tumours of the pancreas may develop which secrete vast quantities of these hormones. Although glucagon, pancreatic polypeptide and somatostatin have important functions in healthy individuals, in patients with pancreatic failure it is only the lack of insulin that appears to have a major effect upon metabolism.

Details of the many varieties of insulin now available for the control of diabetic hyperglycaemia may be found in standard medical texts and monographs. Patients undergoing partial or total pancreatectomy for carcinoma or pancreatitis who did not experience endocrine deficiency before operation frequently become very labile diabetics during the first few months after operation and it is advisable to control their diabetes with repeated injections of soluble insulin. Some patients never become sufficiently stable to be controlled by preparations with prolonged action.

8

Intravenous nutrients

The basic requirements to maintain body composition have been delineated in Chapter 1 and further consideration of the requirements in disease are to be found in Chapters 6 and 7. In this chapter the content of available solutions of amino acids, carbohydrates, fat, trace elements and vitamins is discussed with particular reference to these requirements.

AMINO ACIDS

Proteins are complex molecules built from many amino acids which have the basic formula $R.CH(NH_2).COOH$ where R is an organic compound. The structure of some of the amino acids found in the body is shown in Figure 8.1. The simplest amino acid is glycine, where R = H. The carbon chain can increase in length and in alanine, a three–carbon chain amino acid, $R = CH_3$. More complex amino acids may have branched side chains, such as isoleucine, and others contain benzine rings, such as tyrosine. The amino acids in a protein are linked by the peptide bond CONH which is formed by the condensation of the amine radicle of one amino acid and the carbonyl radicle of the other:

$$COOH + NH_2 \longrightarrow CONH + H_2O$$

If this condensation involves only two amino acids, the substance formed is called a dipeptide, A tripeptide contains three amino acids and two peptide bonds

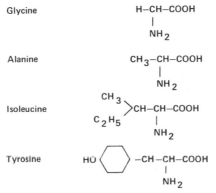

Fig. 8.1 The basic structure of some human amino acids

and molecules consisting of several amino acids are called polypeptides. Proteins are usually extremely complex structures composed of several polypeptide chains with cross−linking between the individual amino acids in these chains.

Human proteins are made from 21 amino acids shown in Table 8.1. Cysteine is the reduced form of cystine containing one more hydrogen atom and glutamine is the amide of glutamic acid. Other close derivatives of these amino acids such as methylhistidine and hydroxyproline have not been included. Amino acids exist in two isomeric forms, the dextro (d−) and laevo (l−) forms. Rose (1949) demonstrated that with the exception of small quantities of d−methionine and d−phenylalanine, the body can utilise only the l−isomers for the synthesis of protein when given by mouth. Subsequent studies suggest that utilisation of infused d−methionine may be negligible (Tweedle et al 1977). The majority of naturally occurring amino acids in food are l−isomers. In this book, any reference to an amino acid implies the l−isomer of that acid unless stated to the contrary.

Table 8.1 Amino acids found in human protein

Alanine	Methionine
Arginine	Ornithine
Aspartic acid	Phenylalanine
Citrulline	Proline
Cysteine/Cystine	Serine
Glutamic acid/ Glutamine	Taurine
Glycine	Threonine
Histidine	Tryptophane
Isoleucine	Tyrosine
Leucine	Valine
Lysine	

In addition to being required for the structural protein of the lean body mass described in Chapter 1, these amino acids are also required for circulating proteins such as haemoglobin, thyroxine, pepsin, albumin, histamine and humoral antibodies. Many of these amino acids can be synthesised in a healthy individual by amination of the appropriate keto acid or by transamination between keto acid and amino acid but following deprivation studies in healthy young volunteers and in various animals it was concluded that eight amino acids (Table 8.2) could not be synthesised in man (Rose 1949). As they must be included in the diet, these amino acids are usually called essential amino acids.

Having established the daily requirement for each essential amino acid, Rose suggested that a safe minimum requirement should be twice the highest require-

Table 8.2 Essential amino acid requirements in healthy adults (g/d). After Rose (1949)

Tryptophane	0.5
Phenylalanine*	2.2
Lysine	1.6
Threonine	1.0
Valine	1.6
Methionine[†]	2.2
Leucine	2.2
Isoleucine	1.4

* in the absense of tyrosine
[†] in the absence of cysteine

ment found in any of the healthy volunteers that he studied and these are the figures shown in Table 8.2. Nevertheless, Rose was aware that he was studying healthy volunteers using a method of investigation that was not particularly accurate and which has been strongly criticised (Hegsted 1964). He emphasised that 'safe' should not be considered to be synonymous with 'optimum' and that these quantities should only be considered as provisional until more data became available. Thirty years later certain features have became apparent that demonstrate the wisdom of Rose's caution.

Non−essential amino acids should be synthesised in the body by amination or transamination but the latter process requires an additional supply of amino acids, sometimes of essential amino acids. Cysteine may be synthesised from methionine and tyrosine from phenylalanine but this increases the requirement for methionine and phenylalanine. A mixture of non−essential amino acids was found to be more effective in maintaining nitrogen balance than glycine alone (Swenseid et al 1959). This suggests that the synthesis of some amino acids from glycine alone or other endogenous sources of amines was less efficient than the provision of these so−called non-essential amino acids. Arginine and histidine were found to be essential in the diet of some animals, but Rose (1949), although clearly suspicious, was unable to confirm this in man. Subsequent studies have shown that the ability to synthesise histidine is very limited in neonates and young children and insufficient for optimal regeneration of tissue (Holt 1967, Bergstrom et al 1970). Solutions of amino acids are toxic when infused in large doses in experimental animals and in man. The major biochemical feature of this toxicity is hyperammonaemia and this may be reduced or prevented by the inclusion of arginine in the mixture (Najarian & Harper 1952). This protective effect probably depends upon an increased rate of synthesis of urea (Winitz et al 1956), suggesting that the ability to synthesise arginine from keto acids or other amino acids may not be adequate for the optimal function of the urea cycle. However, a similar effect has not been observed with ornithine or citrulline, the two other amino acids which are components of the urea cycle. Unfortunately, as might be expected, arginine has little if any beneficial effect in patients with hepatic precoma (Fahey 1957). In these patients lack of components of the cycle is unlikely to be an important factor, hyperammonaemia being a consequence of failure of metabolism within the cycle due to inadequate concentrations of the necessary enzymes. It has been suggested that synthesis of proline, alanine and cysteine may be inadequate for the demands of the young infant (Jurgens & Dolip 1968, Sturman et al 1970, Harries et al 1971). Following major operations the ability of the liver to synthesise cysteine from methionine and tyrosine from phenylalanine may be impaired (Dale et al 1977) and similar observations have been made in patients suffering from postoperative sepsis (Groves et al 1974), experimental sandfly fever (Wannemacher et al 1972) and battle injuries (Levenson et al 1955).

Although healthy young volunteers may be able to synthesise amino acids from keto acids and other amino acids, the studies described above suggest that this ability may be compromised in many patients. It would seem wise to abandon the concept of 'essential' and 'non−essential' amino acids.

The toxicities, imbalances and antagonisms that may be induced by individual amino acids were reviewed by Harper & Rogers (1965) and oral studies have demonstrated that excessive quantities of glycine may have a particularly deleterious effect (Swenseid et al 1960). Large quantities of glycine are excreted in the urine when excessive amounts are infused in patients (Tweedle et al 1972). Glutamic acid is another amino acid that has been blamed for toxic reactions. Many doctors consider its ingestion to be responsible for the 'Chinese Restaurant Syndrome' (Ghadimi et al 1971) and previous studies have shown that it may induce vomiting when infused in dogs (Madden et al 1945). As the majority of ingested glutamic acid is converted to alanine in the gastro–intestinal mucosa and absorbed as such, presumably the body has little difficulty in resynthesising the large quantities that are found in muscle (Furst et al 1978). Nevertheless, previous studies of oral feeding have suggested that nitrogen balance can be improved by including glutamic acid in the mixture of amino acids (Rechigl et al 1957, Swenseid et al 1959). In addition to being used for synthesis of protein or excreted unutilised by the kidneys, excessive quantities of amino acids may be deaminated and their carbon skeletons converted into components of the tricarboxylic acid cycle as shown in Figure 8.2. The amine radicles are converted into urea.

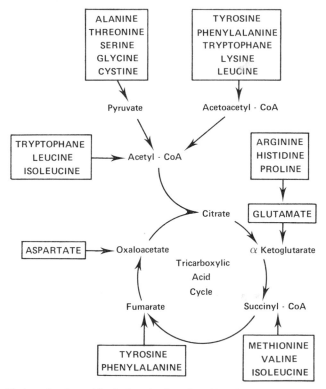

Fig. 8.2 The oxidation of amino acids via the tricarboxylic acid cycle

Some solutions of amino acids contain peptides. These solutions are prepared by hydrolysis of protein (the reverse of the condensation reaction forming the peptide link described at the beginning of the chapter). Not only is the amino acid content of the solution determined by the amino acid content of the protein, but the hydrolysis of the protein is incomplete so that the solution contains as much as 30% of the amino acid in the form of peptides. The utilisation of these peptides is controversial. It has been suggested that the amount of peptides un-utilised is of little significance (Christensen & Lynch 1946) and subsequent stud-ies of nitrogen balance failed to show any difference between the efficacy of the same hydrolysate when compared with modern solutions containing amino acids alone (Tweedle et al 1972). However, studies using different hydrolysates suggested that large quantities of the infused peptides are excreted in the urine (Freeman & MacLean 1971, Long et al 1976). Hydrolysates were no longer used in Great Britain and their use in the rest of Europe is decreasing rapidly. However, large quantities are still being used in North America and other countries.

What is the relevance of this knowledge to the doctor who must choose from a bewildering variety of solutions of amino acids that are now available? Because of doubts about their utilisation, solutions containing peptides or d–isomers of amino acids should not be used. Solutions that contain large quantities of glycine and possibly glutamic acid should not be used for fear of inducing toxicity. As the ability to synthesise so called 'non–essential 'amino acids may be impaired, it is advisable to choose a solution that contains as many of the amino acids shown in Table 8.1 as possible. Unfortunately, it is extremely difficult to manufacture a solution containing all these amino acids without precipitation of the more insolu-ble amino acids cysteine and tyrosine. This tendency increases with increasing concentration and some of the more concentrated solutions do not contain any of these amino acids. Nevertheless, deficiency states due to lack of these amino acids in infusions have not been described.

Although lack of or an insufficient quantity of an amino acid may not produce clinical evidence of a deficiency state, it may affect protein metabolism in gener-al and the doctor should appreciate that solutions containing equivalent total quantities of amino acids or nitrogen may differ considerably in their content of individual amino acids. The optimal composition of these solutions is unknown. Much of the information that has been gained from oral studies may have little relevance to intravenous requirements as the pattern of amino acids released into the bloodstream by the liver differs greatly from that ingested (Elwyn 1970). More information is becoming available from studies of amino acid concentrations in the blood and muscle and their uptake and excretion by individual organs. It is likely that amino acid requirements will differ during health, starvation or spe-cific disease. The possible role of solutions of particular composition in the treat-ment of renal or hepatic failure is discussed in Chapter 7.

The Maillard reaction
When solutions of amino acids are mixed with glucose or fructose, some of the amino acids react with the hexoses. Under suitable conditions the amino group will react with an aldehyde (glucose) or ketone (fructose) group to form a so-called 'Schiff base'. These bases are brown in colour and the reaction is sometimes known as the 'browning reaction'. The extent of this reaction depends upon the length of storage, the temperature and the pH of the solution (Hodges et al 1963, El Ode et al 1966). The loss of amino acids is small if the solution is stored at room temperature and the pH is less than 6 but the loss is much greater if

the mixtures are sterilised by autoclaving. Although amino acid content is reduced by this reaction, there is no evidence that the bases formed are toxic or have an inhibitory effect on the remaining amino acid content (Freidman & Kline 1950). Mixtures of amino acids and glucose or fructose can be prepared by mixing solutions of both substrates which have been sterilised by separate autoclaving or by sterile filtration of the mixture. The reaction can also be prevented by the addition of the reducing agent sodium metabisulphite before autoclaving, but this substance may produce toxic products following reactions with the amino acids (see below under cholestasis). Some amino acid solutions contain ethanol, sorbitol or xylitol which do not react in this manner during autoclaving. However, these alcohols also have undesirable side effects (see below). Furthermore, the quantity of these substances that are added to the amino acid is insufficient to meet non−protein energy requirements (see below). It should be noted that many solutions of amino acids that do not contain hexoses are slightly yellow in colour unless bleached with sodium metabisulphite and so are solutions of glucose and fructose.

CARBOHYDRATES

Carbohydrates are compounds which have the general formula $C_x(H_2O)_y$ but the term is frequently extended to the products of oxidation and reduction of true carbohydrates. Thus, sorbitol which is a polyhydric alcohol with the formula $C_6H_{14}O_6$ is considered to be a carbohydrate. The term sugar is often loosely applied to all carbohydrates but should be reserved for monosaccharides and oligosaccharides. Monosaccharides are used for intravenous infusion and oligosaccharides are constituents of some enteral preparations.

Monosaccharides

Monosaccharides cannot be split further by hydrolysis and according to the length of their carbon chain they are subdivided into pentoses and hexoses etc. Their general formula is $[C(H_2O)]_n$ and the hexoses glucose and fructose, which are important in intravenous nutrition, have the formula $C_6H_{12}O_6$. Like amino acids, sugars can exist as laevo (l−) or dextro (d−) isomers and in the case of sugars, unlike that of amino acids, the great majority of naturally occurring sugars are dextrorotatory. Thus solutions of glucose for infusion are d−glucose and in North America the term dextrose is commonly used for such solutions.

Glucose

Glucose is the natural source of carbohydrate energy in man and the majority of the carbohydrate that is derived from food reaches peripheral organs as glucose. Because of the difficulties experienced with the Maillard reaction during autoclaving (see above) and the need to provide exogenous insulin when large quantities of glucose are infused, many doctors and many manufacturers have attempted to substitute other carbohydrates for intravenous feeding. There have been many claims that these substitutes are superior to glucose when infused intravenously. However, as discussed below, these deductions and arguments have been based upon false concepts and the substitutes are potentially dangerous in scvcrcly ill patients (Froesch 1974, Krebs 1978, Newton et al 1978, Zollner 1978).

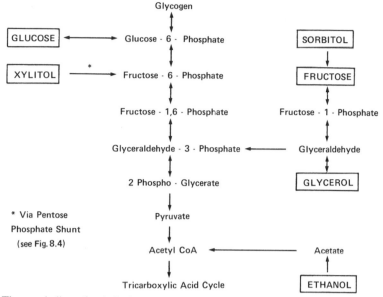

Fig. 8.3 The metabolism of carbohydrates used for intravenous nutrition

The important role of glucose in homeostasis and the need to provide glucose from endogenous protein during starvation and injury have been discussed in Chapter 3. The metabolic pathway of glucose is shown in Figure 8.3. It enters the glycolytic pathway where it is phosphorylated to glucose−6−phosphate. The entry of glucose from the bloodstream into fat cells requires insulin and insulin also increases glucose uptake by the liver and muscles and the formation of glycogen. However, during excerise, muscles take up glucose even in the absence of insulin (Froesch 1974). The pyruvate produced by glycolysis is oxidised to water and carbon dioxide in the tricarboxylic acid cycle yielding much more energy or can be used for resynthesis of glucose by the glucose−alanine cycle or the Cori cycle as described in Chapter 3. If the intake of glucose is in excess of immediate requirements, it is stored as glycogen or converted into depot fat. The maximum uptake of glucose from the blood is about 1−1.5 g/kg per h (Newton et al 1978, Zollner 1978) which is in excess of the energy requirements of any patient. Glucose for intravenous infusion is commercially available in 5% (isotonic), 10%, 20% and 40% solutions. The 20% solution is used most commonly for intravenous feeding and minerals that cannot be included in solutions of amino acids are frequently added to this solution. The potential metabolic complications that can occur during or following the intravenous infusion of these solutions are hypoglycaemia, hyperglycaemia, glycosuria, hyperosmolar coma and hypokalaemia and are discussed below.

Fructose

The majority of the fructose that enters the blood either by infusion or following ingestion is removed by the liver (Froesch 1974, Krebs 1978). The first step in the metabolism of fructose is also that of phosphorylation (Fig. 8.3). However, the phosphorylation of fructose and its subsequent metabolism appears to be unregulated when compared to the very carefully regulated metabolism of glucose (Thoren 1962, Froesch 1974). Fructose reaching muscle or adipose tissue is phosphorylated to fructose−6−phosphate, but the quantity is small compared to that metabolised in the liver.

The rapid removal of fructose from the blood without the need for insulin has led to suggestions that it is an ideal substrate for intravenous feeding in the stressed patient. Like glucose its maximum rate of clearance is about 1−1.5 g/kg per h (Newton et al 1978, Zollner 1978). However, after infusion of fructose there is an increase in the concentration of glucose in the blood and isotopic studies in rats using ^{14}C−labelled fructose have shown that after a small period of time most of the radioactivity appears in glucose in the blood (Froesch 1974). This glucose requires insulin for its utilisation. Consequently, the concept of fructose being independent of insulin for its utilisation is fallacious. Moreover, the rapid utilisation of fructose may produce potentially dangerous changes in metabolism. Large increases in the plasma concentrations of lactic and uric acids may occur (Sahebjami & Scalettar 1971). In healthy individuals, the lactic acidosis induced by the infusion of fructose may be insignificant and transient but many of the patients who receive parenteral nutrients have some degree of lactic acidosis before intravenous feeding is begun (Newton et al 1978). Any further increase induced by intravenous infusion should be avoided if possible. The other major disadvantage of fructose as an intravenous substrate is the depletion of adenine nucleotides that occurs in the liver (Woods et al 1970).

Alcohols

Alcohols are organic compounds that contain hydroxyl (OH) groups which are linked to carbon atoms. In addition to the monohydric alcohol, ethanol, the polyhydric alcohols (polyols) glycerol, sorbitol and xylitol are used for intravenous feeding.

Ethanol (C_2H_5OH)

The value of ethanol in reducing the breakdown of protein has been known for a long time (Atwater & Benedict 1896). The major advantage of ethanol in this respect is its high calorific value (7 kcal/g) when compared with the other carbohydrates. The metabolism of ethanol is controlled by the enzyme alcohol dehydrogenase which is found almost exclusively in the liver. Although a stimulant in very low concentrations, alcohol is toxic to many tissues and in particular to the central nervous system. Man is not the only animal who may be rendered incapable of rational action by alcohol (Krebs & Perkins 1970). The protective action of hepatic oxidation of alcohol requires nicotinamide adenine dinucleotide (NAD) as a co−enzyme in addition to alcohol dehydrogenase. This co−enzyme is also required for the oxidation of sorbitol (see below) and it is unwise to infuse these substrates at the same time.

That there is a maximum rate for the hepatic detoxification of ethanol is well known. The average rate in healthy males is 7.3 g/h and 5.3 g/h in females (Widmark 1952). If the maximum rate is exceeded and the concentration of ethanol increases, there is an osmotic diuresis in addition to the effects upon the central nervous system. Nevertheless, when infused at a concentration of 4% in quantities not exceeding 1.5 g/kg per d, no adverse effects were noted during prolonged intravenous feeding for up to 7 months and the concentration of ethanol in the blood did not exceed 30 mg/100 ml (Coats 1972).

Sorbitol $(C_6H_{14}O_6)$

Sorbitol is the polyhydric alcohol formed by the reduction of fructose and in the body the first step in its metabolism is oxidation to fructose.

This reaction is catalysed by the enzyme sorbitol dehydrogenase and the co-enzyme NAD is also required (see under ethanol above). Like alcohol dehydrogenase, sorbitol dehydrogenase is found predominantly in the liver. The subsequent metabolism of sorbitol is the same as that of fructose and the compounds share the same undesirable metabolic phenomena. However, the additional atom of hydrogen contained in sorbitol increases the tendency to lactic acidosis. This may be a particularly grave problem when sorbitol is infused with ethanol. Both substrates compete for the co-enzyme NAD and large quantities of NADH are formed:

$$\text{Sorbitol} + \text{NAD} \longrightarrow \text{Fructose} + \text{NADH}$$

Further oxidation of the substrates requires the provision of corresponding quantities of NAD. This can be achieved by converting pyruvic acid into lactic acid:

$$\text{Pyruvic acid} + \text{NADH} \longrightarrow \text{Lactic acid} + \text{NAD}$$

Sorbitol can be converted directly to glucose under the control of the enzyme aldose reductase (Hers 1955) but the quantity converted by this route is very small. The concentration of glucose in the blood does increase after infusion of sorbitol but this is by means of the pathway shown for fructose in Figure 8.3. The glucose formed from sorbitol, like that formed from fructose, requires insulin for its further utilisation and sorbitol is not independent of insulin as a source of energy. If sorbitol is infused more rapidly than its metabolism to glycogen, glucose or lactate, than its concentration in the blood increases and it is a potent diuretic (Lee et al 1972).

Xylitol $(C_5H_{12}O_5)$

Xylitol is the most recent polyol to be investigated. Like sorbitol, the initial step in its metabolism is oxidation and this reaction is probably under the control of the same dehydrogenase as sorbitol. The pentose, d-xylulose, is produced by this oxidation (Fig. 8.4) and this undergoes phosphorylation to xylulose-5-phosphate which then enters the pentose phosphate pathway to be converted into fructose-6-phosphate. Like sorbitol, the major site for the initial oxidation under the influence of the dehydrogenase is in the liver. Like fructose and sorbitol, there appears to be very little control of the rate of the initial stages of metabolism of xylitol and large quantities of lactic acid may be produced. The glucose produced from the metabolism of xylitol, like that from fructose and sorbitol, requires insulin for its further utilisation. In addition to the undesirable production of lactic acid, infusion of xylitol, like fructose and sorbitol, may also produce an

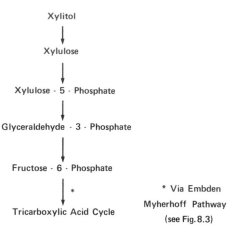

Fig. 8.4 The metabolism of xylitol by the pentose phosphate pathway

increase in the concentration of uric acid in the blood (Donahoe & Powers 1970). Following the infusion of a 20% solution of xylitol in Australia a number of fatal reactions were observed (Thomas et al 1970, Birch 1971). The patients suffered from liver and renal damage and were severely acidotic. Consequently, the intravenous infusion of xylitol has been prohibited in Australia, Great Britain and the United States of America. However, large quantities are still used in other European countries, particularly in Germany.

Glycerol ($C_3H_8O_3$)
Glycerol is a component of fat emulsions. A small quantity is available in the free form and additional quantities may be released by hydrolysis of the triglycerides. It has been suggested that this content of glycerol is the major factor in the reduction of protein breakdown induced by infusion of fat emulsion (Brennan et al 1975). Glycerol joins the Embden–Myerhof pathway as triose phosphate (Fig. 8.3) and is ultimately oxidised in the tricarboxylic acid cycle. Although the infusion of moderate quantities of a dilute solution appear to produce no adverse effects, infusion of quantities sufficient to satisfy energy requirements produces severe toxic reactions (Sloviter 1958) and it cannot be used for this purpose. The quantity of glycerol that is added to stabilise fat emulsions and that produced by hydrolysis of the contained triglycerides does not induce toxicity.

FATS

Fats or triglycerides are esters of fatty acids and glycerol (Fig. 8.5). Although the glycerol is common to all fats, the fatty acids show considerable variation. Fatty

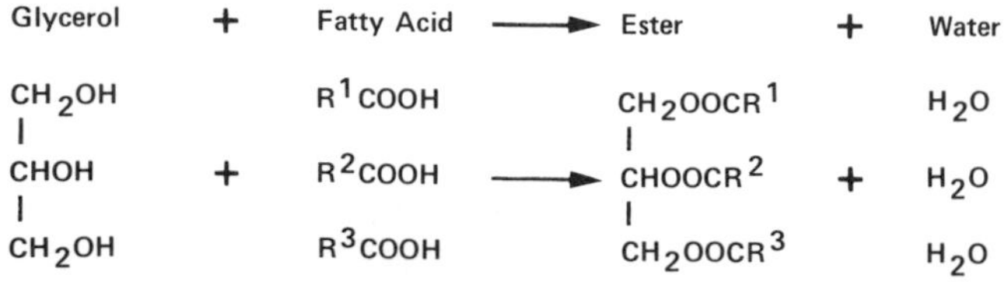

Glycerol	+	Fatty Acid	⟶	Ester	+	Water
CH_2OH		R^1COOH		CH_2OOCR^1		H_2O
$CHOH$	+	R^2COOH	⟶	$CHOOCR^2$	+	H_2O
CH_2OH		R^3COOH		CH_2OOCR^3		H_2O

Fig. 8.5 The formation of triglycerides by the esterification of fatty acids and glycerol

Table 8.3 The composition of fatty acids in ingested triglycerides

	Carbon chain length	Examples
Short chain	Less than 6	butyric acid (4 C)
Medium chain	6–12	caprylic acid (8 C)
		capric acid (10 C)
Long chain	More than 12	palmitic acid (16 C)
		stearic acid (18 C)

acids ingested by humans are subdivided into short, medium or long chain fatty acids according to the length of their carbon chain (Table 8.3). The fatty acid composition of triglycerides in human nutrition was thought to be insignificant, until it was demonstrated that certain fattly acids (so–called 'essential fatty acids') were required in the diet (Burr & Burr 1930). Some, such as stearic acid, are completely saturated with hydrogen, but others such as oleic acid are unsaturated (Fig. 8.6). Oleic acid is said to be monosaturated as it contains one double–bond carbon linkage. Other fatty acids, such as linoleic and linolenic acid, are polyunsaturated. Animals are unable to synthesise fatty acids, such as linoleic and linolenic acid, which have double-bond carbon linkage proximal to the ninth carbon atom in the chain. Consequently, it should be noted that man is not only unable to synthesise linoleic and linolenic acids but is also unable to synthesise linolenic from linoleic acid. The formulae of these fatty acids are now indicated by the notation shown in Figures 8.6 and 8.7. The number preceding the colon is the length of the carbon chain, the number following the colon is the number of double bonds, and the number following omega is the position of the double bond nearest to the terminal methyl group (CH₃).

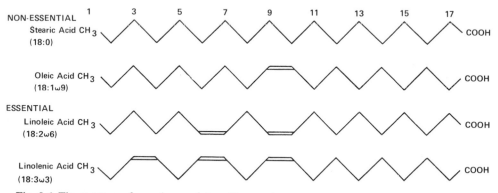

Fig. 8.6 The structure of some human fatty acids

Although much is known about essential fatty acid deficiency in experimental animals, our knowledge of its nature and occurrence in man is scanty but its incidence is increasing, particularly following long-term intravenous feeding without fat emulsions (Wene et al 1975, Riella et al 1975). The principle signs of essential fatty acid deficiency in experimental animals are diminished growth, failure of reproduction and dermatitis. Signs of deficiency occur more rapidly when there is a demand for increased tissue synthesis such as during pregnancy or following starvation. In man dermatitis is the major feature but there has been evidence to suggest that wound healing may be affected (Caldwell et al 1972) and that water loss from burned skin may be decreased by the application of linoleic acid (Jelenko et al 1975). As these polyunsaturated fatty acids are essential components of cellular and intracellular membranes, these features are to be expected. Although the membranes of adipose cells contain polyunsaturated fatty acids, the fat stored within the cell contains predominantly saturated fatty acids with 16–18 carbon atoms. Structural fat, such as the grey matter of the brain, contains 20% of its fatty acids as polyunsaturated essential fatty acids with 18–22 carbon atoms. Further chain elongation and desaturation of linoleic and linolenic acids in the body produces arachidonic and docosahexaenoic acids respectively (Fig. 8.7) and these higher homologues may be the most significant fatty acids in cell membranes. Little is known of the ability of man and other animals to carry out chain elongation and desaturation, but the process is limited in the rat and may not occur at all in the cat (Crawford & Hassam 1976). Linoleic and arachidonic acids are the precursors of prostaglandins.

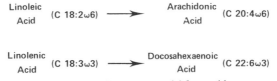

Fig. 8.7 The elongation and desaturation of human essential fatty acids

The quantity of essential fatty acids required by man in health and disease is uncertain. When there is insufficient linoleic acid (18: 2ω6) in the diet the concentration of arachidonic acid (20: 40ω6) in plasma is very low. In such circumstances, elongation and desaturation of oleic acid (18:1ω9) to 5, 8, 11–eicosatrienoic acid (20:3ω9) occurs. The presence of this abnormal acid in the plasma is indicative of essential fatty acid deficiency and the triene/tetraene ratio (20:3/20:4) in the plasma has proved to be a very sensitive indicator of essential fatty acid deficiency. If this ratio is less than 0.4 essential fatty acid deficiency is unlikely but it has been suggested recently that the upper limit in healthy individuals is 0.3 (Holman 1975). In the absence of linoleic acid in the diet, this ratio alters within a few days (Wene et al 1975) and dermatitis is usually obvious when it reaches 3.0. In prolonged, severe deficiency the ratio may approach 20.0. On the basis of clinical observations in infants it was concluded that the quantity of essential fatty acids in the diet should contribute at least 1% of the total energy content of the diet (Hansen et al 1963). A similar conclusion was reached from analysis of the triene/tetraene ratio in infants and experimental animals (Holman 1976). If this requirement is applicable to a healthy adult requiring an intake of 10.5 MJ/d (2 500 kcal/d) then the diet should contain 3 g of linoleic acid. Wolfram & Zollner (1971) suggest that the average daily requirement for a healthy adult is 7 g of linoleic acid.

There is ample evidence that the clinical and biochemical manifestations of essential fatty acids in the diet can be easily reversed and prevented by intravenous infusion of fat emulsions (Collins et al 1971, Caldwell et al 1972, Helmkamp et al 1973). If intravenous infusion is inappropriate, sufficient essential fatty acid may be absorbed from sunflower oil rubbed into the skin (Press et al 1974).

Little is known of the requirement in disease but recent studies have suggested that after severe injury these requirements may increase dramatically and that as much as 50 g of linoleic acid per day is necessary to restore the concentrations of linoleic acid and arachidonic acid in plasma to normal levels (Wolfram et al 1978).

As emphasised in Chapter 1, fat is an ideal source of energy yielding 39 kJ (9.3 kcal) for every gram that is oxidised. Emulsions of fat for intravenous infusion are nearly isotonic but oxidation of their substrates yields quantities of energy that are comparable to the quantities released by the oxidation of highly concentrated solutions of carbohydrate. In Table 8.4 the initial solute load produced by 1 litre of the fat emulsion Intralipid® (the most commonly used fat emulsion in Europe and the only emulsion used in North America) is compared with that produced by equicalorific and equivolaemic quantities of glucose. Although complete utilisation of either substrate results in the excretion of the hydrogen atoms as water and the carbon atoms as carbon dioxide without any change in osmolarity, utilisation may not be so rapid and fatal complications may develop from the injudicious use of hypertonic solutions of glucose (see below).

Table 8.4 The energy and solute content of intravenous carbohydrate and fat solutions

Energy content (MJ)	(kcal)	Substrate	Concentration (%)	Volume (ml)	Solute load (mosmol)
239	1000	Intralipid®	10	1000	280
272	1140	Glucose	30	1000	2100
478	2000	Intralipid®	20	1000	330
455	1900	Glucose	50	1000	3800

If the fat is infused as the sole source of energy in healthy subjects the extent of protein conservation observed when compared to starvation is less than might be expected as a consequence of the total energy intake (Brennan & Moore 1973). The protein conservation observed appears to be due to the free and esterified glycerol contained in the emulsion (Brennan et al 1975). Similarly, when infused as the sole source of energy after truncal vagotomy and pyloroplasty, fat emulsion had no significant effect on protein conservation (Craig et al 1977). When infused as the sole substrate, any protein–sparing probably reflects a reduction in gluconeogenic requirements from protein due to the effect of the glycerol. However, when infused in conjunction with amino acids and glucose, there is ample evidence from studies involving indirect calorimetry that the fatty acids contained in the emulsion are also utilised (Reid 1967, Tweedle & Johnston 1971). Although indirect calorimetry is being used with increasing frequency in intensive care units, it is not available to monitor the rate of utilisation of intravenous substrates in the majority of patients. Utilisation of fat emulsions can also be demonstrated by isotopic studies (Eckart et al 1973) but such investigations require sophisticated equipment and the patient is subjected to unnecessary irradiation. Clearance of the infused fat from the blood can be measured (Hallberg 1965) and is frequently assumed to reflect utilisation. It can be measured in the laboratory by nephelometry and is a useful clinical observation. If there is obvious incomplete clearance of fat emulsion from the serum of a specimen of venous blood obtained 3 hours after infusion of fat has been stopped, then it may be assumed that more fat is being infused than the patient can utilise.

Table 8.5 The composition of intravenous fat emulsions (g/l)

	Lipiphysan®	Lipofundin®	Intralipid®	Lipofundin–S®
Vegetable oil				
Cottonseed	150	100		
Soya bean			100 or 200	100 or 200
Polyhydric alcohol				
Sorbitol	50	50		
Xylitol				50
Glycerol			25	
Emulsifier				
Soya bean lecithin	20			
Soya bean phosphatide		7.5		7.5 or 15
Egg–yolk phosphatide			12	

The composition of four commercially available emulsions of fat for in-travenous infusion is shown in Table 8.5. The basic composition is very similar, each containing a vegetable oil, an emulsifier and an alcohol to render the solution isotonic. Nevertheless, the differences in the individual components appears to be very important in terms of toxicity. Studies in man and in experimental animals have demonstrated that emulsions prepared from cottonseed oil may be toxic (Hallberg et al 1966, Hakansson 1968) causing gastro–intestinal haemorrhage, anaemia, jaundice and centrolobular necrosis of the liver. However, further comparative studies with Intralipid® and Lipofundin–S®, both of which are prepared from soya bean oil, showed that similar haemorrhagic complications followed infusion of Lipofundin–S® (Jacobson & Wretlind 1970), suggesting that other factors such as differences in emulsifying agents, polyhydric alcohols or particle size may be important. The major portion of ingested fat consists of long–chain triglyceride and the fatty acid composition of soya bean oil (Table 8.6) is purely long–chain. Medium–chain triglycerides contribute less than 5% of the

Table 8.6 Fatty acid composition of soya bean oil emulsion (Intralipid)®

Palmitic acid (C16)	9%
Stearic acid (C18)	3%
Oleic acid (C18 ω1)	26%
Linoleic acid (C18 ω2)	54%
Linolenic acid (C18 ω3)	8%

normal diet but they are more soluble in water and are more rapidly oxidized than long–chain acids (Scheig 1968). When infused intravenously, they appear to be utilised more rapidly than long chain triglycerides (Eckart et al 1980, Sailer & Muller 1980). In the future these triglycerides and water–soluble short–chain monoglycerides (Birkhahn et al 1979) may have a limited role as a source of in-travenous energy.

Toxicity

Intralipid® became available commercially in 1962 and it and the other fat emulsions shown in Table 8.5 have been developed in Europe. However, the first emulsion to be produced commercially was Lipomul® which was developed in the United States of America and which became available about 1947. Unfortunately, although the initial results of clinical investigation were encouraging, the emulsion proved to be toxic in routine use and was withdrawn. As a consequence of this experience, clinicians have been alert to recognise any possible complication following the infusion of the emulsions shown in Table 8.5. In some cases, it has been impossible to assert that the observed phenomenon was due to infusion of fat and in many cases the clinical features would suggest an alternative cause. It has already been emphasised that the composition of the fat emulsions shown in Table 8.5 differs and that these differences may have pronounced effects upon potential toxicity. In the following account of metabolic complications following intravenous feeding, comments concerning fat emulsions refer mainly to Intralipid®.

METABOLIC COMPLICATIONS

The possibility that the patient's condition may be made worse or that he might even die as a consequence of ill–judged treatment should always be considered before starting intravenous feeding. This possibility becomes more likely as the problems of respiratory, circulatory and nutritional support become more complex. Unfortunately, human frailty dictates that the occasional infusion of incorrect quantities of solutions, minerals and drugs is inevitable. Experience has shown that such incidents are more likely to occur when several solutions or pharmocological agents are being given at the same time, as usually pertains during intravenous feeding, and such incidents are more likely to occur when the doctor or nurse is unfamiliar with the technique. Many patients require little more than the infusion of isotonic saline solutions to enable their natural homeostatic mechanisms to restore their altered physiology to normal. However, inadequate therapy may also result in avoidable morbidity and mortality and, when indicated, fear of inducing complications should not deter the clinician from feeding a patient intravenously.

Hydrogen ion imbalance

Acidosis commonly occurs in patients who require intravenous feeding and it is not always obvious whether this is mainly a consequence of the patient's disease or injury or mainly a consequence of intravenous feeding. However, there are many potential causes of acidosis in parenteral nutrients (Table 8.7). Although

Table 8.7 Potential causes of acidosis

1. Free hydrogen ions (pH)
2. Titrable acidity
3. Excess cationic amino acids (lysine and arginine)
4. Excess glycine
5. Excess methionine and cystine
6. Ammonium ions (casein hydrolysates)
7. Phosphate ions and phosphatides
8. Ketones
9. Lactic acidosis (fructose, sorbitol and ethanol)

the quantity of free hydrogen ions present in solutions of amino acids is small as indicated by their pH, their potential for inducing acidosis is much greater. These solutions are buffers and their titrable acidity is often in excess of 50 mmol/l (Tweedle 1974). Hydrogen ions may also be released by metabolism of the amino acids. Solutions containing an excess of cationic amino acids such as lysine and arginine can produce hyperchloraemic acidosis (Heird et al 1972a). Hyperammonaemia may occur following the infusion of solutions containing large quantities of glycine (Heird et al 1972b) and the infusion of casein hydrolysates which contain large quantities of ammonium ions (Johnson et al, 1972). These patients may become acidotic due to the hydrogen ions released when ammonia is converted to urea in the liver. Catabolism of the sulphur–containing amino acids methionine and cystine produces sulphuric acid. Some solutions of amino acids contain large quantities of phosphate ions and phosphoric acid may also be produced by metabolism of the phosphatides in fat emulsions. In addition to containing a small quantity of free fatty acids, the metabolism of fat emulsions produces large quantities of ketones. Although solutions of amino acids and fat emulsions may contribute to metabolic acidosis, this contribution is very small when compared to that which may occur following the infusion of fructose, sorbitol or ethanol (discussed in detail above).

Hyperglycaemia and hypoglycaemia

The use of hypertonic solutions of any type of carbohydrate may produce hyperglycaemia, particularly in the stressed patient with increased secretion of catabolic hormones (see Ch. 3 for further details). If highly concentrated solutions (40 or 50%) are used, the patient may die from hyperglycaemic, hyperosmolar coma (Meng et al 1969, Dudrick et al 1972). Although coma and death is fortunately rare even when solutions of this concentration are used it is not uncommon to observe hyperglycaemia and glycosuria in patients receiving less concentrated solutions (20%). The renal excretion of glucose requires water and the osmotic diuresis produces dehydration. The amount of insulin required to control the blood glucose concentration may vary from hour to hour in seriously ill patients and may increase dramatically with the onset of septicaemia. However, this syndrome usually develops over a period of days and should be recognised before the patient's condition deteriorates. When it occurs, the condition usually responds rapidly to treatment with insulin and water. If the patient is unable to drink water, hypotonic or isotonic solutions should be infused. Insulin requirements during infusion of concentrated solutions of glucose are discussed in greater detail below.

Hypoglycaemia is an uncommon observation following intravenous feeding but it occurs occasionally if the infusion of highly concentrated solutions of carbohydrates is stopped suddenly without further oral or intravenous of substrate. Endogenous secretion of insulin usually responds rapidly to changes in the blood glucose concentration, but presumably on these occasions secretion has continued at a rate that is now excessive. It is a wise precaution to continue infusion with isotonic solutions of glucose for a few hours after stopping infusion of concentrated solutions.

Electrolyte disturbances

The causes, clinical signs and treatment of excessive or inadequate quantities of electrolytes and minerals have been discussed in Chapter 2 but certain abnormalities are commonly associated with intravenous feeding and are discussed below. Although some solutions of amino acids are deliberately manufactured with a low content of electrolytes and minerals, many contain considerable quantities. Unfortunately, it is not possible to produce a solution that contains all the daily requirements of these substances in one container. Such a mixture is unstable and complex salts of calcium, magnesium, phosphate and other ions precipitate. These substances may also be added during manufacture or before infusion to solutions of glucose.

Hyponatraemia

The solutions of amino acids and carbohydrates used in parenteral nutrition are hypertonic and some retention of water and an expansion of the extracellular volume usually occurs producing a dilutional hyponatraemia. Patients requiring intravenous feeding may be sodium–deficient if they have lost gastro–intestinal secretions, but the majority are not. The hyponatraemia usually corrects itself when the infusion of nutrients is stopped and the kidneys excrete the excess water.

Hypokalaemia

The concentration of potassium in the blood may vary according to disease or injury, but it may be reduced dramatically by infusion of concentrated solutions of carbohydrate and insulin, entering the cell with glucose. Potassium requirements during infusion of concentrated solutions of glucose are discussed in greater detail below.

Hypophosphataemia

Hypophosphataemia, like hypokalaemia, may occur during the infusion of concentrated solutions of glucose. The depletion of organic phosphates in the red blood cell can be fatal (see Ch. 2). Phosphate requirements during infusion of concentrated solutions of glucose are discussed below. It would be beneficial if all solutions of amino acids contained more phosphate and fewer chloride ions. Although the phosphorus content of Intralipid® is organic in nature, hypophosphataemia has not been observed when this emulsion has been a component of the intravenous nutrients.

Hypocalcaemia and hypomagnesaemia

Some solutions of amino acids do not contain calcium or magnesium and if these elements are not included in the other solutions used, hypocalcaemia and hypomagnesaemia may develop. Patients who require intravenous feeding are frequently hypoalbuminaemic and the concentration of ionised calcium in the blood may be normal but the total concentration, which is usually measured in the laboratory, is low due to a reduction in protein–bound calcium. In such patients, infusion of calcium is unneccessary and will not alter the total concentration.

Trace element deficiency

The importance of the seven elements known to be required in trace quantities in the human diet has been discussed in Chapter 1. The measurement of these elements in the laboratory is often difficult and expensive. Consequently, less data are available for consideration than have been collected for elements such as sodium that are required in large amounts. Furthermore, much of the data that has been collected has been restricted to measurement of concentrations in the blood and occasionally in tissue. Few studies have been made involving daily balances. The figures given in Table 1.4 for the weekly requirements of these elements may require modification when more data are available, particularly in disease and after injury. Deficiencies of iodine may occur in patients being fed intravenously at home who have no intake over several months, but deficiency is rare in patients who require prolonged parenteral nutrition in hospital. Deficiency of fluorine, cobalt and manganese during parenteral nutrition has not been reported.

Deficiency of iron is a common finding in many patients requiring intravenous feeding. In some patients with anaemia, transfusion of blood may be required in addition to the infusion of parenteral iron. Some clinicians prefer to correct major deficits by intravenous infusion of a quantity of iron that has been calculated to restore the concentration in the serum to normal levels, others prefer to restore the concentration more slowly by intramuscular injections. So called 'total dose infusion' may cause anaphylaxis (Bonnar 1965). The anaemia of many ill patients fails to respond to iron infusion, presumably due to the effects of toxins and anoxia upon the bone marrow. Although iron is included in some commercially available preparations of trace elements, it is relatively insoluble and its inclusion may necessitate modification of the other contents.

Severe deficiency of copper may cause anaemia and leucopenia (Karpel & Peden 1972, Dunlap et al 1974). However, a significant fall in serum concentration in patients with increased losses only occurs after two or three weeks of intravenous feeding (Lowry et al 1979) and clinical deficiency may only occur after several months of inadequate intake.

Zinc deficiency is the most commonly recognised trace element deficiency occurring during intravenous feeding. Although it is the cutaneous manifestations of alopecia and peri–oral, perinasal and peri–anal dermatitis that are often recognised first by the doctor (Kay et al 1976) the patient may also suffer from diarrhoea and mental depression. There is often secondary infection of the skin lesions which fails to respond to appropriate antimicrobial treatment. Some patients lose their sense of taste (Henkin et al 1975). These features may occur during anabolic recovery from severe illness. As is the case with copper deficiency significant falls in serum concentration occur after two or three weeks of parenteral nutrition (Lowry et al 1979) but clinical features occur after more prolonged inadequate intake. Changes in serum concentration may be difficult to interpret as nearly all the zinc in the blood is bound to various proteins. The response to treatment is often dramatic, the skin lesions disappearing in two or three days. Patients who lose their hair may be reassured that it will grow again. As much as 1.2 mmol/d has been infused intravenously in treating deficient patients (Kay et al 1976) but zinc is toxic if given in massive quantities (Brocks et al 1977).

Vitamin deficiency

Overt deficiency of vitamins during intravenous feeding is a rare occurrence because the majority of clinicians are aware of the dangers of vitamin deficiency and ensure that commercially available mixtures of water–and fat–soluble vitamins are given. With the exception of patients suffering from obstructive jaundice, deficiency of fat–soluble vitamins during intravenous feeding is uncommon even in patients who have not been given supplements. The quantity of vitamin A and D stored in the liver is probably sufficient to meet the requirements of most patients for nearly a year. Although deficiencies of other water–soluble vitamins such as thiamine may occur during intravenous feeding (Blennow 1975), folate deficiency has been the most commonly observed deficiency. A prospective, controlled trial showed that plasma folate concentrations fell rapidly after starting intravenous feeding without supplementation, 8 out of 10 patients developed megaloblastic anaemia and 3 of these patients developed thrombocytopenia or leucopenia as well (Wardrop et al 1975). The changes observed responded to treatment with 500 μg/d of folic acid given intravenously. Although infusion of ethanol was initially considered to be the cause, similar changes were observed in patients who were fed intravenously without alcohol (Wardrop et al 1975, Ibbotson et al 1975). It is possible that some other factor unrelated to parenteral nutrition may have been responsible for the folate deficiency. In a similar study, folate concentration in the red blood cell was below the normal range in 4 out of 11 surgical patients who were critically ill but the serum folate concentration was within the normal range (Bradley et al 1978). Both concentrations rose in the majority of these patients during parenteral nutrition when they were given 15 mg folic acid by intramuscular injection each week.

Erythropoietic function

Anaemia is a common observation in patients receiving parenteral nutrients and in the great majority is unrelated to the therapy. As discussed above, it is often unresponsive to treatment with iron. Isotopic studies have demonstrated normal red cell survival following infusion of fat emulsion made from cottonseed oil and soya bean oil (Upjohn et al 1957, Jacobson 1969) and there is no convincing evidence that fat emulsions have any effect upon erythropoiesis. Anaemia following infusion of cottonseed oil emulsions is probably due to gastro–intestinal haemorrhage (Hallberg et al 1966, Hakansson 1968). There have been numerous studies of the effect of different fat emulsions upon coagulation and fibrinolysis and the conclusions reached have been inconsistent and contradictory. Hypercoagulability due to a direct thromboplastic effect of soya bean oil emulsion was reported by Amris et al (1964) but subsequent studies have failed to confirm this (Reid & Ingram 1967, Cronberg & Nilsson 1967, Kapp et al 1971). Although soya bean oil emulsion appears to produce a reduction in platelet adhesiveness that lasts for a few hours after the infusion has been stopped (Kapp et al 1971) prolonged infusion is without effect upon the platelet count (Jacobson 1969).

Intravenous infusion of solutions of amino acids and carbohydrates has not been associated with any effect upon the erythropoietic system other than the possible effect of alcohol discussed above (Wardrop et al 1975).

Hepatic function

Many patients requiring parenteral nutrition have evidence of hepatic dysfunction and, as is the case with other metabolic disturbance observed in such patients, it is often very difficult to determine the cause. Undoubtedly the early cottonseed oil emulsions were toxic to the liver (Preston et al 1957, Watkin 1957) and prolonged infusion of all types of fat emulsion is associated with the deposition of fat pigment in the liver and other reticulo–endothelial tissue (Lawson 1965). The significance of this pigment is uncertain. Although many investigators have attributed abnormal hepatic function following infusion of fat emulsion in man to the deposition of this pigment, Thompson (1976), who has studied the phenomenon extensively, considers this to be unlikely as there is no correlation in either man or in experimental animals between the occurrence of abnormal hepatic function and the deposition or otherwise of the pigment in the liver.

Fatty infiltration of the liver is more likely to occur during intravenous feeding with concentrated carbohydrate solutions. When the glycogen stores are full, carbohydrate infused in excess of immediate energy requirement is converted to triglyceride in the liver. This is particularly likely to occur in septic patients (Kaminski et al 1980). Surprisingly, fatty infiltration of the liver may improve following infusion of fat emulsions in patients who have been deprived of fat for many months (Jeejeebhoy et al 1973, Freeman 1978). Deposition of fat in the liver is a common feature of essential fatty acid deficiency.

Abnormal elevations of the serum concentrations of bilirubin, alkaline phosphatase and aspartate serum transferase have recently been observed during parenteral and enteral nutrition in a group of patients who had no other apparent cause for these changes (Tweedle et al 1979). These changes have subsequently been observed in patients who had previously normal hepatic function, who had not undergone anaesthesia, operation or radiation, who had no evidence of sepsis and who were not suffering from malignant disease. During these studies, it has become apparent that these changes can be observed following intravenous or enteral infusion of a wide variety of commercial products including amino acids, carbohydrates and fat emulsions. These features exclude toxicity due to degradation of tryptophane as a cause of the hepatic dysfunction (Grant et al 1977). Changes in the concentrations of these enzymes have been shown to coincide with intrahepatic cholestasis and with periportal infiltration by round cells and occasionally with proliferation of bile ducts (Sitges–Creus et al 1977). Similar histological and biochemical changes are found in drug-induced cholestasis (Sherlock 1968) but a common constituent cannot be found in the parenteral and enteral products infused in these patients. Although the cause of this hepatic dysfunction remains obscure, the enzyme concentrations often returned to within the normal range before stopping the parenteral or enteral infusion and permanent dysfunction has not been observed. These alterations in enzyme concentrations are disturbing and further investigation is required to identify the cause. Nevertheless, they appear to be transient and there has been no evidence that they produce or are associated with deleterious phenomena within the patient. Accordingly, parenteral or enteral nutrition should not be witheld from malnourished patients for fear of inducing these changes.

The use of special solutions of amino acids in the treatment of patients with hepatic failure is discussed in detail in Chapter 7.

Pulmonary function

The infusion of 500 ml of a 10% solution of soya bean oil emulsion over a 4–hour period produced a significant decrease in the pulmonary diffusion capacity of 6 out of 10 healthy young men. However, the extent of the reduction was related to the increase in the concentration of the plasma lipids and was no greater than that observed during post–prandial lipaemia. The reduction was thought to be due to either an alteration in blood viscosity or to interference with transport of oxygen across the membrane of the erythrocyte (Greene 1976). The pulmonary diffusion capacity of patients with burns who were given a 10% soya bean oil emulsion did not alter and there was no significant change in ventilatory capacity or peripheral oxygen concentration in these patients, some of whom were given 5 g/kg per d of fat emulsion (Wilmore et al 1973).

Many patients who require intravenous feeding develop clinical and radiological signs of pulmonary congestion and in some the changes resolve when the infusion is stopped, suggesting that the infusion may have been responsible. Occasional cases have been attributed specifically to infusion of fat emulsion (Guignier et al 1975) but it is impossible to identify with certainty the solution responsible when others have been infused either concomitantly with the emulsion or immediately preceding it. Similar changes may be produced by infusion of excessive quantities of isotonic saline solution. Four infants who were infused with large quantities of a 20% soya bean oil emulsion were found to have pulmonary capillaries and alveolar macrophages laden with fat at post mortem. Although caution must be exercised in equating the finding of intravascular lipid at post mortem with intravenous infusion of fat emulsion it was concluded that this was a factor in the aetiology (Barson et al 1978). In a subsequent investigation, 8 pre–term infants who were infused with 20% soya bean oil emulsion at a maximum rate of 8 g/kg per d were also found to have pulmonary capillaries distended with fat globules. Analysis of lung homogenates from these infants showed a very high concentration of linoleic acid and a lower concentration of palmitic acid than found in the lungs of other pre–term infants who had not been infused with fat emulsion, suggesting that the fat accumulated in the lungs was from the fat emulsion (Levene et al 1980). These infants died from causes unrelated to intravenous infusion and there is no evidence to indicate whether the accumulation is reversible. The infants were infused with a 20% emulsion whose particle size is slightly larger than that of the 10% solution. The mean particle size of the 20% solution is 0.16 μm and that of the 10% solution 0.13 μm but naturally occurring chylomicrons of ingested fat have mean diameters of 0.5–1 μm (Jones et al 1962, Kay & Robinson 1962). Emboli from fluorocarbon emulsions will form if the particle size exceeds 6 μm (Fujita et al 1971).

It has recently become apparent that the infusion of very large quantities of carbohydrates may seriously embarrass pulmonary function (Askanazi et al

1980a). The ultimate fate of the infused carbohydrate varies (see below) but regardless of this there is an increased production of carbon dioxide which may produce respiratory distress in a patient with marginal pulmonary reserve.

SELECTION OF PARENTERAL NUTRIENTS

The foregoing account of the general requirements of various nutrients, the complications that may ensue following their infusion, the specific deficits and altered metabolism of individual patients, the experience of the clinician and the equipment and the assistance that is available to him may all influence the selection of parenteral nutrients. The initial studies of parenteral nutrition in man revealed that the improvement in nitrogen balance that followed the infusion of protein hydrolysates was increased if glucose was also infused (Elman 1939). Furthermore, the timing of this infusion was important, concomitant infusion of both solutions producing a greater improvement in nitrogen balance than that observed if the protein was infused in the morning and the glucose in the afternoon. These features have subsequently been confirmed in many studies and the need to infuse sufficient quantities of non–protein energy with amino acids is a basic principle in parenteral nutrition. It is presumed that failure to provide sufficient non–protein energy and, in particular, failure to provide sufficient glucose results in the breakdown of the infused amino acids with the production of glucose, the amine radicle being excreted as urea. Although Gamble (1947) demonstrated that the daily provision of 100 g of glucose reduced protein breakdown during starvation, contrary to what is often stated, he did not believe that this was the maximum conservation that could be achieved. Gamble was primarily concerned with preventing fatal dehydration in individuals on life–rafts who had meagre provisions and his comments were confined to the provision of glucose alone. He was aware that greater conservation could be achieved in hospital by the provision of protein and large quantities of non–protein energy, but suggested that this was unneccessary in the majority of patients.

It has been suggested that 'for protein synthesis to occur maximally during the

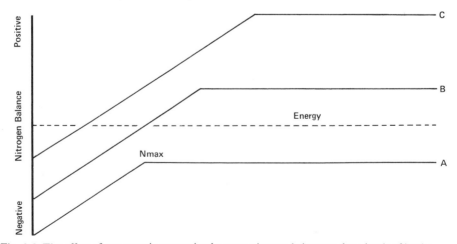

Fig. 8.8 The effect of non-protein energy intake upon nitrogen balance at three levels of intake

anabolic phase of convalescence, a calorie/nitrogen ratio of 200 (85 kJ/g N) is necessary' (Moore 1959). This is the typical ratio that is obtained from normal diets. Subsequent studies have suggested that to achieve the absolute utilisation for a given quantity of intravenous nitrogen after injury, it is necessary to give at least double this quantity (Johnston & Clark 1972). There is a limit to the improvement in nitrogen balance that may be induced by increasing the intake in non-protein energy. At this point (Nmax, Fig. 8.8) all the infused nitrogen is being used for protein and any further improvement in nitrogen balance can only be achieved by infusing a greater quantity of nitrogen (B and C, Fig. 8.8). If the intake of nitrogen is inadequate, positive balance is impossible, regardless of the intake of non−protein energy (A, Fig. 8.8). As discussed in Chapter 3, following severe injury or sepsis the hormonal milieu may discourage protein synthesis and a positive nitrogen balance may be impossible to achieve, regardless of intake. Most clinicians agree that a calorie/nitrogen ratio of 200–250 (85–105 kJ/g N) is suitable for the majority of patients, but it should be remembered that certain patients require predominantly proteins and others predominantly energy (Table 3.1).

Table 8.8 The determination of the components of an intravenous regimen

1. Select quantity of amino acid required
2. Select amino acid solution (profile)
3. Select quantity of non−protein energy required (energy/nitrogen ratio)
4. Select carbohydrate/fat content of non−protein energy requirement
5. Select single−bottle, multiple−bottle or plastic bag technique
6. Select initial insulin requirement
7. Select vitamin and mineral additives

The basic steps in selecting the parenteral nutrients to be infused are shown in Table 8.8. Having decided upon the quantity of amino acids required, the solution should be selected according to the criteria discussed above. Ideally this choice should be based upon the content of individual amino acids. The quantity of non−protein energy required is then determined and the next major decision to be reached is the relative quantities of glucose and fat emulsion to be included.

Non-protein energy

For many years some clinicians relied entirely upon glucose as the source of non−protein energy during parenteral nutrition, because of a lack of an available alternative substrate (Dudrick et al 1972) or because of the need to prevent hypoglycaemia during treatment with large quantities of insulin (Hinton et al 1971). Others used approximately equal calorific quantities of glucose and fat emulsion (Tweedle & Johnston 1971, Wretlind 1972). Both types of regime produced beneficial clinical and biochemical results in the majority of patients. Nevertheless the ability of individual patients to clear infused fat from the blood appears to vary. Patients who have undergone prolonged starvation may be given as much as 70% of their non-protein energy requirements as fat, but a few patients who have sepsis are unable to clear the blood of fat infused at a dose of 2 g/kg per d.

Some comparative studies have suggested that fat is as effective as glucose or other carbohydrates as a source of non-protein energy in the maintenance of nitrogen balance. Gazzaniga et al (1975) found no difference in the nitrogen balance of two groups of nine patients with a variety of surgical disorders and a similar observation was made following partial gastractomy in nine patients (Bark et al 1976). In an elegant cross–over study of 27 patients with gastro–intestinal dysfunction, no alteration in nitrogen balance was observed when the patient's intake of non–protein energy was changed from glucose to predominantly fat (83% of the energy) or vice versa (Jeejeebhoy et al 1976). However, in patients with burns who were given non–protein energy in 12 different combinations of fat and glucose, urea excretion was inversely proportional to the intake of glucose and increasing the intake of fat appeared to have no effect. If glucose was infused to meet the metabolic expenditure of the patients, there was no further improvement in nitrogen balance unless exogenous insulin was also provided (Long et al 1977). It was concluded that in starving patients, equicalorific quantities of fat and glucose had a similar effect upon nitrogen balance when either was infused with amino acids but that after major trauma and sepsis the first priority is to provide sufficient glucose to satisfy the demands of metabolic expenditure.

These results might suggest that in the severely injured or septic patient, a major aspect of treatment should be an attempt to reduce the increased gluconeogenesis by infusion of large quantities of glucose. Isotopic studies revealed the maximum suppression of gluconeogenesis was achieved by the infusion of glucose at 4 mg/kg per min (approximately 84 kJ/kg per d or 20 kcal/kg per d) in healthy individuals (Wolfe et al 1979) and at 7 mg/kg per min (approximately 146 kJ/kg per d or 35 kcal/kg per d) in postoperative patients requiring parenteral nutrition (Wolfe et al 1980). Glucose infused in excess of these rates was not oxidised and was probably converted to fat. An important finding in these studies was that there was no correlation between the rate of clearance of glucose from the blood and the rate of oxidation. In many previous studies of so–called 'glucose utilisation', the clearance from the blood was assumed to reflect oxidation. Although these studies have emphasised the importance of supplying large quantities of glucose to severely injured and septic patients, breakdown of endogenous triglyceride was still observed in this type of patient when glucose was infused at nearly twice the rate required to satisfy energy expenditure (Askanazi et al 1980b). The mean respiratory quotient of these patients increased from 0.76 to 0.90 indicating that large quantities of infused glucose were being oxidised but oxidation of endogenous fat was continuing, the excess glucose being converted into glycogen. These findings contrasted considerably with those recorded in nutritionally depleted patients without injury or sepsis, in whom the mean respiratory quotient rose from 0.83 to 1.05, indicating that the excess glucose was converted to fat with no evidence of net breakdown of fat. Infusion of large quantities of glucose produces a corresponding increase in the secretion of insulin which inhibits oxidation of fat. However, the effect of increased secretion of insulin induced by infusion of large quantities of glucose in severely injured patients appears to be dominated by a large increase in the secretion of catecholamines (Carpentier et al 1979). When nutritionally impoverished patients were given total parenteral nutrition with large quantities of glucose, their oxygen consumption rose by only 3% but that of the septic patients increased by 29% (Askanazi et al 1980b). The corresponding increases in carbon dioxide production were 32% and

56% respectively. It was suggested that the increased production of carbon dioxide might precipitate respiratory distress in patients with compromised pulmonary function and might prove to be a critical factor in weaning a patient from ventilatory support. The oxidation of equicalorific quantities of fat emulsions would produce less carbon dioxide.

Table 8.9 The theoretical ideal intravenous substrate for the provision of energy

---
 1. Utilised by all tissues
 2. No hormones required for utilisation
 3. No metabolic or physiological side effects
 4. High renal threshold
 5. High calorific value
 6. Non-irritant to tissues
 7. Stable in solution
 8. No reaction with plastic
 9. No reaction with other solutions or additives
10. Will not support microbial growth
11. No interference with laboratory estimations

How do these findings influence the choice of substrate for parenteral nutrition? The features that would be found in an ideal substrate are shown in Table 8.9. It is apparent that it is impossible to fulfil all the requirements of this ideal concept. By providing non–protein energy as a mixture of fat and glucose it is possible to avoid essential fatty acid deficiency and to reduce the chances of inducing complications such as fatty infiltration of the liver, hyperglycaemia and respiratory distress. In nutritionally impoverished patients who do not have the altered metabolism of injury or sepsis it would seem appropiate to supply non–protein energy as approximately equal quantities of glucose and fat as occurs in most ingested diets. It has been emphasised that 'when we are forced to do something artificial we must aim at remaining as close as possible to the natural situation' (Krebs 1978). There is insufficient knowledge about substrate oxidation in severely injured or septic patients and further investigations are required involving infusion of substrates labelled with isotopes and indirect calorimetery. At present it would appear advisable to administer the major proportion of the non-protein energy requirement of these patients as glucose. However, fat emulsion should be given at regular intervals to reduce the risk of essential fatty acid deficiency and the clinician should be well aware of the potential dangers of hyperglycaemia and the need to provide sufficient quantities of insulin (see below).

Single–bottle regimens

Having decided that the patient requires feeding intravenously many doctors use a standard solution prepared commercially in a single bottle for all their patients regardless of individual requirements. Many do this out of ignorance and it is evident that nutrition does not receive due regard in the curricula of medical schools and other higher institutions. However, some doctors are well aware that these solutions are inadequate in many respects and that their use compels an inflexible approach to intravenous feeding in many respects, but continue to use them. They argue that such a method offers an approximation of the basic requirements to the majority of patients without exposing them to the risks of injudicious therapy by the inexperienced. There is little doubt that many patients have benefited from the use of these solutions but, because of the impossibility of mixing all the nutritive requirements of even a healthy individual in a single bottle, the use of these solutions will always indicate inferior treatment. Furthermore, in some patients there may be inherent dangers involved in their use due to their content.

The majority of these single–bottle solutions consist of a mixture of amino acids and one or more carbohydrates. Certain amino acids such as cystine and tyrosine may be absent or included in inadequate concentration due to problems involving solubility and precipitation of electrolyte complexes as discussed above. In many of the solutions the content of carbohydrate is inadequate and the nitrogen/non–protein energy ratio is too low to ensure adequate utilisation of the infused amino acids. In most solutions, sorbitol is used as the source of non–protein energy so that the solution can be autoclaved without inducing the Maillard reaction (see above). The metabolism of sorbitol may induce dangerous lactic acidosis and this danger is increased by solutions that contain both sorbitol and ethanol (see above). Although ethanol has a higher calorific value than other carbohydrates the osmolarity of these solutions is often in excess of 1000 mosmol/l and they should be infused into a central vein. Sorbitol and alcohol are also potent diuretics. These solutions frequently contain inadequate quantities of electrolytes, particularly phosphate ions, and of trace elements. Water–and fat–soluble vitamins must be provided as required for all patients being fed intravenously.

There have been few detailed studies of the use of these solutions, probably because they are not often used in teaching hospitals where the majority of investigations are performed. In one excellent study a solution containing large quantities of sorbitol and alcohol was infused for 10 days in patients with inflammatory bowel disease or upper gastro–intestinal obstruction and following major operations upon the gastro–intestinal tract (Wells & Smits 1978). The solutions were infused at a constant rate by means of an infusion pump into a central vein. When the solution was infused at a rate of 50 ml/kg per d the urinary losses of nutrients were 9.5% of the infused sorbitol, 2.9% of the amino acids and less than 0.5% of the ethanol. Osmotic dehydration was not observed. The mean lactate concentration in the blood increased from 1.5 mmol/l to 2.5 mmol/l and the contribution of ammonia to the total urinary nitrogen content increased from 7.1% to 12%. It was concluded that with adequate monitoring before and during infusion the likelihood of inducing lactic acidosis of sufficient severity to endanger the patient was slight but that these solutions should not be used in patients with acidosis. During this study large supplements of potassium and phosphorus were required and the concentration of magnesium in the serum fell as the solution did not contain this element.

A recent development in Europe is the commercial production of mixtures of amino acids, carbohydrates and fat emulsion. Although the three primary substrates have been mixed in this manner for many years in Montpellier (Solassol & Joyeux 1976) there are potential dangers in this technique (discussed below in greater detail). The major problem is to maintain the stability of the fat emulsion and it is often necessary to exclude amino acids such as histidine, arginine and cystine from the solution. Even then separation of the fat emulsion may occur after short periods of storage (Wenzel 1972).

It is evident that single–bottle regimens cannot provide all the nutritional requirements of a healthy individual and that this system is inflexible in the face of differing requirements. A more flexible approach is provided by the use of multiple–bottle or plastic bag regimens. In Great Britain the majority of hospitals use the multiple–bottle technique but as adequate facilities become available for the mixing of solutions under sterile conditions in the pharmacy, the use of plastic bags is increasing rapidly and it is likely that this technique will eventually become predominant.

Multiple–bottle regimens

Although it is impossible to mix all the nutritional requirements of an individual in one bottle, it is possible to provide them in a series of bottles and this is the basis of this technique. However, the composition of each bottle does not vary and so whilst it is possible to alter the intake by suitable selection from the different solutions available, infinite variation is not available and it may be impossible to provide the precise requirements, Nevertheless, this technique allows a very close approximation to the precise requirements to be made and does not place any restriction upon the doctor in his choice of substrate to provide non–protein energy. As in the other systems, it is necessary to provide trace elements and vitamins. Sometimes these supplements may be added to some of the solutions. However, in many cases the additives may be incompatible with the solution and expert advice should be available from the pharmacist.

A convenient method of displaying the contents of the regimen and instructions to the nursing staff about the method of infusion are shown in Figure 8.9. A 'V type' intravenous infusion set is used and the two columns indicate the solutions to be infused in each line. In this method, the amino acids are infused synchronously with a supply of non–protein energy to ensure optimal utilisation. The sequence and time of infusion is selected to suit the work of the unit. It is

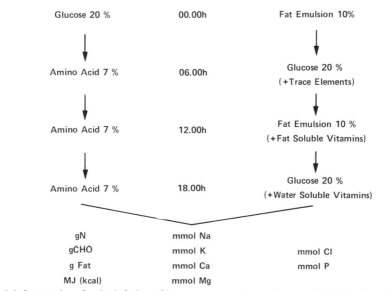

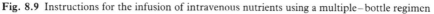

Fig. 8.9 Instructions for the infusion of intravenous nutrients using a multiple–bottle regimen

inconvenient to ask the nurses to change the bottles when they are changing shifts. When possible, solutions containing additives should be infused during the daytime so that pharmacists and doctors are readily available to answer any queries. If fat emulsions are not infused for two or three hours before the phlebotomist draws blood, there is less likelihood of exogenous fat in the blood interfering with biochemical and haematological investigations. All the solutions of glucose shown in Figure 8.9 will contain added electrolytes. Some commercial solutions of glucose are now available which contain a variety of added electrolytes and there are also a variety of commercially available mixtures of trace elements and vitamins. Vitlipid®, a commercial preparation of fat–soluble vitamin, can be added to the fat emulsion Intralipid® without disturbing its emulsification. Having selected the components of the regimen, the doctor should calculate the basic contents and record them as shown in Figure 8.9.

A multiple–bottle regimen involves more work for the clinician in selecting appropriate components and then calculating the total content of the various nutrients. A regimen of the composition shown in Figure 8.9 will also necessitate giving the patient insulin to control hyperglycaemia and glycosuria. However, a much greater burden falls upon the nurse who is constantly adjusting the clamps upon the infusion sets to ensure synchronous infusion of the amino acid solutions and the non–protein energy substrate. This may prove particularly difficult when fat emulsions and amino acid solutions are being infused as there is a large difference in their specific gravity. Many of the patients requiring intravenous feeding also require infusion of antibiotics and monitoring of central venous pressure and arterial blood pressure. On the intensive care unit it is not unknown for the nurse to be controlling seven or eight infusion sets in one patient.

Plastic bags
The use of plastic containers in which the nutritional requirements of each patient can be mixed is theoretically the most appealing system. However, there are a number of practical problems, some of which may prove to be insurmountable. In order to use this technique it is necessary to mix the constituents under a laminar flow hood in a sterile room which should not be used for any other purpose. The pharmacist must not only have a detailed knowledge of the compatibilities of the various nutrients but must also have some knowledge of bacteriology and be adequately trained in aseptic technique. Cap, mask, gown and gloves should be worn during mixing and regular bacteriological assessment of the mixtures and of the room and contents should be made. Solutions may be mixed in plastic bags that contain 1 or 3 litres. The larger bag offers the simplest method of intravenous feeding for the nurse but supplying the nutrients in three bags may allow the pharmacist to alter the composition of individual bags, so avoiding incompatibilities. However, each bag should contain amino acids and a source of non–protein energy. In some hospitals, standard solutions are mixed in this manner but differ from single–bottle solutions in having glucose as their source of carbohydrate energy. When the facilities and expertise are available to mix a solution that is particularly appropriate for an individual patient, it seems inappropriate to prepare standard solutions. The solutions should not be mixed more than 24 hours before infusion, and may be stored in a refrigerator on the ward or in

the pharmacy after mixing. In future it may be possible to store these mixtures by freezing and thawing before use in a microwave oven (Klim & Hardy 1980).

When using this technique, it is necessary to provide all or nearly all the non-protein energy requirement in the form of glucose. It is very difficult to prepare an emulsion of fat suitable for intravenous infusion that remains stable. If mixed with other substances, the components of the emulsion may separate into individual layers and the droplets of fat, which were originally similar to naturally occurring chylomicrons, may coalesce. Although amino acids, carbohydrates and fat emulsions have been mixed and infused without complications (Solassol & Joyeux 1976) many pharmacists and doctors have attempted this but have been unable to prepare a solution that is stable, particularly if storage is necessary (Gove et al 1979). Consequently, if fat emulsion is infused to prevent essential fatty acid deficiency or to provide a source of energy in an isotonic solution, it must be infused separately. As the emulsion is isotonic, it may be infused into a peripheral vein.

Insulin requirements

Insulin may be given intermittently by intramuscular injection as a bolus dose or continually in the infusion or by separate infusion using a pump. The safest method is probably to add the insulin to the solution to be infused as this ensures that the patient is given exogenous insulin only when receiving exogenous glucose. Some insulin may be absorbed by the container and consequently the requirement may be a little greater when insulin is given in this manner. When insulin is given by subcutaneous or intramuscular injection, there may be inconsistent absorption into the blood and the patient is subjected to the inconvenience of repeated injections. Severely injured patients and those with sepsis may have rapidly changing requirements for insulin due to changes in the secretion of the antagonistic hormones glucagon, cortisol and catecholamines. These two methods do not allow for such changes and in this type of patient, separate infusion using a pump offers greater control.

The amount of insulin required may vary considerably from patient to patient. Many patients who are suffering from nutritional depletion without injury or sepsis can be given as much as 300 g of glucose per day intravenously as a 10% solution without requiring exogenous insulin. The majority of patients who are infused with a 20% solution will develop unacceptable hyperglycaemia and glycosuria during infusion without insulin, regardless of the total daily intake. Patients who have undergone severe injury or major operations and particularly those who have sepsis frequently require large quantities of insulin when infused with a 10% solution. In most patients it is advisable to provide one unit of insulin for 4 g of glucose. The values shown in Table 8.10 are calculated on this basis.

Table 8.10 Intravenous feeding with glucose and insulin

	Glucose		Energy		Insulin
Volume (l)	Concentration (%)	Quantity (g)	MJ	kcal	iu
2	20	400	6.7	1600	100
1.5	40	600	10.0	2400	150
1	50	500	8.4	2000	125

The volumes and concentrations of the solutions shown are often used each day during intravenous feeding. Two litres of a 20% solution of glucose do not provide sufficient non–protein energy for the majority of patients, but this quantity is frequently infused in combination with fat emulsion. One litre of a 50% solution is frequently used in patients with acute renal failure as a method of providing a large quantity of energy in a small quantity of fluid. In the severely injured patient insulin requirements may increase so that more than one unit of insulin is required for each gram of glucose. By infusing 50 ml/h of a 50% solution of glucose containing initially 120 units of insulin in each litre, Hinton et al (1971) were able to reduce considerably the catabolic response to injury in burned patients. In some patients, as much as 600 units each day were required to control hyperglycaemia and glycosuria. Frequent estimations of the concentration of glucose in the blood and urine are needed to establish the requirement for insulin during the first day of treatment with large quantities of glucose. Large quantities of potassium and phosphorous are also required (see below).

Having started infusion with one unit of insulin being given for every 4 g of glucose, most doctors instruct the nurses to alter the intake of insulin according to a 'sliding scale' which is based upon the concentration of glucose in the blood and urine. It is advisable to construct such scales so that there is a tendency for the patient to be hyperglycaemic rather than hypoglycaemic. When using this technique, many doctors rely predominantly upon the results of the 'Clinitest' for the concentration of glucose in the urine and one or possibly two random measurements in the blood. This can be extremely dangerous in severely ill patients who may have fluctuating urine production and infrequent passing of urine. In these patients the concentration of glucose in the urine passed may be unrepresentative of the concentration that now exists in the patient's blood. Such mistakes can be avoided if the patient has a catheter inserted into the bladder and the concentration of glucose in the urine is tested every hour. However, another potential mishap may occur due to failure to recognise that the 'Clinitest' examination fails to indicate by how much the concentration in the urine may exceed 2%. In some patients it may be as high as 10% and these patients may receive an inadequate quantity of insulin as a consequence.

In many units the practice of predicting requirement upon the concentration in the urine has become obsolescent following the introduction of a number of simple methods that allow rapid and reasonably accurate estimations of the concentrations in the blood. These estimations are easily performed by nurses from drops of blood obtained by pricking the tip of a finger with a needle (Webb et al 1980). In this way it is possible to obtain more accurate control of the concentration of blood glucose by frequent estimations and appropriate adjustments of the infusion of insulin (Woolfson 1980). In the severely ill patient in an intensive care unit hourly estimations may be warranted. A typical scale for controlling the concentrations of blood glucose by this technique is shown in Table 8.11. This scale has been designed to maintain the concentration in the range of 6–11 mmol/l. This range is a little higher than that observed in healthy individuals, but ensures that patients are unlikely to become hypoglycaemic. Even at the upper end of the range, few patients exhibit glycosuria but in patients who have a low renal threshold and unacceptable glycosuria, the scale can be modified

Table 8.11 Insulin requirements during intravenous feeding

Blood glucose (mmol/l)	Insulin (iu/h)
0–3	None
3–5	Reduce by 2
5–7	Reduce by 1
7–11	Same as previously
11–15	Increase by 2
> 15	Increase by 4
Start at 4 iu/h	

to prevent this. However, such modification does increase the chance of the patient becoming hypoglycaemic. The scale shown is for use in a patient who is not intolerant to glucose and who is receiving approximately 400 g of glucose per day. If the rate of glucose infusion is greater, it is necessary to start the infusion of insulin at a correspondingly higher rate. If it is known that the patient is intolerant to glucose due to severe injury the initial rate of infusion of insulin may also be increased but the patient should be observed very closely during the first hour of infusion to ensure that he does not become hypoglycaemic. When patients are infused with large quantities of glucose and insulin, the nursing staff must be able to recognise the clinical features of hypoglycaemia and know what action is required to reverse it.

Potassium and phosphorous requirements

The electrolyte and mineral requirements of patients requiring intravenous feeding have been discussed above and in Chapter 2. However, patients who are fed intravenously with large quantities of carbohydrates and insulin have an increased requirement for potassium and inorganic phosphorous. As glucose enters the cell under the influence of insulin, so too do potassium and phosphate ions and dangerous hypokalaemia and hypophosphataemia may ensue. The amount of potassium and phosphorous required varies and the concentration in the blood should be measured at least twice on the first day of infusion. If 400 g of glucose are given each day, most patients require at least 100 mmol KCl and 20 mmol KH_2PO_4.

Additives

The number of additives that are made to intravenous solutions has increased considerably during the last decade. In addition to insulin, potassium and phosphorous discussed above, all the elements and vitamins shown in Tables 1.4 and 1.6 may be added to these solutions. Many of these components may interact with other drugs or with the solutions to which they are added (D'Arcy & Griffin 1974) and it is advisable for these additives to be made in the pharmacy by an experienced pharmacist. The dangers of introducing organisms to the solution have been discussed above. It should be remembered that some patients who require intravenous feeding may be able to drink and absorb a small quantity of fluid containing the trace elements or vitamins required. The incidence of trace element deficiency of sufficient severity to cause symptoms and signs is extremely low and many patients who require intravenous feeding for short periods of time (one or two weeks) do not require these supplements if they have been well nourished previously. In some hospitals pharmacists prepare mixtures of trace elements, in others commercial preparations are used. Supplements may be given daily or weekly. As discussed above, the fat–soluble vitamin complex Vitilipid® may be added to the fat emulsion Intralipid®. Not all water–soluble vitamin plexes contain all the vitamins shown in Table 1.6. Information concerning the fate of water–soluble vitamins is inadequate, but it is known that they are excreted in the urine if the concentration in the plasma exceeds the renal threshold. Consequently it is advantageous to infuse these compounds over a period of hours each day rather than to give them intravenously as a bolus injection. Some of the water–soluble vitamins may be denatured by amino acids and by ultraviolet light. They should not be added to solutions of amino acids and the container to which they are added should be covered with a bag to exclude the light.

PERIPHERAL INFUSION OF AMINO ACIDS

The importance of providing adequate quantities of non-protein energy to ensure optimal utilisation of the infused amino acids has been discussed above and this basic concept of total parenteral nutrition is recognised by all experienced clinicians. When optimal utilisation has been achieved, a further improvement in protein balance can only be achieved by increasing the intake of amino acids. Many patients who do not require total parenteral nutrition using hypertonic solutions infused into a central vein do not receive any protein for three to five days. Blackburn and his colleagues (1973a, b) achieved near–positive nitrogen balance following the peripheral infusion of amino acids alone. It was suggested that non-protein energy was provided predominantly from oxidation of fat and ketones and that ketosis was beneficial (Blackburn et al 1973b, Lancet 1973, 1975). Furthermore, it was suggested that the inclusion of glucose in the infusion should be avoided as this would stimulate secretion of insulin and depress mobilisation of fat and lipolysis.

Nitrogen balance and ketosis
In patients who have undergone prolonged starvation, ketones can account for 60% of cerebral oxygen consumption with considerable saving of protein breakdown for gluconeogenesis (Owen et al 1967). However, during infusion of amino acids without glucose in healthy subjects and surgical patients the concentration of ketones in the blood is usually less than 2 mmol/l compared with 7.84 mmol after prolonged starvation. The contribution of ketones to cerebral energy consumption will be only 210 kJ/d (50 kcal/d) at a concentration in the blood of 2 mmol/l (Tweedle 1980b). If this quantity of energy must be provided by gluconeogenesis, approximately 25 g of protein must be broken down and the importance of this mechanism in reducing protein breakdown during prolonged starvation is evident. However, patients receiving 3 litres of isotonic fluid each day after operation receive four times this quantity of energy as glucose.

Nitrogen balance and insulin concentration
Insulin is an anabolic hormone that increases the transport of amino acids and other nutrients into cells and their incorporation into protein (Manchester 1968,

1970). Hence an increase in its concentration would appear to be beneficial to protein metabolism although depressing mobilisation of fat. Infusion of amino acids stimulates secretion of insulin and in most studies of peripheral infusion of amino acids the concentration of insulin in the blood has been considerably greater than that usually observed during prolonged starvation (Tweedle 1980b). Concentrations of that magnitude are inhibitory to the development of a moderate ketosis. In most studies the addition of glucose to the infusion has produced a small increase in the concentration of serum insulin.

GLUCOSE, AMINO ACIDS OR TOTAL PARENTERAL NUTRITION?

Although in the initial study (Blackburn et al 1973a, b) the nitrogen balance of the patients receiving amino acids alone was better than that of the patients receiving amino acids and glucose, the differences appeared to be due to the greater intake of nitrogen in the patients who received amino acids alone. Other studies of peripheral infusion of amino acids have confirmed Elman's original observation (1939) that the addition of glucose improves the nitrogen balance. Positive nitrogen balance was achieved during infusion of amino acids alone in only three out of 15 studies, although many of the patients received large intakes of nitrogen (Tweedle 1980b). Although peripheral infusion of amino acids produces an improvement in nitrogen balance compared to that observed following infusion of isotonic solutions of glucose, the difference is small and is difficult to justify on a financial basis. The hypothesis that infusion of amino acids will maintain the concentrations of 'visceral proteins' (Bistrian & Blackburn 1974) that are responsible for immunocompetence (Law et al 1973) is attractive but remains to be established. Peripheral infusion of solutions of amino acids requires less knowledge and expertise than that required for total parenteral nutrition and the complications are likely to be less frequent and less severe. Although a particular role for this type of therapy may emerge in the future, it must be emphasised that it is not a substitute for total parenteral nutrition.

NUTRITIONAL TEAMS

Doctors visiting other countries frequently observe that the number of patients receiving nutritional support in other European countries and in North America is much higher that in Great Britain, particularly by the intravenous route. Such an observation does not necessarily imply inadequate care in Great Britain. The potential benefits that might accrue from more frequent use of nutritional support have been discussed in Chapter 3 and those benefits must be weighed against the potential complications of intravenous feeding discussed in this chapter and of enteral feeding discussed in the next chapter. The details shown in Table 8.12 are from one surgeon's gastro–enterological practice in a British teaching hospital (Tweedle 1981). The number of patients requiring nutritional support in a general surgical practice in a district general hospital will be considerably less. If the great majority of the patients requiring nutritional support within a hospital are treated within one unit, then the expertise required to provide that support can be developed within that unit. In many hospitals, the patients who require nutri-

Table 8.12 The site of disease and route of infusion in patients requiring nutritional support (1977–79)

	Benign	Malignant	Total	Naso–enteral	Parenteral	Total*	%
Oesophagus	47	9	56	5	2	7	12.5
Stomach	64	50	114	5	5	10	8.8
Duodenum	95	1	96	1	6	6	6.3
Biliary system	191	9	200	3	8	8	4.0
Pancreas	62	25	87	9	17	19	21.8
Large bowel	232	45	277	5	1	6	2.2
	691	139	830	28	39	57	6.9

*Some patients received nutritional support by enteral and parental routes

tional support are dispersed throughout the hospital. The formation of a team of people with specialised knowledge who will visit these patients upon request may be beneficial in such institutions. In addition to providing the combined expertise of a group of individuals a team should also be able to provide assistance when a clinician is ill or on vacation. The frequency with which the team will meet will be governed by the number of patients that it is supervising. Upon the ward, it is essential that all decisions concerning the patient's care are made by the doctors and nurses responsible for his care. The members of the team should offer advice and assistance but they cannot replace and should not attempt to replace the patient's attendants upon the ward. Effective communication is crucial and in addition to regular discussion between the ward staff and the nutritional team, adequate information should be inserted at frequent intervals in the patient's notes.

The size and composition of the team will reflect the requirements within the hospital, but ideally it will contain two or three doctors (Table 8.13). If the group is too large it may spend too much time in internal debate. The consequences of bureaucracy can be overwhelming and it is advisable to appoint a director. It is helpful to have a physician and a surgeon in the team and one of them should have sufficient knowledge of gastro–enterology to make decisions such as the choice of enteral or parenteral routes for feeding. An anaesthetist is often a valuable member, usually being particularly adept at inserting catheters into central veins. Anaesthetists are also more aware than others of the potential dangers of excessive intravenous infusion to the lungs and heart. Although the advice of biochemists, bacteriologists and radiologists should be readily available, their specialised knowledge is not required in the majority of patients and it is wasteful of their time to include them.

Table 8.13 The composition of a nutritional team

Essential	Non-essential
Physician (? gastro-enterologist)	Biochemist
Surgeon (? gastro-enterologist)	Bacteriologist
Anaesthetist (with an interest in intensive care)	Radiologist
Pharmacist	Stomatherapist
Dietitian	Statistician
Nutrition nurse	

The non–medical members of the group may reflect the differing policies within the hospital concerning parenteral and enteral feeding. A dietitian is an obvious requirement, but their role varies. Some dietitians consider that they should act purely in an advisory capacity upon the ward or in the out–patient department. Others prepare solutions for enteral feeding upon the ward or in the diet kitchen. In many hospitals the expert knowledge of the dietitian is wasted in the time–consuming and fatuous exercise of advising patients how to lose weight. If all the patients requiring intravenous feeding receive peripheral infusions of commercially available solutions without additives, a pharmacist is unnecessary. If all the patients receive solutions which are mixed in the pharmacy according to their individual requirements, a pharmacist is an essential member. Most teams contain at least one nurse. In many countries they are called 'IV nurses' but as enteral feeding has become more popular and their knowledge and expertise are more extensive than implied by this term, it would be preferable to refer to them as nutrition nurses. These nurses must undertake the potentially sensitive role of advising colleagues who may be senior to them about the potential hazards of enteral and parenteral feeding. Their work may be considerable, particularly important aspects including the routine care of intravenous catheters and ensuring that the infusion set is changed daily. The incidence of infection during intravenous feeding may be influenced by this nurse (Freeman et al 1972). The nurse should ascertain whether patients receiving enteral nutrients have diarrhoea and whether patients receiving parenteral nutrients have glycosuria and should take appropriate action if either of these complications occur. In many hospitals these nurses assess the nutritional status of the patient by anthropometry and immunocompetence by cutaneous hypersensitivity to a variety of allergens. If a nurse is unavailable or too busy to perform anthopometric measurements, these may be performed by the dietitian but legal considerations may prevent the dietitian from performing assessment of delayed hypersensitivity. Many patients requiring nutritional support have stomata, fistulae and abscesses and some teams contain a stomatherapist. Although collection of aspirates and exudates may be a difficult and important feature of the nutritional assessment, the major function of the group is to provide advice and assistance in the nutritional care of the patient and it may be a waste of valuable time for the stomatherapist to attend regular meetings. Nevertheless, if the hospital does not contain a stomatherapist it may prove beneficial to train the nutrition nurse how to manage these stomata. Analysis of data recorded during nutritional support may indicate deficiencies in nutritional support in addition to providing material for teaching and research. It is advisable to discuss how the data should be recorded with a statistician. The task of recording this information usually falls upon the nurse.

9

Intravenous infusion

The equipment that may be required to infuse electrolyte or nutrient solutions into peripheral or central veins is discussed in this chapter. The sites of access to peripheral and central veins are described and the septic and physical complications of these methods are compared. The physiological and metabolic consequences of intravenous infusion are discussed in Chapters 2, 3, 4 and 8.

CONTAINERS

When the Medicines Commission submitted their 'Interim report on heat–sterilised fluids for parenteral administration' to the Secretary of State in 1972 (usually referred to as the Rosenheim Report after its chairman), the total usage of intravenous fluids in Great Britain was 10 million containers per year, nearly half of which was manufactured in hospitals (Medicines Commission 1972). This report and the Clothier Report (1972) had a profound influence upon the supply of intravenous solutions in Great Britain and manufacture of intravenous fluids in hospitals has fallen dramatically. The Rosenheim Committee also approved the increasing use of plastic containers for intravenous fluids which was evident at that time and which subsequently has superseded the use of glass containers in most hospitals. The major requirements of an ideal container for intravenous fluids are shown in Table 9.1. The glass and plastic containers presently available have different advantages, but unfortunately no container satisfies all the requirements shown in Table 9.1. The majority of plastic containers are manufactured from polyvinyl chloride and there is little doubt that bacterial contamination is less

Table 9.1 The requirements of an ideal container

Effective sterilisation
Effective closure
Maintain sterility
No interaction with contents
No leakage of particles into contents
Visual inspection
Easy storage and transport
Unrestricted flow of contents
Easy suspension
Easy, sterile connection of infusion set
Effective mixing of additives
Low cost

likely to occur in these containers than in glass bottles. This feature, more than any other, is responsible for the increasing use of plastic containers. Bacterial contamination during manufacture is a rare but potentially devastating occurrence (Clothier Report 1972, Maki et al 1976a).

Glass containers

Bottles can be made from many varieties of glass, each with different characteristics. Bottles for intravenous solutions should conform to the appropriate British Standard. Their composition is dictated by the requirement to withstand autoclaving so that their contents are maintained at a temperature of 115°C for 30 minutes as suggested by the British Pharmacopoeia. Hairline cracks in the bottles that may be undetectable can develop during the sterilisation process but the major problem arises in the method of closure. The usual method of closure is by inserting a synthetic or natural rubber plug which is held in place by metal caps and rings. These plugs have different coefficients of expansion from the bottles and some bottles (particularly those that are re–used) may have small defects due to chipping of the lips. Consequently, contamination of the contents may occur during the sterilisation process. Some manufacturers cool the bottles by spraying with cold water to shorten the time taken and to lessen the risks of injury produced by opening sterilizer doors under pressure. In the past, spray cooling of inadequately closed or cracked bottles with unsterile water has been the major cause of contamination (Beverley et al 1973) and the Rosenheim Committee were particularly concerned about this practice, which fortunately is only in limited use (Medicines Commission 1972).

Bottles are the most fragile containers and the most likely to undergo damage during transit and storage (Myers 1974). Some types of glass are attacked by alkaline solutions and cannot be used to contain solutions of sodium bicarbonate. Another serious disadvantage of bottles is the high particle counts that are found in their contents (Garvan & Gunner 1971). These particles come from both the glass and the rubber plug and high counts are likely to be found in inadequately washed bottles that are being re–used. Bottles afford better visual inspection of their contents and more accurate assessment of the volume remaining during infusion than plastic containers. However, the Rosenheim Committee emphasised that visual inspection cannot give a positive indication of sterility or of contamination and lack of transparency is not therefore in itself a hazard (Medicines Commission 1972).

Bottles are the most stable of the containers in use and can be stored individually on shelves, but glass is denser than plastic. The flow of solution from the container is unrestricted if an airway is used but it is impossible to compress the contents and rapid flow can only be achieved by using a roller pump. The necessity of using an airway is an additional potential source of contamination and, using an infusion without an alarm system, a potential source of intravenous air embolism. The routine use of infusion sets containing microbial filters would considerably diminish the danger of extrinsic contamination by inadequately filtered air. Most bottles now contain an integral metal or plastic loop for attaching it to a drip stand but some require an additional cage for suspension. It is physically more easy to insert an infusion set into a glass bottle than into a plastic bag but there may be a greater risk of contamination of the contents by air particles from the rubber plug. Similarly it is easier to mix additives in a bottle but the risk of contamination is greater. Even when re-used the cost of bottles is greater than plastic containers.

Plastic containers

Plastic containers may be made from polyvinyl chloride or from polyethylene. Containers made of either material are cheaper, lighter and less fragile than those made of glass. As the closure parts of the majority of the containers are an integral part made from the same material and are usually smaller than those of glass bottles, contamination during the sterilisation process is less likely. Not all plastic containers will withstand heating of their contents to 115°C for 30 minutes. The Rosenheim Committee suggested that sterilisation could be achieved by other combinations of time and temperature but it is apparent that adequate sterilisation cannot be achieved by prolonged exposure to heat if the temperature is not sufficiently high.

Polyvinyl chloride

These containers are usually made in the form of a bag by welding two sheets of polyvinyl chloride and the polymers and plasticizers used are flexible and transparent. The polyvinyl chloride is permeable to water and the storage life of these containers is reduced by the small reduction in volume that may occur (McDonald 1974). Under normal conditions up to 2% water loss can occur each month from the unprotected bag. Some bags are made with an impermeable over-wrap to reduce this loss and these also reduce the risk of contamination due to seam failure or pin-holing (the description usually applied to very small defects in the plastic sheet). The major potential disadvantage in the use of polyvinyl chloride bags is the finding of toxic chemicals in their contents (Jaeger & Rubin 1972). Small quantities of phthallate salts used to soften the polymers may leach from the plastic into the fluid. The particle counts within solutions contained in polyvinyl chloride bags are greater than those found in polythene containers but much less than those found in glass bottles.

Polyvinyl chloride bags allow visual inspection of their contents when the over-wrap has been removed. However, their flexibility does not allow any accuracy in assessing the volume of fluid left in the bag. The bags are lighter than glass bottles but are difficult to store individually on a shelf. Flexibility of the bags allows unrestricted but different flow rates when compared with glass bottles in the laboratory (Furber et al 1978). However, laboratory studies may be irrelevant in clinical practice as flow rates during infusion in patients are very different and vary from minute to minute (Collin et al 1973). The bags do not require an airway and flow rates can be increased by external pneumatic compression.

Sterile insertion ports under tear-off seals allow easy insertion of infusion sets without the need for preliminary swabbing with antiseptics. This is less likely to produce bacterial contamination than may occur during insertion through rubber plugs, but particles of plastic may still be introduced. An additional port is produced for the mixing of additives but the bag may be pierced from inside by the needle if the addition is not made with care. Mixing within the bag may be incomplete and this may be potentially dangerous with additives such as potassium salts. Where possible, patients requiring such supplements should be infused with appropriate fluids which already contain the required supplement added during manufacture.

Polythene

Polythene containers can be manufactured to withstand the temperatures required for adequate sterilisation but unfortunately high density polythene must be used which is less pliable and more opaque than polyvinyl chloride. The entry and additive ports are also more difficult to manufacture and it is not possible to print the contents and instructions for use on the container which must be labelled after sterilisation, thereby excluding the possibility of using an overwrap. These features render the polythene container more prone to inadequate sterilisation than polyvinyl chloride containers. However, there is no loss of content due to permeability and an over–wrap is unnecessary in this respect. Polythene is also less permeable to carbon dioxide than polyvinyl chloride and consequently is an ideal substance for containing solutions of sodium bicarbonate. Although these containers are more opaque than those made of polyvinyl chloride and visual inspection for clarity of content is less efficient, these containers have the lowest particle counts when measured with a Coulter counter and leaching of plasticisers does not occur. Polythene containers are lighter than glass bottles but heavier than polyvinyl chloride containers. Some which are shaped like a bottle can be stored individually on a shelf, but others cannot because of a suspensory ring which is an integral part of the container. The major problem encountered in the use of polythene containers is distorted flow and incomplete emptying due to the rigidity of the container (Furber et al 1978). This problem could be overcome by the use of an airway (see above under glass bottles). This rigidity also prevents compression of the container and rapid infusion in a emergency can only be achieved by an infusion pump. Some polythene containers are manufactured without an additive port and additives can only be introduced into the solution by direct puncture of the container with potential contamination of the contents. However, mixing of the additives is more efficient than in polyvinyl chloride bags and absorption is far less.

INTRAVENOUS INFUSION SETS

(Administration set, giving set, drip set, and IV line are alternative titles given to this piece of equipment).

Considerable thought and development have produced major changes in the design of containers, pumps and catheters used for intravenous infusion. By comparison, very little effort appears to have been expended upon the requirements of the infusion set since those made of plastic superseded the old sets made of a mixture of rubber and glass tubing. At the present time the Department of Health and Social Security recognises only two approved suppliers of infusion sets for the intravenous infusion of blood, parenteral nutrients and standard solutions of glucose and electrolytes. These sets were designed in the era preceding the use of infusion pumps. It is likely that changes in their design will be made in the near fu-

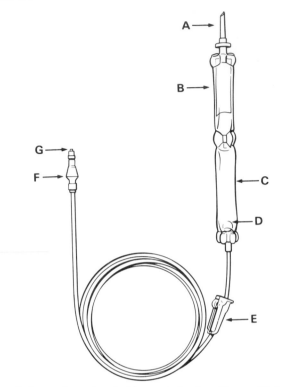

Fig. 9.1 Blood transfusion set (reproduced with permission from Travenol Laboratories Ltd)
A — piercing pin, B — filter chamber, C — drip chamber, D — ball valve, E — roller-clamp,
F — drug injection port, G — Luer connector

ture which will make them more suitable for use with infusion pumps. The basic design of an intravenous infusion set for blood transfusion is shown in Figure 9.1.

The piercing pin may be made of plastic or metal. Those made of plastic must be sufficiently sturdy to enable insertion through the rubber stoppers of bottles. The pin should be long enough to pierce the rubber stopper of the bottle or the entry port of the plastic container but excessive length increases the risk of unintentional piercing of the wall of a plastic container.

Infusion sets for transfusing blood (usually referred to as blood sets) differ from those used for infusing other solutions (usually referred to as solution sets) in having two chambers rather than one. The upper chamber contains a filter with a pore size of 170–230 μm. These filters will remove large particles of rubber and plastic and macro–aggregates of blood cells and platelets that would form emboli in the lungs upon intravenous infusion. However, there are many doctors who emphasise that much smaller aggregates may pass through these filters during transfusion and may be an important factor in the development of post–traumatic pulmonary insufficiency (see Ch. 7). For this reason, many doctors use filters with a much smaller pore size when transfusing patients with large quantities of blood (see below).

In many hospitals blood sets are used routinely for all intravenous infusions. Blood sets are more expensive than solution sets, but such a practice ensures that an inexperienced nurse does not transfuse unfiltered blood into the patient. After the transfusion is complete, the infusion set should be changed before infusing other solutions. In particular, it is important not to infuse solutions of glucose after blood as large aggregates may form in the tubing distal to the filter. The filter may also become blocked with aggregates and the infusion may stop with subsequent clotting in the intravenous cannula.

The lower chamber of a blood set is similar to the drip chamber of a solution set but is usually longer so that it can be used as a manual pump in emergency. It contains a ball valve for this purpose. The drip chamber of a solution set allows a visual inspection of the rate of infusion. There are usually about 20 drops per ml but the size may vary according to the viscosity and specific gravity of the fluid, disturbance of the infusion set and movement of the patient. The sensors of infusion pumps are fastened to this chamber and may slide down, recording incorrectly and stopping the infusion (see below).

A clamp is used to compress the plastic tube to control the rate of flow. Unfortunately the plastic tube distorts with use and this produces a poor control of the rate of flow. Between the end of the plastic tubing and the Luer connection there

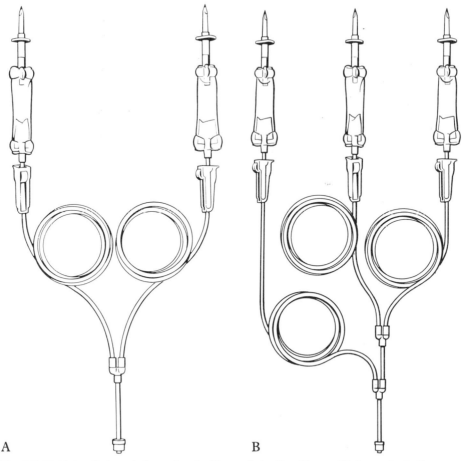

A   B

Fig. 9.2 Multiple infusion sets (reproduced with permission from Travenol Laboratories Ltd)

is a short piece of rubber tubing which is usually called the drug injection port. This is a potentially weak point in the infusion set and many injection ports have disrupted when massive transfusion under pressure has been required. It would be preferable in future if intravenous injections of drugs were made through adequately designed injection ports incorporated into cannulae (see below) The injection ports of the infusion set have also been used to allow simultaneous infusion of other solutions by inserting a needle from the other infusion set into the injection port. This is usually referred to as 'piggy-backing'. It is a potential source of infection and unnecessary as V and W infusion sets are now available to allow simultaneous infusion of two or three solutions without prior mixing in the container (Fig. 9.2). The use of intravenous antibiotics and other drugs is increasing rapidly, particularly in patients requiring intensive care. Some of these drugs must be mixed with comparatively large quantities of fluids (as much as 200 ml). Some are already prepared by the manufacturer in small bottles and smaller, simpler infusion sets than those described above have been designed for their infusion.

An alternative method of coping with this problem is shown in Figure 9.3. These infusion sets contain valves which are closed by the greater head of pressure produced by raising the second container above the height of the first container. When the fluid in the second container (which contains the antibiotic or other

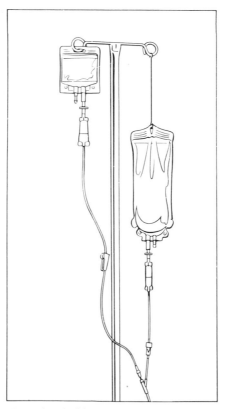

Fig. 9.3 Valved infusion set (reproduced with permission from Travenol Laboratories Ltd)

drug) has been infused, the valve opens and the fluid from the first container is now infused. Drugs in solution may also be added to burettes incorporated in the infusion set. Burettes also allow precise control of infusion rate but they are likely to become contaminated (Duma et al 1971).

The Luer connections of the present generation of infusion sets are designed as either a simple taper or incorporating a lock. Although a lock has the advantage of a secure connection, particularly when an infusion pump is being used, it is more difficult to connect and disconnect and unintentional rotation of the Luer connection on the hub of the cannula may provoke thrombophlebitis.

FILTERS

The filters incorporated into intravenous infusion sets (170–230 μm) are designed to remove macro–aggregates of components of human blood. Other types of filters may be inserted between the container and the intravenous cannula. At present there are two types of filter inserted in this manner, blood microfilters and microbial filters. The names given to these filters indicate their primary function but in addition, the filters also remove particulate matter according to their pore size.

Blood microfilters

It has been known for many years that within a few hours of storage, micro–aggregates of platelets, red and white corpuscles and fibrin can be identified in blood (Fantus & Schirmer 1938). The number of aggregates formed is proportional to the length of time that the blood is stored (Solis et al 1974). During the first week of storage, micro–aggregates of platelets predominate and during the second week leucocytes form an increasing component. The possible role of these micro–aggregates in the production of post–traumatic pulmonary insufficiency has been recognised during the last decade (Allardyce et al 1969, Ljungqvist 1973).

A number of microfilters have been developed to remove micro–aggregates that will pass easily through the 170–230 μm filters incorporated into blood sets. The filters contain a variety of screens and foreign surfaces made of nylon, polyurethrane, Dacron and other polyesters (Table 9.2). Some filters rely predominately upon the pore size of their screens, where others rely mainly upon adsorption onto foreign surfaces. Those that have layers of screens with a decreas-

Table 9.2 Blood microfilters

Type	Pore size (μm)	Filter	Company
Bentley PFF 100®	20	Polyurethane foam	Bentley
Biotest®	10	Nylon mesh	Biotest Folex
Fenwal®	20	Polyester foam and nylon fibre	Travenol
Intersept®	20	Polyester screen and Dacron fibre	Johnson & Johnson
Pall Ultipor®	40	Polyester screen	Pall Biomedical
Swank IL 200®	25	Dacron fibre	Extracorporeal

ing pore size are more effective than those that have a single screen. The pore size shown in Table 9.2 is that of the smallest element of the filter. According to the material used and the method of construction, the efficiency of a filter may deteriorate after transfusion has begun or show an initial improvement. Ultimately, all filters become blocked and must be changed. This may occur after transfusion of 3–10 units of blood depending on the length of time for which the blood has been stored and the type of filter used.

It is comparatively easy to demonstrate in vitro the effect of different filters upon the content of stored blood (Marshall et al 1976) and there have been a few studies of their effect during extracorporeal circulation (Hill et al 1970, Patterson & Twichell 1971). In an important prospective study of 54 patients requiring transfusion of 10 or more units of blood following major injury, there was a highly significant decrease in the incidence of post–traumatic pulmonary insufficiency in the patients who were transfused with blood that had passed through a 40 μm filter (Reul et al 1974). Post–traumatic pulmonary insufficiency developed in 7 out of 17 patients receiving unfiltered blood compared with only 2 out of 27 patients transfused with filtered blood. Biopsies of the lungs showed micro–aggregates composed of platelets, cell membranes and fibrin deposits in the precapillary arterioles of 4 out of 5 patients transfused with unfiltered blood, but no micro–aggregates were found in 5 patients transfused with filtered blood. Further studies of this type are required to establish the role of these filters in the prevention of post–traumatic pulmonary insufficiency with particular reference to the quantity of blood transfused and the length of time that it has been stored.

Microbial filters

As their name implies these filters were designed to remove organisms during infusion but in addition they also remove particles greater than their pore size and reduce the risk of air embolism. The earlier designs (Table 9.3) had a pore size of 0.45 μm which was small enough to remove fungi and most bacteria but Pseudomonas, *E. coli* and other Gram–negative bacteria begin to pass through the filter after six hours of infusion (Maki 1976b). Filters with a pore size of 0.22 μm remove all bacteria and fungi (Rusmin et al 1975). Particles of paper, cotton, flax, glass, fibreglass, rubber and plastic have been identified in the contaminants removed by these filters during intravenous infusion (Myers 1972).

Table 9.3 Antimicrobial filters

Type	Pore size (μm)	Manufacturer
Final Filter®	0.45	Travenol
Pall Ultipor®	0.22	Pall Biomedical
IVEX–2®	0.22	Abbott
Millex–GS®	0.22	Millipore SA

The rate of infusion is considerably reduced by all filters, but the reduction is particularly severe when using the filter with the lower pore size. The reduction in flow increases dramatically with an increase in the viscosity of the fluid (Collin et al 1973) and concentrated solutions of glucose and amino acids required for intravenous feeding must be infused under pressure using an infusion pump. It is not possible to infuse fat emulsions, blood or plasma through a microbial filter.

Even during routine infusion of isotonic solutions, the first generation of microbial filters became blocked so rapidly that it was sometimes necessary to change the filter six times in a day. This blockage was not due to the extraction of particles from the solution, but to air bubbles. A recent development is the production of microbial filters with a pore size of 0.22 μm which incorporate a hydrophobic filter through which the air bubbles are expelled. Although these new models are less bulky than the original models, improvements in design have produced a considerable increase in the surface area of the filter. In spite of these improvements, it is still necessary to infuse viscous solutions under pressure.

The filters are inserted between the distal end of the infusion set and the intravenous cannula. This is the logical site, as it appears unlikely that a microbial filter can be incorporated into the hub of an intravenous cannula. Some filter sets include an injection port in the tubing distal to the filter so that blood, plasma or fat emulsion can be infused without removing the filter.

The ability of these filters to remove organisms and particles from contaminated solutions has been clearly demonstrated in the laboratory and in clinical practice and it has been shown that 'during extensive intravenous therapy a patient may receive between 100 000 and 2 000 000 particles greater than 1 μm (Myers 1972). However, there has been no reduction in the incidence of infective complications and conflicting reports of the incidence of phlebitis following the use of these filters during intravenous infusion of isotonic solutions. Although in one controlled study in Great Britain there was no difference in the incidence of phlebitis (Collin et al 1973), in two controlled studies performed in the same institution in the United States of America the incidence was two and a half times as great in the patients receiving unfiltered solutions as in those receiving filtered solutions (De Luca et al 1975, Bivins et al 1979). The possible consequences of phlebitis are discussed later in this chapter.

Controlled studies of the use of antimicrobial filters in patients being fed intravenously have not been performed, but in an uncontrolled study the incidence of sepsis was four times as great in the patients who had a filter included in the infusion system than in those who did not (Freeman & Litton 1974). The increase in the incidence of sepsis was attributed to an increased incidence of manipulations of the infusion system (particularly of the cannula) by the nurses in order to change blocked filters. Although filters remove contaminants, their use produces an increase of 10% in the incidence of extrinsic contamination (Miller & Grogan 1973). This increase in extrinsic contamination could be avoided if the filter was incorporated into the distal end of the infusion set but blood, plasma and fat emulsions could not be infused through this set.

Many drugs are extracted from solution by microbial filters due to filtration and to binding and they can be used to reduce the incidence of phlebitis induced by infusion of solutions containing particulate antibiotics (Maddox et al 1977). However, this mechanism inevitably reduces the quantity of drug infused and not enough is known about how much of a particular drug is removed by different filters and whether this quantity is influenced by different preparations of the same drug. In ill patients in whom the precise quantity of drug infused may be critical, it is necessary to inject the drug into the infusion system distal to the filter.

CATHETERS

Plastic catheters for intravenous infusion were introduced by Zimmerman (1945). The initial stimulus for their development was the requirement for long catheters to be inserted into the central veins. More recently the use of short catheters (usually referred to as cannulae) for infusion into peripheral veins has become standard practice and the use of needles of stainless steel has almost been abandoned. During this time, many varieties of catheters and cannulae have been developed which differ in length, internal and external diameter and in their composition (Tables 9.4 to 9.7). This variation in design has come about due to differing requirements and to advances in manufacturing technology.

Table 9.4 Catheters inserted through the needle

Name	Material	Diameter (G)	Length (cm)	Manufacturer
Drum Cartridge®	PE	14	71.1	Abbott
EZ Cath®*	PTFE or PVC	14–18	8–36	Deseret
Intrasil®*	Silicone	14–17	50.8–55.9	Travenol
Subclavian T®	PTFE	14–18	9–16	British Viggo

*Inserted through a split needle which may be removed

Originally, intravenous catheters were introduced by the cut–down technique. However, this technique is associated with a high incidence of local and systemic infection (Maki 1976a) and the vein becomes thrombosed and obliterated, particularly if ligated distal to the point of insertion of the catheter. For routine purposes, this technique of insertion has been replaced by catheters and cannulae that are inserted through or over a steel needle. The earlier designs were all of the 'through the needle' variety (Fig. 9.4 and Table 9.4) and this type has been associated with catheter embolism due to the sharp edge of the needle cutting through the plastic catheter, usually during insertion. (Wellmann et al 1968). This type of accident usually occurs when an inexperienced doctor is unable to advance the catheter through the needle. If it proves impossible to advance the catheter to the required distance, the procedure should be abandoned and the catheter and the needle should be withdrawn simultaneously. In spite of such precautions, the incidence of complications produced by the use of this type of cathe-

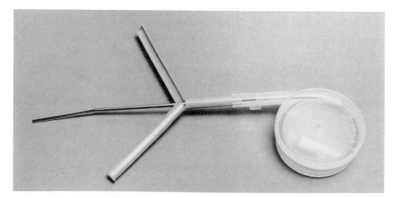

Fig. 9.4 Intravenous catheter of the 'through the needle' variety

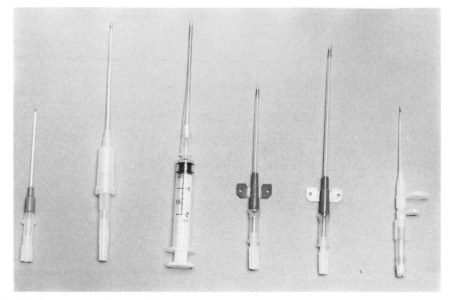

Fig. 9.5 Intravenous catheters of the 'over the needle' variety

ter led the Department of Health and Social Security to issue a warning against their use (John 1972). Certainly this is a very serious complication; 13 of the 37 cases reported by Wellmann et al (1968) died as a consequence of the accident. Consequently, the use of catheters inserted over a needle (Fig. 9.5 and Table 9.5) has increased considerably during the last decade. An advantage of this type of catheter is that the smallest possible hole is made in the wall of the vein. A disadvantage of the 'over the needle' variety is the requirement for the catheter to be composed of more rigid material that will withstand the force required for insertion through the tissues and the end of the catheter must be tapered. These features make the catheter more likely to traumatise the vessel wall and produce thrombophlebitis (Jones & Craig 1972).

Table 9.5 Cannulae inserted over the needle

Name	Material	Diameter (G)	Length (cm)	Manufacturer
A–Cath®	PTFE	14–20	3.2–14	Bard
Abbocath T®	FEP	14–22	3.2–14	Abbot
Angiocath®	PTFE	14–22	2.5–13.3	Deseret
Intranule®	PP	13–18	6–12	Vygon (UK)
Medicut®	PP	12–22	2.2–4.5	Sherwood
Trocaflon®	PTFE	14–16	6–9	Vygon (UK)
Venflon®	PTFE	14–21	2.5–4.5	Vygon (UK)

Alternative methods of introduction have been devised to avoid the disadvantages of these two basic techniques, whilst retaining their advantages. Some catheters may be inserted through a needle that splits in half. Although this lessens the chance of the needle tip cutting through the catheter after insertion, it does not reduce the chance of this happening during insertion. Another technique is to insert a guide wire in the manner first described by Seldinger (1953). The

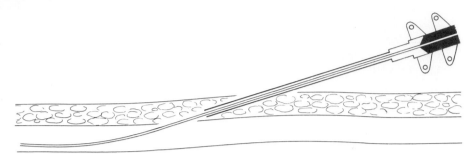

Fig. 9.6 Intravenous catheter inserted through a cannula

safest technique is to insert the catheter through a short cannula (Forman & Powell 1969). Using this technique, a short 'over the needle' cannula is inserted into the vein. The needle is removed and a catheter is inserted through the cannula and advanced to the required length. The more rigid cannula may then he withdrawn from the vein, but can with benefit be left with its tip in the subcutaneous tissue so as to prevent kinking of the less rigid intravenous catheter at the site of exit from the skin (Fig. 9.6). A number of manufacturers have designed cannulae and catheters of compatible internal and external diameters to facilitate this technique (Fig. 9.7 and Table 9.6).

Table 9.6 Catheters inserted through a cannula

Name	Material	Diameter (G)	Length (cm)	Manufacturer
Advanset®	PTFE	14–18	22.9–61	Bard
Centrasil®	Silicone	16	21.6	Travenol
Leader–Cath®	PE	14–20	8–25	Vygon (U.K.)
Long–line®	PE	12–16	5–8	Vygon (U.K.)
Nutricath–S®	Silicone	12–13	35–60	Vygon (U.K.)

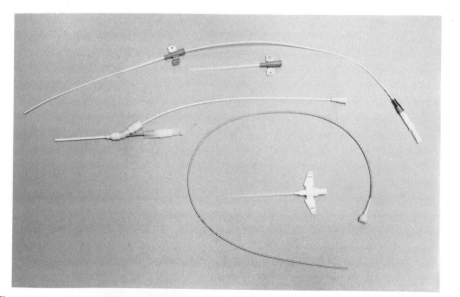

Fig. 9.7 Intravenous catheters inserted through cannulae

The hubs of cannulae and catheters differ in design. Some of the larger catheters have hubs that can be removed and then re–inserted. This feature is particularly useful when it is intended to create a subcutaneous tunnel between the point of entry of the catheter into the vein and the site of exit from the skin. The hub is a potentially weak point in the catheter and may split. Although the usual consequence is failure of infusion and the need to change the catheter, air embolism may occur (Armstrong et al 1977). The hubs of some cannulae are designed to include injection ports to allow intravenous injections to be made through the cannula. These ports may become contaminated (Oberhammer 1980) and should only be incorporated into the cannula when they can be disinfected. An advantage of some catheters is the inclusion of a small, transparent bulb on the end of the needle which fills with blood to indicate successful insertion into the vein, a phenomenon usually referred to as flashback. All cannulae and catheters should be radio–opaque.

Although plastic cannulae have largely replaced steel needles for peripheral venous infusion, the incidence of septicaemia appears to be much lower when steel needles are used (Maki 1976a), although a controlled trial has not been performed. Unfortunately the older type of steel needle provided for transfusion of blood was difficult to fix to the skin and the newer 'butterfly' or 'scalp vein' needles (Table 9.7) do not allow rapid infusion. Nevertheless Maki (1976) has suggested that for elective infusions, steel needles should be used whenever feasible, in preference to plastic catheters.

Table 9.7 Butterfly or scalp vein needles

Name	Diameter (G)	Manufacturer
Butterfly®	14–27	Abbott
E–Z Set®	16–27	Deseret
Medi–Wing®	14–25	Argyle
Venoflux®	14–27	Vygon (U.K.)

Plastic cannulae and catheters may be made of polyvinyl chloride, polyethylene, polypropylene, teflon and siliconised rubber. Each substance has different chemical and physical characteristics which may be advantageous or disadvantageous according to the requirement for its use. The great majority of catheters used for central intravenous infusion are made of polyvinyl chloride, polyethylene or polypropylene which have the advantage of being cheap but which produce a much greater incidence of phlebitis than the more pliable but more expensive catheters made of siliconised rubber. A few catheters and cannulae have been made of polyurethane and nylon but catheters made of these materials have been found to have no advantage over catheters made of the materials discussed below.

Polyvinyl chloride (PVC)

The use of polyvinyl chloride in the manufacture of plastic bags for infusion solutions has been discussed above. The polymerisation of vinyl chloride produces a hard plastic which must be softened by the inclusion of phthallate salts. These salts leach out of the plastic during use and, in addition to any potential toxicity, the loss of the phthallate salts hardens the catheter. Consequently catheters made of polyvinyl chloride are particularly likely to produce thrombosis and phlebitis (Jones & Craig 1972). These irritative properties can be reduced to some extent by siliconisation of the surface of the catheter. The incidence of thrombophlebitis, bacterial contamination of the tip of the catheter and septicaemia is related to the length of time the catheter is in the vein (Maki 1976a). Cannulae made of polyvinyl chloride may be suitable for short–term infusions into peripheral veins, but the infusion site should be changed every 48 hours.

Polyethylene (PE)
Polyethylene is much softer than polyvinyl chloride and incorporation of softeners is not required. Although the surface of these catheters can be siliconised and they are less likely to produce thrombophlebitis than those made of polyvinyl chloride (Jones & Craig 1972), a sleeve of fibrin may envelope the catheter within 24 hours of its insertion (Hoshal et al 1971). Bacteria may proliferate in these sleeves and thrombosis in the central veins may occur.

Polypropylene (PP)
Polypropylene has a similar basic structure to that of polyethylene and the physical and chemical characteristics of cannulae made of these materials are also very similar.

Teflon (PTFE, FEP)
There are two varieties of teflon, polytetrafluorethylene (PTFE) and fluoroethylene propylene (FEP). Teflon is a very stable substance and consequently its rigidity cannot be reduced by the incorporation of phthallate salts. Although it is less likely to produce thrombo-phlebitis than polyvinyl chloride (Jones & Craig 1972) and polyethylene (Dinley 1976), the material still provokes the formation of sleeves of fibrin around the catheter (Hoshal et al 1971). Cannulae made of fluoroethylene propylene appear to be less likely to produce venous complications than those of polytetrafluoroethylene (Dinley 1976).

Siliconised rubber (silicone elastomer, silastic)
Catheters made of siliconised rubber induce far less reaction than those made of polyethylene (Welch et al 1974) and there is little doubt that catheters made of this material are the most suitable of those available at the present time for insertion into the central veins. Unfortunately, these catheters are more expensive than their plastic counterparts. This type of catheter should always be used when it is expected that intravenous feeding will be required for a month or more. In many hospitals these catheters are used routinely for all patients requiring intravenous feeding. The cost of the catheter is a minor item when compared with the overall cost of feeding a patient intravenously for a week. Furthermore catheters made from siliconised rubber require changing at less frequent intervals than plastic catheters so that there is little if any difference in cost. When these catheters are brought out to the skin surface through a subcutaneous tunnel (see below under central venous catheterisation) they remain patent, uninfected and in the correct position for 1–30 months (Riella & Scribner 1976) and it is standard practice to

use them in patients who require intravenous feeding for prolonged periods in the home.

INTRAVENOUS CONTROLLERS, PUMPS AND REGULATORS

There are three categories of equipment commonly used to control the rate of infusion from bottles and plastic containers:
- a. controllers
- b. pumps
- c. regulators

These devices may be stood on the top of bedside lockers or clamped to drip–stands or beds. Electric power may be obtained from the mains or from rechargeable batteries. The battery life depends upon the flow rate and will last for 2 to 30 hours. Controllers and pumps for intravenous infusion in the hospital usually weigh between 3 and 6 kg and cannot be carried by the patient by means of a shoulder strap. Small, lightweight infusion pumps that lack the sophistication of these pumps have been developed for use during parenteral nutrition in the home. Intravenous infusion by gravity feeding is sufficiently accurate for the majority of patients but in those requiring accurate and steady rates of infusion changes in fluid viscosity, drop size, drip rate, height of container above the patient and changes in venous pressure due to movement of the patient produce unacceptable inaccuracies for the infusion of certain solutions or drugs (Collin et al 1973, Flack & Whyte 1974).

Controllers

These units do not pump the solution into the patient. The solution is infused by gravity and consequently the container must be elevated to a sufficient height above the patient. Flow rates of about 5–70 drops per minute may be selected and if the flow is interrupted due to some failure in the infusion line, clogging of the cannula or infiltration into the tissues, the control unit cuts off the flow and visual and audible alarms are activated. This type of device is very sensitive and changes in the patient's posture may be sufficient to activate the alarm unnecessarily. Controllers and peristaltic pumps regulate the infusion by monitoring the rate at which drops of fluid traverse the drip chamber in the infusion set. An optical sensor is clipped on to the drip chamber. The level of the fluid in the drip chamber must be adjusted so that the sensor can distinguish drops of fluid from the meniscus. Unfortunately, the sensor may slip down the chamber and will then register the fluid in the chamber as continuous infusion and the alarms will be activated. If the infusion is accidentally disturbed and the level of the meniscus in the drip chamber momentarily crosses the sensing device, it will be incorrectly recorded as a drop. Both the controller and the peristaltic pumps regulate drop rate and not the volume infused. Drop size varies according to the type of infusion set being used and according to the rate of infusion. The manufacturers frequently state that their controllers are accurate to within 1 or 2% of the selected drop rate. The actual rate may differ by more than 20%, particularly at high rates of infusion. However, although the true rate may differ considerably from that selected, when once selected the rate of infusion is regular (Rithalia & Tinker 1978).

Peristaltic pumps

Peristaltic pumps share many of the disadvantages of the controllers discussed above, particularly with regard to the optical sensor. However, because the solution is pumped into the vein rather than relying on gravity, a greater range of infusion from 1 to 99 drops per minute is available. If isotonic crystalloidal solutions are being infused the maximum rate of infusion is approximately 400 ml/min. These pumps are more accurate than simple drop rate controllers, the actual rate of infusion usually being within 5% of the selected rate, but at low rates of infusion the rate of infusion may be irregular over short periods of time (Rithalia & Tinker 1978). Peristaltic pumps develop high pressures and if distal obstruction occurs at low rates of infusion it may take many minutes before sufficient back pressure develops to activate the alarm. Because of these problems neither the controller nor the peristaltic pump afford the precise control of infusion rates that may be required for the infusion of drugs.

Volumetric pumps

Because of the difficulties in obtaining very accurate rates of infusion using peristaltic pumps discussed above, a different type of pump that would infuse a specified volume in a given time was developed. These pumps contain disposable cassettes of known volume which can be filled and emptied according to movements of a piston and an inlet and outlet valve. A potential disadvantage in using this type of pump rather than a peristaltic pump is the necessity of attaching the infusion tubing to the cassette. There has been no evidence that septic complications are more frequent when using this type of pump, but the cassette must be changed each day. It is possible to purchase casettes that are an integral part of an infusion set, thereby reducing this slight risk of infection.

Regulators

In addition to electrically powered, expensive controllers and pumps, a number of manufacturers have recently developed small, inexpensive regulators which offer greater control than the clamps that are a component of standard infusion sets (Table 9.8). These regulators may be incorporated into the infusion sets or inserted between the infusion set and the cannula. Although they appear to give better control of the rate of infusion than that afforded by standard clamps, their accuracy is far lower than that of controllers and pumps. They rely upon gravity and Helix® and Dial-a-flow® (Table 9.8) are very susceptible to changes in the height of the container above the patient and to changes in venous pressure. Isoflux® contains a proportionating valve which reduces the variations in flow induced by changes in the height of the container and in venous pressure. These effects are particularly evident at low rates of infusion and regulators are not suf-

Table 9.8 Regulators

Type	Range (ml/h)	Manufacturer
Isoflux®	10–400	Van Leer
Helix®	3–200	Van Leer
Dial–a–Flow 30®	5–250	Simonsen & Weel

ficiently accurate to control the infusion of intravenous drugs. Lacking sensors and alarms, regulators are unable to compensate for these variations in flow. Until the results of controlled trials are available, the role of these appliances is uncertain but they may prove to be particularly useful in busy wards in which a number of patients require intravenous feeding.

PERIPHERAL VENOUS CATHETERISATION

The erection of a peripheral venous infusion is one of the common procedures performed in all varieties of units in hospitals. This is frequently done very badly by the most junior doctor who is in a hurry to insert the cannula using inappropriate materials under inadequate circumstances. It is surprising how few doctors have received any instruction of how to insert a cannula into a peripheral vein and to assemble the infusion set. As it is usually accepted that due to continued practice anaesthetists are the most skilled in this technique, it would seem appropriate that all medical students receive some formal tuition when they are studying anaesthesia.

If a patient requires intravenous infusion, this therapy may be required for longer than was originally anticipated and it may be required on more than one occasion. In spite of adequate technique, venous thrombosis may follow catheterisation and it is sensible to start at the most peripheral site and proceed in a proximal direction when further sites are required. If there is any possibility that the patient may require haemodialysis it is important to discuss the problem with the renal physician and surgeon who may stipulate that certain sites should be reserved for the creation of arteriovenous shunts. As infusion in the lower limb is associated with a high incidence of complications, particularly those of a thrombo–embolic nature (Schulte 1969) it should only be used as a last resort. The ideal site is a vein on the back of the hand but if this overlies the wrist the cannula may be dislodged unless the wrist is immobilised. If the veins on the back of the hand are unsuitable, the veins of the forearm are to be preferred to those at the elbow which require immobilisation of the joint after insertion of the cannula. The vein should be chosen when the limb is warm and dependent and after application of a tourniquet. It is surprising how often a vein on the back of the hand which may have been considered too small proves to be suitable after the hand has been immersed in warm water for a few minutes. Veins with tributaries or bifurcations are less mobile and easier to puncture, particularly in the elderly.

After selecting the site for cannulation, a brief explanation of the procedure to be undertaken should be given to the patient. The skin should be cleansed with alcohol around the site of insertion and it is advisable to shave the area in the hirsute. Very few doctors use local anaesthesia before inserting an intravenous cannula. A small quantity (0.2 ml) of 2% lignocaine adequately anaesthetises the skin and it is the puncture of the skin by the needle and overlying cannula that is the most painful feature of intravenous cannulation. For this reason some doctors make a tiny incision in the skin with a scalpel blade. After injection of the anaesthetic, the needle and its cannula should be examined to ensure that they are patent and one can easily be removed from the other. The smallest cannula that is suitable for the required infusion should be selected.

A tourniquet should now be applied proximal to the site of insertion. Although the rubber band type of tourniquet is very convenient for this purpose and is easily released, injudicious application may result in arterial flow into the limb being stopped. If a sphygmomanometer is used, the cuff should be inflated to a pressure of 40 mmHg. The patient should then flex and extend the fingers to pump the veins full of blood. Small veins will often dilate if tapped with a finger. When the vein is suitably distended it should be stretched between the tourniquet proximally and the doctor's hand distally.

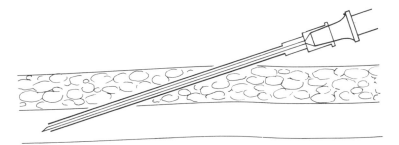

Fig. 9.8 The insertion of an intravenous cannula

Before the needle is inserted it is advisable to ensure that the nurse has primed the infusion set and has prepared some adhesive tape to fix the cannula hub to the skin. The skin should be punctured distal to the site of entry into the vein and if possible the cannula advanced for a few millimetres in the subcutaneous tissue before piercing the vein (Fig. 9.8). The easiest point at which to pierce the vein is in the angle of a bifurcation but this may produce a local haematoma. It is easier to insert the cannula from above the vein than from the side and the bevel of the needle should be orientated accordingly. That the needle and cannula have pierced the vein is confirmed by aspiration or flashback into the bulb. The needle is then withdrawn and the cannula advanced proximally in the vein. It is easier to advance the cannula into the vein if the cuff of the sphygmanometer is still inflated, but there is a greater tendency for leakage of blood to occur from the point of insertion into the vein and from the end of the cannula. This leakage may be controlled by pressure over the point of insertion into the vein. If it is impossible to advance the cannula, the needle should not be re–inserted as this may transect the cannula (Fig. 9.9) with disastrous consequences (Wellmann et al 1968). When the cannula has been inserted to the required depth the cuff of the sphygmomanometer should be deflated and the infusion set connected. The cannula

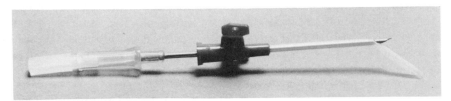

Fig. 9.9 The transection of an intravenous cannula. Although this occurs more frequently when cannulae of the 'through the needle' type are used, it may also occur with cannulae of the 'over the needle' variety as shown here

should be fixed to the skin with tape and a sterile dressing applied over the puncture site in the skin.

CENTRAL VENOUS CATHETERISATION

Catheters may be inserted into the central venous system through veins draining into the superior vena cave or the inferior vena cava. Complications following the insertion of catheters into the inferior vena cava through an approach to the long saphenous vein anterior to the medial malleolus or the long saphenous or femoral veins at the groin are common (Brucke et al 1966, Schulte 1969) and the incidence of pulmonary embolism is high. This method of introducing catheters into the central veins should only be used as a last resort. Catheters may be inserted into the superior vena cava through the basilic, cephalic, subclavian, external and internal jugular veins.

The insertion of a catheter into a central vein is a potentially dangerous procedure and in particular it may allow the entry of bacteria into the bloodstream. The procedure should only be performed when there is an incontrovertible requirement and the catheter should be inserted by an experienced doctor or under expert supervision. It should not be undertaken by an inexperienced doctor without supervision. The insertion should be performed in an aseptic manner. If necessary, the skin overlying the point of access should be shaved and it should always be disinfected. Sterile towels should be draped around this area and the doctor should have scrubbed his hands and be wearing gloves and a mask. Ideally, this procedure should be performed in the operating theatre with full aseptic technique. A co−operative patient makes the procedure much easier to perform and the patient should be given an adequate explanation of what is involved. Anxious patients may be given diazepam (5−10 mg intravenously according to the response). Puncture of the basilic vein at the elbow may be performed without local anaesthesia but the needles required are large and few doctors would relish undergoing the procedure themselves without local anaesthesia. Insertion of catheters at other sites should always be preceded by adequate infiltration of local anaesthetic.

There is disagreement concerning the ideal point for the tip of the central venous catheter when it is being used for intravenous feeding. Some believe that it should be in the right atrium where the nutrients mix with the large volume of blood returning to the heart. However, there have been several episodes of cardiac perforation when the more rigid type of catheter has been used (see above), the majority of patients dying of this complication (Thomas 1969), and the sino−atrial node and the myocardium may be irritated by the hypertonic solutions used for intravenous feeding. Nevertheless, the superior vena cava may also be perforated by a rigid catheter. Such mishaps may be avoided by the use of catheters made of siliconised rubber. When the central veins are catheterised in order to measure central venous pressure, it is unnecessary to advance the catheter beyond the brachiocephalic vein. It would be beneficial if all catheters were marked so that the distance to which they had been inserted could be easily ascertained.

Provided that certain important safety features have been confirmed, the position of the tip of the catheter can be deduced by electrocardiography (Brockle

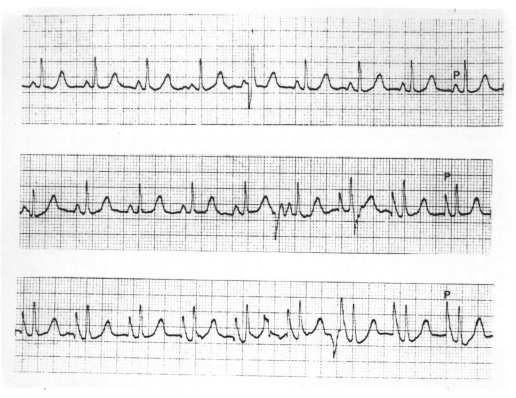

Fig. 9.10 Endocardial electrocardiogram obtained by advancing a saline–filled catheter from the right external jugular vein into the right atrium

hurst et al 1967). If the catheter is filled with saline and its lumen connected to the active electrode of the electrocardiograph by means of a sterile wire it will record a tracing as shown in Figure 9.10. As the catheter is advanced down the superior vena cava and approaches the opening into the right atrium the P wave in particular and also the T wave increase in size. In the right atrium the P wave becomes very large and ultimately, when the tip of the catheter is immediately adjacent to the sino–atrial node, the P wave is taller than the QRS complex as shown in Figure 9.10. Before using this technique it is essential to ensure that the design of the electrocardiographic equipment is such that there is no chance of an electrical short developing between the power supply and the active electrode. Such an occurrence could produce asystole or cardiac arrythmia. Diathermy should not be used during the insertion of the catheter.

Basilic vein
The basilic vein at the elbow offers the simplest access of any vein in the body. Every doctor has obtained venous blood from this site and the insertion of a catheter into the vein is not much more difficult. Nevertheless, there are potential difficulties and occasional serious complications. It is not always possible to advance the catheter beyond the shoulder, even when the arm is abducted to a right angle with the trunk. When this has been accomplished, greater difficulty may be

experienced in advancing the tip of the catheter into the required position in the superior vena cava. The tip of the catheter may often be found in the subscapular, subclavian, external or internal jugular or brachiocephalic veins of the same side and even in the brachiocephalic, subclavian or jugular veins of the opposite side. If the catheter is pushed too far, the tip may pass through the right atrium of the heart into the inferior vena cava or turn back on itself in the superior vena cava. The opening of the superior vena cava into the right atrium is about 40 cm from the right elbow and 45 cm from the left. Only isotonic solutions of electrolytes or glucose should be infused slowly through the catheter until the correct positioning of its tip has been verified radiologically. If the tip of the catheter is incorrectly positioned, it may be possible to manipulate it into the correct position in the superior vena cava or to withdraw the catheter so that its tip lies in the subclavian vein, but sometimes the catheter must be removed and another inserted, usually in the opposite arm. Manipulation of an incorrectly positioned catheter increases the risk of phlebitis and infection and if performed by an inexperienced doctor through a needle, a portion of the catheter may be transected and pass into the circulation (see above). In 54 patients receiving total parenteral nutrition for 3–5 days the tip of the catheter was initially positioned incorrectly by this technique in six patients and it was necessary to remove the catheter and insert another in two of these patients (Tweedle 1974). Phlebitis developed during infusion in five patients and the catheter had to be replaced in three of these patients. Catheters inserted at this site are particularly prone to kinking when the elbow is flexed. This can be prevented by splinting the elbow but prolonged immobilisation of joints should be avoided. In spite of these problems, the introduction of a catheter into a central vein by this route is simple and the incidence of serious complications is lower than those associated with other sites of access. It is the ideal approach to the central veins for the inexperienced.

Cephalic vein

The cephalic vein may be punctured by a needle at the elbow and a catheter advanced in a similar manner to that described above following puncture of the basilic vein. However, the majority of catheters are introduced into the cephalic vein after surgical exposure in the deltopectoral groove and sepsis and thrombosis are more common following this procedure (Maki 1976). The same problem of advancing the catheter is experienced as in the approach through the basilic vein but it is often more difficult to advance the catheter into the subclavian vein due to angulation of the cephalic vein as it passes through the clavipectoral fascia. The opening of the superior vena cava in the right atrium is about 25 cm from the usual site of puncture of the vein on the right and about 30 cm on the left.

Subclavian vein

The veins of the neck are in close apposition to many important structures which may be damaged during faulty catheterisation with considerable morbidity and mortality. Before attempting to catheterise these veins it is necessary to be familiar with their anatomy (Figure 9.11). The subclavian veins begin at the outer border of the first rib and end behind the sternoclavicular joint where they join the internal jugular veins to form the brachiocephalic veins. Both veins arch upwards

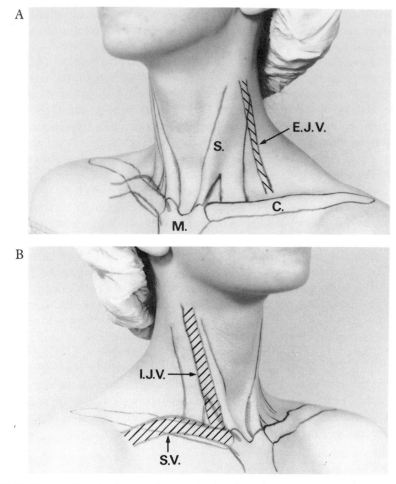

Fig. 9.11 The superficial landmarks of the great veins of the chest and neck

E.J.V. — External jugular vein, I.J.V. — Internal jugular vein, S.V. — Subclavian vein, S.C.M. — Sterno–cleidomastoid muscle, C. — Clavicle, M. — Manubrium

in their course behind the clavicle and the subclavius muscle. The dome of the pleura lies below and behind the vein and the artery is above and behind. On the right side the dome of the pleura is a little lower and on the left side the thoracic duct enters the brachiocephalic vein at its origin so that complications of catheterisation are less likely to occur on the right.

A catheter can be inserted into the subclavian vein from below or from above the clavicle. The infraclavicular approach first described by Aubaniac (1952) is to be preferred to the supraclavicular approach described by Yoffa (1965) as there is less likelihood of damaging the pleura or lung due to the more oblique angle of approach with the needle. Furthermore, as the site of puncture is more lateral with the infraclavicular approach, there is less chance of damaging the thoracic duct on the left and the lymphatic trunk on the right and the subclavian artery is less closely applied to the vein at its lateral extremity. Catheters inserted by the infraclavicular route appear to cause less inconvenience to the patient and sweat does not collect at the site of insertion. As discussed below, the risk of damaging the pleura and the subclavian artery is a little lower using the infraclavicular approach. When performed by a doctor with some experience of the technique, insertion of a catheter into a subclavian vein offers the greatest rate of successful cannulation and it can be performed more rapidly than cannulation of central veins at other sites. The supraclavicular approach may be more rapid than the infraclavicular approach and when urgent resuscitation is required, the doctor may insert a catheter by this method without hindering colleagues who require access to the chest or abdomen.

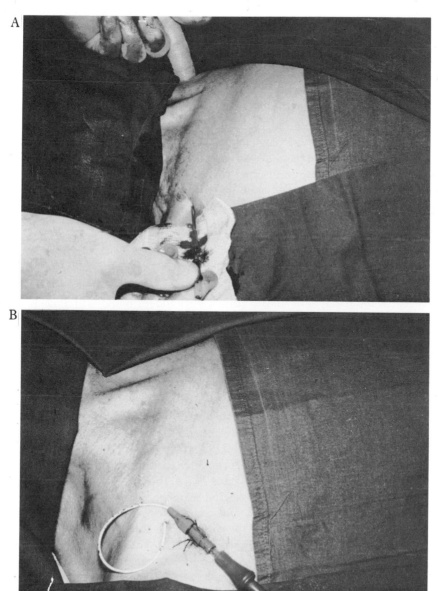

Fig. 9.12 Catheterisation of the subclavian vein by the infraclavicular route

a. Infraclavicular approach

The patient should be supine with the arms by the side and the shoulders raised slightly towards the head to increase the space between the first rib and the clavicle. The body should be tilted a little in the head–down position so that the veins are engorged with blood and the risk of inducing cerebral air embolism is reduced. The head should be turned in the opposite direction. After the usual preparation of the skin and injection of local anaesthetic, the needle should be inserted through the skin immediately below the junction of the lateral third and the medial two thirds of the calvicle. It should be advanced so that its tip is aimed at the scalene tubercle on the first rib which may be palpated by the tip of the index finger of the other hand (Fig. 9.12). Thus the point of the needle is directed slightly superior to the termination of the vein behind the sternoclavicular joint and should penetrate the vein behind the middle third of the clavicle. The needle must pass through the subcutaneous tissue including the platysma and the subclavius muscle before penetrating the vein. The vein is at a depth of 3–6 cm from the site of puncture of the skin. That the vein has been entered is confirmed by aspiration with the syringe. If the needle is maintained closely applied to the clavicle during its insertion, damage to the pleura or artery is unlikely. When the vein has been entered, the cannula or catheter can be advanced and the needle withdrawn. A catheter can be inserted through the cannula if required and the cannula withdrawn so that its tip lies outside the vein but within the subcutaneous tissues. When the catheter is being advanced, it is advisable to turn the patient's head towards the side of insertion and to press on the internal jugular vein as this lessens the chance of the catheter entering this rather than the brachiocephalic vein. The opening of the superior vena cava into the right atrium is 15–20 cm from the site of puncture of the skin on the right and 20–25 cm on the left. If the infusion system is connected to the catheter and the container is lowered to below the height of the patient's shoulder, blood will flow back if the catheter is in the vein. However, the rate of infusion should only be sufficient to prevent clotting within the catheter until its position has been identified radiologically.

b. Supraclavicular approach

The patient should be placed in a similar position to that described above for the infraclavicular approach. When the head is turned towards the opposite shoulder, the sternomastoid muscle becomes prominent and the lateral border of its clavicular head should clearly be identified by palpation and inspection. The needle should puncture the skin in the angle formed by the medial third of the clavicle and the lateral border of the clavicular head of this muscle. The tip of the needle should be at an angle of 45° with the saggital plane pointed towards the posterior aspect of the sternoclavicular joint. In comparison with the infraclavicular approach, there is less tissue between the vein and the skin and the vein is usually 2–3 cm distant from the site of puncture of the skin. When the vein has been punctured, the catheter should be advanced using the same precautions discussed above for the infraclavicular approach. The opening of the superior vena cava into the right atrium is 15–20 cm from the site of puncture of the skin on the right and 20–25 cm on the left.

External jugular vein

The external jugular vein is formed by the confluence of the posterior auricular vein and the retromandibular vein below the angle of the jaw. It runs downwards in a superficial plane passing obliquely over the sternomastoid muscle into the posterior triangle of the neck where it pierces the deep cervical fascia above the mid–point of the clavicle to empty into the subclavian vein (Fig. 9.11). The patient should be positioned as described above for puncture of the subclavian vein. The vein is usually easy to identify and may be distended by compression above the clavicle or by asking the patient to exhale against a closed glottis (Valsalva manoeuvre). The vein may be punctured at any point but it is usual to puncture the skin about the mid-point of its crossing the sternomastoid muscle (Fig. 9.13). There is a valve immediately proximal to the entrance of the vein and it is often difficult to negotiate this valve with the tip of the catheter. Sometimes this may be achieved by abducting the arm at a right angle to the trunk. The entrance of the superior vena cava into the right atrium is 15–20 cm from the usual site of puncture on the right and 20–25 cm on the left. This vein has a thin wall and can be perforated easily by the tip of short rigid cannulae particularly when the patient moves his head. Patients are frequently irritated by catheters inserted in the neck and this is not an ideal site for prolonged catheterisation in a conscious patient. However, it is comparatively easy to insert a catheter in this vein and it is frequently used during anaesthesia and for urgent resuscitation. The pleura and the subclavian and carotid arteries are unlikely to be damaged by insertion of a catheter into this vein.

Internal jugular vein

The internal jugular vein emerges from the base of the skull behind the internal carotid artery and as it runs downwards it comes to lie lateral to the internal and common carotid arteries beneath the sternomastoid muscle. It joins the subclavian vein to form the brachiocephalic vein behind the sternoclavicular joint (Fig. 9.11). The patient should be positioned as described above for puncture of the subclavian vein. The internal jugular vein cannot be seen and before attempting to insert a wide bore needle and catheter, it is often useful to verify its position by aspiration with a fine bore needle. The proximity of the carotid arteries makes many doctors apprehensive when attempting to insert a catheter into this vein and it should not be attempted by the inexperienced. However, those who use this vein regularly argue that it is ideal (Daily et al 1969, Jernigan et al 1970). The right side is preferable to the left as the superior vena cava, brachiocephalic and internal jugular veins are in line and there is less risk of damaging the lymph channel on that side. The internal jugular vein may be punctured from three sites:

a. Posterior border of sternocleidomastoid muscle

The patient should be lying with his head rotated to the opposite side. The carotid artery (and overlying internal jugular vein) are palpated with the finger of the opposite hand and the needle is inserted in the angle made by the external jugular vein and the posterior border of the sternomastoid muscle. It should be directed downwards and at an angle of 30° with the skin in the direction of the medial bor-

A

B

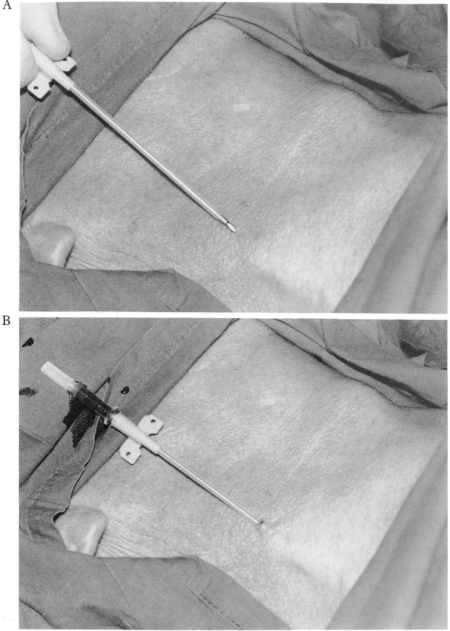

Fig. 9.13 Catheterisation of the external jugular vein

der of the clavicular head of the sternomastoid muscle. When inserting the needle it is useful to remember that the terminal portion of this vein lies behind the triangle formed by the medial end of the clavicle and the sternal and clavicular heads of the sternocleidomastoid muscle. Using this route the vein is usually punctured 3–4 cm beneath the skin.

C

D

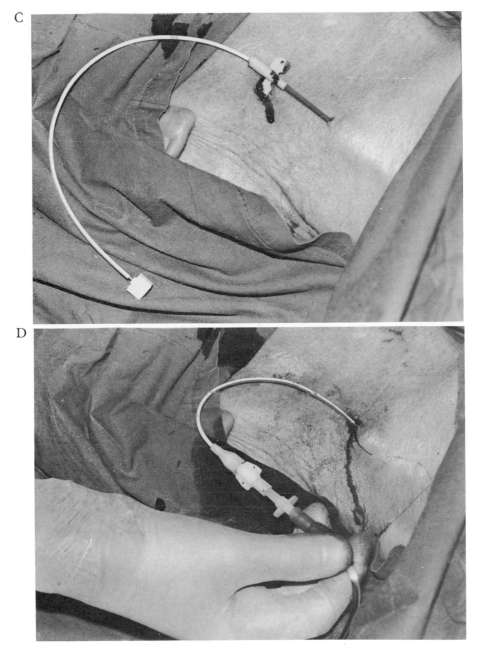

b. Anterior border of sternocleidomastoid muscle
The patient should be lying with his neck well extended by placing a pillow between his shoulders and the head should be rotated towards the opposite side. The needle should be inserted at the anterior border of the sternocleido-mastoid muscle at the level of the thyroid cartilage. It should be inserted la-

A

B

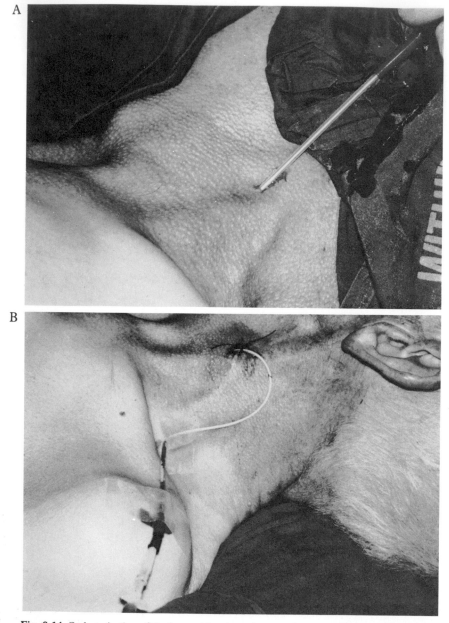

Fig. 9.14 Catheterisation of the internal jugular vein

teral to the common carotid artery which should be palpated with the finger of the
opposite hand and the needle directed towards the nipple on the same side
(Fig. 9.14). The vein is usually punctured 2–3 cm beneath the skin. Although
this approach is more direct than the posterior approach, the catheter emerges
from the anterior triangle of the neck which may be very inconvenient and uncomfortable.

c. Origin of sternocleidomastoid muscle

The internal jugular vein may be punctured at its distal extremity by a needle inserted between the sternal and clavicular heads of the sternocleidomastoid muscle. The patient should be lying with the neck slightly flexed and the head rotated towards the opposite side. The common carotid artery can be palpated within this triangle and the vein lies lateral to it. Although the vein is comparatively superficial at this point it may prove very difficult to puncture. As catheters inserted at this site are inconvenient and uncomfortable and there is a greater risk of damaging lymphatic trunks and pleura, this site is the least suitable for catheterisation of the central veins.

Subcutaneous tunnels

There is evidence to suggest that a large number of patients who develop septicaemia following catheterisation of the central veins are infected by organisms which migrate along the subcutaneous track between the site of puncture of the skin and the vein (see below). Many studies have shown that the incidence of infective complications is related to the length of time that the catheter has been inserted and the complication was a particular problem in patients who required prolonged intravenous feeding to survive, sometimes for the rest of their lives. The incidence of infective complications in this type of patient who manages his own parenteral nutrition in the home has been greatly reduced by creating subcutaneous tunnels so that there is a considerable distance (15–20 cm) between the entrance of the catheter through the skin and the vein (Broviac et al 1973). Although the technique was developed for catheters inserted into the subclavian vein by the infraclavicular approach (Fig. 9.12) it may also be used for catheters inserted into this vein by the supraclavicular approach and into the external and internal jugular veins. Movement of the catheter within the tunnel may be restricted by a cuff of Dacron. This cuff may be important in preventing the migration of organisms along the tunnel (Broviac et al 1973, Powell–Tuck 1980). The catheter may be brought out on the lateral or medial aspect of the thoracic wall. Females with large breasts often find that it is more difficult to connect and disconnect infusion systems when the catheter is brought out laterally. These tunnels were usually created under general anaesthesia in the operating theatre but due to improvements in catheter design with removable hubs many tunnels are now created under local anaesthesia in dressing rooms on the ward. However, strict aseptic technique is essential.

Although there is little doubt that the incidence of septic complications in patients who require prolonged parenteral nutrition in the home has been reduced by this technique, its role in patients requiring less prolonged intravenous feeding in the hospital is less certain and controlled, randomised studies are required. The effect of a subcutaneous tunnel may differ according to its length, the material from which the catheter is made and the type of illness from which the patient is suffering.

SEPSIS

Septicaemia occurring in a patient receiving intravenous infusion may arise from the solution, from the infusion set, from the cannula or catheter, or within the patient. The majority of investigations have concentrated upon the role of cannulae and catheters as this portion of the infusion system appears to be the major cause of septic complications during intravenous infusion. However, in many patients so–called 'catheter–sepsis' has been incorrectly blamed for the origin of the septicaemia when the patient has another, sometimes clinically silent focus. A further difficulty in assessing the incidence and the importance of septic complications of intravenous infusion is in deciding upon the significance of positive microbial cultures in patients who do not exhibit clinical features of sepsis. There are many commensal organisms in the skin such as *Staphyloccus epidermis* and diphtheroids which are not considered to be pathogenic in man and which have been excluded from some analyses. It appears likely that these organisms may become pathogenic in the severely debilitated patient who may be receiving intravenous nutrients. This organism is now isolated more frequently than any other organism from the tips of intravenous cannulae (Sanders & Sheldon 1976, Sitges–Serra et al 1980). However, the significance of positive bacteriological cultures from the tips of catheters is not clear. In one review of 33 studies, the incidence of positive cultures from the catheter varied from 3.8–77% but the incidence of septicaemia varied from 0–18% (Maki et al 1973).

Contamination of solutions during manufacture is fortunately a rare event and delivery of large quantities of these solutions to hospitals should be preventable by the use of suitable methods of inspection at the place of manufacture. The effects of such contamination can be disastrous and because such events are rare may not be considered as the cause of septicaemia in an individual patient (Philips et al 1972). The potential methods by which fluids may be contaminated during manufacture have been discussed above. A much greater potential for contamination of the fluid in the container exists in the increasing requirement for the addition of drugs. Potassium chloride, heparin, antibiotics and a variety of drugs acting on the heart are frequently added to intravenous solutions. Surprisingly there is no clear evidence that such additions are associated with an increase in the incidence of contamination (D'Arcy 1976). Nevertheless, if additives are required, it seems a wise precaution for this to be performed in the pharmacy under sterile conditions.

If all the intravenous drugs required could be prepared in the pharmacy, the incidence of contamination of the infusion set would be reduced but not eliminated. In practice, many drugs must be infused urgently and many pharmacies are unable to meet the large numbers of requests for intravenous preparations. The use of antimicrobial filters does not appear to reduce the incidence of sepsis due to intravenous infusion (see above) and the most practical methods of reducing contamination from this source are to reduce to a minimum the number additives inserted through various parts in the system and to change the infusion set frequently (every 24–48 h). The last step would have considerable economic repercussions and controlled studies are required in large numbers of patients to establish whether such a policy would reduce the incidence of septicaemia due to contamination.

When faced with a patient who has developed septicaemia while being fed intravenously through a central vein, many clinicians would remove the intravenous catheter. In many of these patients the infection has been introduced at the site of catheterisation and in the majority of these the cather is acting as a source of re-infection. If the patient has local inflammation at the site of insertion, *Staphylococcus aureus* is grown from the bloodstream and there is no obvious focus of infection elsewhere in the body then it is highly probable that the catheter is a nidus of infection and should be removed. However, in patients undergoing operations for gastro-intestinal disease who are being fed intravenously, the major cause of septicaemia is septic foci within the gastro-intestinal tract. In these patients the most common organism isolated from the bloodstream is *Escherichia coli* and it is uncommon to isolate this organism from the tip of the catheter. Nevertheless, most cases of septicaemia are due to migration of organisms from the skin to the vein. That direct contamination of the tip of the catheter at the time of insertion is an uncommon cause is suggested by observations that the incidence of septicaemia increases with the length of time that the catheter has been in place, frequently occurring about the third week. If a patient with gastro-intestinal disease develops septicaemia during intravenous feeding and there is no evidence of local inflammation at the site of insertion of the catheter or phlebitis, it is wise to assume that the catheter is not the source of the sepsis and to investigate the patient thoroughly to identify this source. This suspicion is strengthened if an urgent Gram stain of a blood film shows Gram-negative bacilli. In these patients it is usually unnecessary to remove the catheter but if the septicaemia does not respond to such measures as drainage of abscesses and the exhibition of appropriate antibiotics it is wise to remove the catheter. However, in the majority of patients who have failed to respond to these measures, removal of the catheter from the central veins rarely has any effect.

In severely ill patients who have required intravenous feeding for prolonged periods of time, systemic infection with *Candida albicans* may develop (Quie & Curry 1971). Although systemic infection may develop in severely ill patients who are not fed intravenously, the incidence is higher in those who are and can be prevented by instillation of amphotericin (Brennan et al 1972). Intriguingly, the incidence of candidaemia has been far greater in North America than in Europe. Although Candida grows rapidly in mixtures of protein hydrolysates and concentrated carbohydrate solutions that are used more frequently in North America, contamination of intravenous nutrients with Candida is a rare occurrence (Maki 1976). As Candida can frequently be isolated from the skin of patients who have been severely ill for many days, it is likely that the fungus reaches the bloodstream from the site of catheterisation in the same manner as the Staphylococcus. It is often difficult to isolate Candida from the bloodstream and serological tests for antibody titres may take a few days. If retinal lesions are observed (Fishman et al 1972) or blastospores or pseudohyphae identified in blood smears (Portnoy et al 1971) it is advisable to remove the catheter and begin systemic treatment with an antifungal preparation.

If a catheter is removed because it is considered to be the probable cause of septicaemia, the tip should be placed in a sterile container and sent for bacteriological investigation. In addition to obtaining samples of blood from another vein, some doctors also withdraw a specimen of blood for culture through the catheter, hoping to increase the chance of identification of the source of septicaemia. After this the doctor is faced with the dilemma of whether to insert another catheter. If the patient is haemodynamically unstable it may be essential to monitor central venous pressure and there is little choice. If the catheter has been used for intravenous feeding, the majority of patients can withstand the loss of one day's nutrients and it is well worthwhile delaying the re–insertion for 24 h in the hope that adequate levels of antibiotics maintained during this time will reduce the risk of recolonisation of the catheter from organisms in the bloodstream. New catheters should always be inserted at a different site.

There is very little evidence to suggest that the incidence of septicaemia is related to the type of catheter that is used or to the use or otherwise of antimicrobial filters, topical antibiotics or dressings. The creation of subcutaneous tunnels does appear to reduce the incidence of septicaemia, as discussed above. The routine fashioning of subcutaneous tunnels for all central venous catheters would produce impossible demands upon the doctor's time. The incidence of septicaemia from central venous catheterisation is much lower when performed for the recording of central venous pressure than when performed for intravenous feeding and a subcutaneous tunnel is unnecessary for the former purpose. Although it may prove beneficial to insert all central venous catheters for intravenous feeding through a subcutaneous tunnel, it is uncommon to witness septicaemia due to the catheter during the first week.

In many hospitals, a team of doctors, nurses, dietitians and technicians supervise the nutritional requirements of all patients who require specialised enteral or parenteral feeding. The composition of this team and their duties differ from hospital to hospital (Tweedle 1981) but a major role for all teams is to ensure that there is a strict adherence to aseptic technique during the insertion and routine care of the central venous catheter. If the catheter is being used for intravenous feeding it should not be used for occasional measurement of central venous pressure, the giving of intravenous drugs or the taking of blood samples. Although controlled, randomised studies have not been performed, a reduction in the incidence of sepsis has been observed in all the institutions who have established such teams. In one study the incidence of septicaemia due to Candida and Gram–negative organisms fell from 21.2% to zero (Freeman et al 1972).

PHYSICAL COMPLICATIONS

Phlebitis

The commonest complication of peripheral infusion is phlebitis and this will occur when central catheters are inserted through peripheral veins. The incidence of phlebitis is influenced by the pH, the osmolality, the chemical composition of the cannula or catheter (see above) and the length of time it has been inserted. The smallest catheter that is adequate for the required rate of infusion should be selected. There is no clear–cut evidence that the addition of hydrocortisone or heparin to the solution being infused reduces the incidence of phlebitis. The conflicting reports concerning the use of antimicrobial filters has been discussed above. Little is known of the incidence of phlebitis in the central veins. Studies in dogs have demonstrated phlebitis but the major finding was of thrombosis (Welch et al 1974).

Suppurative phlebitis is a rare but frequently lethal infection in the vein, usually produced by *Staphyloccus aureus*. It is more common in patients with burns. In addition to the use of appropriate antibiotics, the vein should be ligated proximal to the affected segment which should be excised (Crane 1960).

Thrombosis

Thrombosis is a common sequel to venepuncture in a peripheral vein. Usually this is of little significance, the thrombosis being restricted to a short segment of vein which becomes a painless, solid cord easily palpable under the skin. Occasionally, the thrombosis extends proximally to involve central veins with profound and sometimes fatal consequences. Although this is particularly likely to occur following insertion of catheters into the veins of the lower limb (Burri & Ahnefeld 1978) it probably occurs more frequently in the upper limb than is often suspected (Ryan et al 1974, Havill & Faracs 1975). The subsequent venous obstruction produces swelling in the affected limb which is distressing to the patient, but the danger lies in progression into the vena cava or embolism into the lungs. The differing thrombogenic properties of catheters of various materials are discussed above.

Pneumothorax and haemothorax

These complications occur most frequently when catheters are inserted into the subclavian vein, particularly by the supraclavicular approach, but may also occur during catheterisation of the internal jugular veins. This complication occurs in about 0.5–2% of attempted venepunctures by these routes but death is uncommon.

Arterial damage

The subclavian artery may be damaged during attempted puncture of the subclavian vein and the carotid arteries during attempted puncture of the internal jugular vein. This complication occurs in about 0.5–1.5% of attempted venepunctures by these routes and is more dangerous than pneumothorax or haemothorax. According to published reports, about one patient in every thousand undergoing attempted catheterisation of the subclavian vein will die from this complication.

Rare complications

The dangers of embolism from fragments of catheters have been stressed above and its particular relationship to the use of catheters inserted through a needle have been emphasised. In some patients thoracotomy has been avoided by transvenous extraction of fragments by a variety of loops, forceps and balloon catheters.

Although air embolism is always a potential danger when catheters are introduced into central veins it is an extremely rare event and usually occurs following puncture of the subclavian vein (Ferrer 1970). Catheters should always be inserted into the subclavian and jugular veins with the patient in the Trendelenburg position.

Cardiac perforation with subsequent pericardial effusion and tamponade is a rare and usually fatal event and is more likely to occur when rigid catheters are used (Henzel & De Weeze 1971). The central veins may also be perforated by the catheter with consequent formation of a haemothorax or hydrothorax.

10

Enteral feeding

If the gastro–intestinal tract is intact, the simplest method of delivering nutrients to its lumen is to ask the patient to ingest them. However, many severely ill patients are anorexic and this may be a particular problem in patients with cancer (De Wys 1977). Abnormalities of taste may contribute to the anorexia experienced by patients with cancer (De Wys & Walters 1975) and to those with zinc deficiency (Hambridge et al 1972). Many patients with partial obstruction in the upper part of the gastro–intestinal tract may be eager to eat but unable to ingest solid food. Many of these patients may be able to ingest partially liquidised food such as minced beef and the majority are able to drink liquid nutrients. If the food must be completely liquidised, the commercial preparations are usually more appealing than a liquidised meal prepared in the hospital. However, some commercial preparations are extremely unpalatable and their taste must be improved by the addition of a variety of flavours. These additions may be made during commercial preparation or by mixing on the ward. Unfortunately, the addition of flavour inevitably increases the osmolarity of the feed, increasing the likelihood of the patient suffering from diarrhoea (see below). Although patients with partial obstruction of the upper gastro–intestinal tract, particularly of the oesophagus, may be unable to drink 100 ml at a time, many are able to maintain a sufficient intake of nutrients by the repeated sipping of smaller quantities throughout the day. If time is taken to explain the problem to the patient, he or she will usually oblige by pouring small quantities from a jug on the bedside locker, particularly when aware that the alternative will involve some method of tube feeding or intravenous feeding.

The indications for nutritional support by either the enteral or parenteral route have been discussed in Chapters 3 and 6. The complications of parental nutrition are more serious than those of enteral nutrition and the utilisation of nutrients is usually more efficient when they are absorbed from the gastro–intestinal tract rather infused into a vein (Tweedle et al 1979). Nutrients infused into the gastro–intestinal tract also have an important trophic effect upon the mucosa (Feldman et al 1973) which is lost during intravenous feeding. The benefits of enteral feeding have been recognised for many years (Masterton et al 1963, McMichael et al 1967) but tube feeding has been used infrequently in the past due to difficulties in the preparation and delivery of an appropriate feed into the appropriate portion of the gastro–intestinal tract. Tube feeding was employed in only 19 patients during a three–month survey performed in 1977 in a teaching hospital containing 854 beds (Tweedle 1980a). It is only during the last three or four years that the technique has become popular with patients, nurses and doctors. This increase in popularity has coincided with improvement in the methods of delivering the feed into the appropriate portion of the gastro–intestinal tract and with the development of commercially prepared nutrients.

NUTRIENTS

A simple approach to the problem of supplying the patient with a well–balanced tube feed is to homogenise the ordinary diet given to the other patients. However, these mixtures are visually unattractive and when infused into the stomach often induce nausea and vomiting. The nasogastric tube frequently blocks when these mixtures are used and it is not possible to infuse them through a narrow gauge tube. An alternative approach is to mix all the nutritional requirements from a variety of commercially available components in a diet kitchen or pharmacy (Woolfson et al 1976, Tweedle et al 1979). The components usually include a protein hydrolysate, a glucose polymer and additional minerals and vitamins. To reduce the osmolarity of the mixture, some non–protein energy can be provided by medium chain triglycerides and essential fatty acids can be supplied by adding one egg yolk to the mixture each day. This method allows much greater flexibility than using commercially prepared mixtures but nurses and dietitians (and sometimes pharmacists) must spend a considerable time in preparing the mixture and supervising its infusion (Woolfson et al 1976). Although the cost of such mixtures is considerably less than elemental diets (Tweedle et al 1979), the cost is now a little more than that of commercially prepared mixtures containing whole protein. Nutrients prepared in the diet kitchen may also be contaminated with bacteria (Casewell & Philips 1978) and consequently, most hospitals now use commercially prepared mixtures.

The requirements for protein, carbohydrate, fat, elements and vitamins in health and disease have been discussed in Chapters 1, 3 and 8. Some specific problems related to the provision of these requirements in tube feeds are discussed below.

During the last decade, it has been recognised that complete hydrolysis of protein to free amino acids is unnecessary for adequate absorption of protein to occur (Silk 1979), much relevant information having been ignored. Rose (1949) had demonstrated that if the same quantity of amino acids was supplied as whole protein, nitrogen balance was improved when compared with that achieved if free amino acids were given. Subsequently, it was shown that dipeptide could be taken up by the enterocyte (Newey & Smyth 1962) and it was emphasised that food is present in the lumen of the small intestine for an insufficient length of time for the liberation of all the free amino acids from the protein (Fisher 1954). Nevertheless, during this time so–called 'chemically defined' or 'elemental' diets were developed in which the protein content was in the form of free amino acids. These diets are more expensive than those containing whole protein or peptides and they are more likely to induce nausea, vomiting and diarrhoea. In spite of the addition of various flavours, elemental diets are very unpalatable to the majority of healthy subjects and patients (Gallagher & Tweedle 1981). In the vast majority of patients, a preparation containing whole protein is preferable as the source of nitrogen. Elemental diets may be useful in a few patients with a severe reduction in capacity for luminal hydrolysis due to disease of the exocrine pancreas or the small bowel syndrome. If whole protein is provided, deficiencies of individual amino acids are unlikely and the amino acids will be l-isomers (see Ch. 8). If elemental diets are used the content of cysteine and methionine may be inadequate. These amino acids contain sulphur and their taste is particularly unpleasant. Commercial preparations containing essential amino acids only have been developed for use in patients with renal failure. Their role has been discussed in detail in Chapter 7.

Carbohydrate
Carbohydrate is the major source of non–protein in enteral feeds. As in intravenous feeding, the low calorific value of glucose (17 kJ/g) is a disadvantage and enteral infusion of large quantities of glucose will induce dumping, abdominal distension and diarrhoea. Consequently the majority of enteral diets contain disaccharides, oligosaccharides and glucose polymers in addition to glucose. In this way an equivalent quantity of energy can be infused in a solution with a lower osmolarity. Hydrolysis of these polymers, disaccharides and oligosaccharides yields predominantly glucose and if this hydrolysis does not occur too quickly, this glucose is absorbed and diarrhoea will not occur. A high proportion of Asian and African subjects have inadequate concentrations of lactase in the brush border of the small intestine to digest lactose in the diet (Simoons 1969) and milk or products made from milk should not be included in enteral feeds for this population. Lactose intolerance is far less common in Europeans, occurring in about 6% of the population in England (Neale 1968). There is insufficient knowledge of the rate of hydrolysis of disaccharides and oligosaccharides but maltose would appear to be an ideal disaccharide for enteral nutrition (McMichael et al 1967, Cook 1973). Regardless of the type of carbohydrate used, hyperglycaemia may occur when carbohydrate is the predominant source of non–protein energy.

Fat
Although the use of fat as a source of non–protein allows an equivalent quantity of energy to be infused in a feed with a lower osmolarity, many feeds prepared commercially or in the diet kitchen do not contain fat. In mixtures prepared in the diet kitchen, fat may form an unattractive layer on top of the mixture. Some fats may induce nausea and any indigested fat in the diet may produce steatorrhoea. This is particularly likely to occur in patients with pancreatic and biliary disease.

The majority of the triglycerides in food are long chain triglycerides, particularly esters of palmitic acid (16 carbon atoms) and stearic acid (18 carbon atoms). Long chain triglycerides cannot be absorbed intact by the small intestine. Under the influence of pancreatic lipase and in the alkaline milieu of the small intestine, the triglycerides undergo total hydrolysis to free fatty acids and glycerol or partial hydrolysis to monoglycerides. They are then absorbed through the brush border as micelles. The formation of micelles requires bile salts. Within the mucosa the majority of monoglycerides, free fatty acids and glycerol undergo re–esterifaction and the triglycerides enter the lymphatic system to reach the circulation via the lymphatic duct. Medium chain triglycerides such as esters of caprylic acid (8 carbon atoms) and capric acid (10 carbon atoms) do not require intraluminal hydrolysis and the formation of micelles for their absorption. They may be absorbed intact by the mucosa of the small intestine in the absence of biliary and pancreatic secretion. In the mucosa the medium chain triglycerides are hydrolysed and the free fatty acids and glycerol enter the portal vein. Medium chain triglycerides from coconut oil are used to provide non–protein energy in some commercially prepared diets. In addition, these diets contain a small quantity of the essential fatty acids, linoleic and linolenic acid.

Non-protein energy/nitrogen ratio
The necessity of supplying sufficient quantities of non–protein energy to ensure adequate utilisation of the source of protein has been discussed in Chapter 8. Many commercial enteral diets are available in differing concentrations. In some diets an increase in the quantity of protein is not accompanied by an increase in the non–protein energy content in order to lessen the increase in osmolarity. In these preparations the non–protein energy/nitrogen ratio may be as low as 500 kJ/g N (120 kcal/g N) and it is likely that much of the protein is broken down for energy. The importance of supplying adequate quantities of non–protein energy with the protein in tube feeds was emphasised by Masterton et al (1963). A syndrome including hypernatraemia, hyperchloraemia, uraemia and dehydration may occur when this type of enteral diet is infused (Kaminski 1976) and it is comparable to the hyperosmolar, non–ketotic coma that may occur following enteral or parenteral infusion of concentrated solutions of glucose.

Minerals and vitamins
All the commercial preparations contain sodium, potassium, chloride and phosphate ions. The majority provide between 40 and 100 mmol of sodium in the quantities given each day and this is usually sufficient for the patients who can be fed enterally. Patients whose daily losses exceed this often require feeding by the intravenous route. In patients with renal failure, the higher intakes may be excessive and the preparations containing little sodium should be used in these patients. Not all the commercial products contain calcium and magnesium and it may be necessary to add these supplements. The iron, trace element and vitamin content of commercial products varies considerably and additional supplements may be required. Although tablets and capsules of iron salts may induce constipation, solutions of iron often have the opposite effect.

CONTAINERS

Commercial nutrients may be supplied as powder in tins or packets or as liquid in cans or bottles. It is possible to infuse some liquid nutrients direct from the bottle but the powder must be mixed with water and then infused from another container.

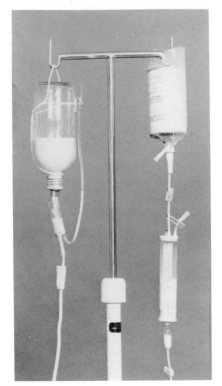

Fig. 10.1 Enteral feeding from a can or Winchester bottle

Cans

If the nutrient in the can is liquid it may be possible to make a hole in the top of the can and to insert a rubber bung which can be pierced by the needle of an infusion set (Fig. 10.1) but there is frequently leakage of the contents between the rubber bung and the rim of the hole. It is not possible to observe how much of the contents remains to be infused and as much as 15% of the volume of the liquid may be left in the can because of the length of the piercing needle of the infusion set. Because of these disadvantages it is likely that this system will be superseded by those discussed below.

Plastic bags

A variety of plastic bags (Fig. 10.2) are available from which enteral nutrients may be infused. Some are extremely pliable, like polyethylene bags in everyday use. Others are less flexible and some are very rigid. All have the advantage of allowing visual inspection of their contents. The majority of plastic containers have a scale printed on the external surface to indicate the volume contained. As they are less distensible and deformable, the volume can be determined more accurately in the rigid containers. The volume of the containers varies. Some have a volume of only 500 ml whereas others will contain 3 litres. The latter variety have sufficient volume to hold the total daily requirement of most patients. However, 3 litres of enteral nutrients weigh more than 3 kg and mobile patients often find this unwieldy and occasionally unmanageable. Some plastic containers

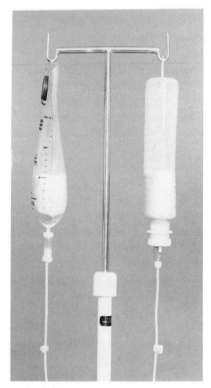

Fig. 10.2 Enteral feeding from plastic bags

have an integral infusion set, others accept standard infusion sets of simplified design for enteral feeding. Enteral nutrients make ideal culture media for bacteria and plastic containers should not be re–used.

Bottles
Enteral nutrients may be infused from Winchester bottles (DHSS codes 4168 and 4169) using a modified bladder irrigation set with a screw connector which fits the bottles (Fig. 10.1). These bottles may be re–used after adequate sterilisation. Some commercial nutrients are now available in bottles to which an infusion set may be attached (Fig. 10.3) by either screwing or clipping the cap of the set to the bottle. If the nutrient does not require dilution, this system offers the simplest and least time–consuming method of preparation and infusion and can easily be managed by the patients as well as the nurses. The infusion set should be changed every day. The bottles may contain 235 ml or 500 ml of nutrients. The latter require less frequent changing, but are not too large to be uncomfortably heavy even when suspended with an infusion pump from the shoulder (see below).

NASO–ENTERAL TUBES

Enteral nutrients may be infused through the standard Ryle's tube used for naso-gastric aspiration after abdominal operations. However, these tubes are uncom-

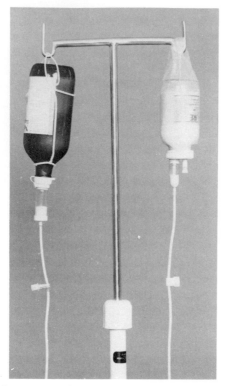

Fig. 10.3 Enteral feeding from commercial bottles

fortable for the patient as they are made of polyvinyl chloride which hardens on contact with digestive juices. A variety of tubes have been designed specifically for naso–enteral feeding (Fig. 10.4). Some are made of polyurethane or silastic which are softer and more pliable than polyvinyl chloride. Some are coated with a special lubricant so that the surface remains slippery during use. Naturally, the smaller the diameter of the tube, the less likely it will be to irritate the nose, pharynx or oesophagus. Very fine bore tubes with an internal diameter of 1 mm have been developed but not all enteral nutrients can be infused through these very fine tubes. Many patients have been fed through the same naso–enteral tube for five or more weeks. Not all the tubes are long enough to reach the duodenum or beyond so that the nutrients must be infused into the stomach (see below). Another disadvantage with some tubes is their radiolucency. It is often a great advantage to be able to discern the entire length of the tube upon X–ray. The incorporation of a small balloon containing mercury at the end of the tube makes regurgitation of the tube much less likely, particularly if the distal end of the tube is beyond the pylorus. The distal end of tubes that contain these weighted balloons are less likely to be regurgitated from the duodenum into the stomach. The nutrient emerges from either a single orifice at the end of the tube or from a number of orifices along the side of the tube. A tube with a single orifice may be more likely to blockage, but too many orifices may also be a disadvantage if infusion into the duodenum is required without infusion into the stomach. The proximal end is usually made with a Luer connection. If naso–enteral tubes were made

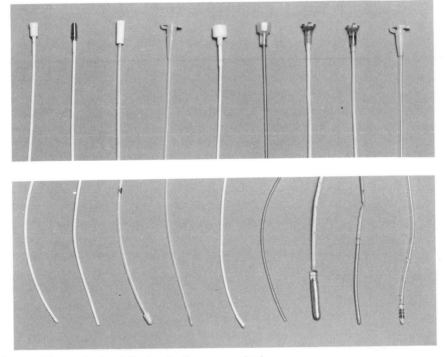

Fig. 10.4 The proximal and distal ends of naso–enteral tubes

with a male connector it would hopefully ensure that inadvertent connection of a naso–enteral infusion system to an intravenous catheter would be very unlikely. However, such a system would require the manufacture of infusion sets and syringes (for aspiration and insufflation) with female connectors. The use of Luer connections incorporating a locking mechanism would lessen the chances of disconnection during infusion but the use of such a mechanism would increase the chances of the tube being pulled out if the infusion system is disturbed accidentally.

Insertion
Enteral nutrients may be infused through tubes inserted through the nose or through those inserted at operation and which enter the gastro–intestinal tract by means of a pharyngostomy, gastrostomy or jejunostomy. Many patients become very apprehensive at the thought of having a tube inserted through the nose. Some argue forcibly that they would prefer to swallow the tube after insertion into the mouth and a few proclaim that they could not tolerate the procedure regardless of the site of insertion. If the tube is inserted through the mouth, inflammation and excoriation of the angle of the mouth begins in a few hours. Very few individuals are unable to tolerate transnasal insertion, particularly after careful explanation of the procedure. It is often useful to show the patient that he or she can breathe adequately through one nostril and to allow the patient to feel the pliability of the tube to be inserted. If possible, the lubricated tube should always be passed with the patient sitting upright. During insertion into the nasopharynx,

the tube should be pushed gently in a horizontal plane, not upwards. When the distal end has reached the nasopharynx, the patient should swallow as the tube is inserted further. At this point it is often useful to rotate the tube and some patients find it easier to swallow the tube with sips of water sucked through a straw. Most naso–enteral tubes have external markings to indicate the length of tube that has been inserted. Although the distance may vary according to the build of the patient, the distance from the incisors to the oesphagogastric junction is usually about 40 cm. If it is intended to infuse the nutrients into the stomach, transnasal insertion of 50 cm is usually sufficient. The tube should never be advanced forcibly against resistance. If resistance is encountered, the tube should be pulled back a little way and further attempts made to advance it to the required distance. If the patient begins to cough violently or to choke the tube may be coiling in the pharynx or it may have entered the larynx. In an unconscious patient, cyanosis may occur. Regardless of the state of consciousness, a fine bore tube may occasionally be inserted into the trachea without any reaction from the patient.

If naso-enteral infusion is required, the tube must be inserted to greater length. Approximately 75 cm is usually sufficient to reach the duodenum. Although feeding tubes, particularly those with a mercury balloon at the end, may pass spontaneously from the stomach into the duodenum after some hours, this occurs in less than half the patients. If the patient's condition permits, it is preferable to insert the tube into the duodenum under radiological observation using an internal guide wire. Many of the manufacturers supply guide wires designed for their tubes. However, these are often very expensive. Most radiological departments have a ready supply of suitable guide wires discarded after arterial catheterisation. After lubrication these wires may be inserted into all but the narrowest tubes, but care must be taken to ensure that the tip of the wire does not protrude through one of the side holes of the tube. Using this technique, it is often possible to insert a feeding tube into the duodenum beyond a gastric fistula and to feed the patient enterally. If it proves impossible to pass a feeding tube through an oesophageal stricture it may be possible to pass a flexible endoscope through the stricture (particularly after dilatation) and to insert a narrow gauge tube into the stomach alongside the endoscope (Atkinson et al 1979). The end of the tube is grasped with biopsy forceps inserted through the biopsy channel and drawn into the distal end of the endoscope during insertion. When the endoscope has been passed into the stomach, the biopsy forceps are pushed into the lumen and the tip of the feeding tube is released before withdrawing the endoscope. A guide wire should not be inserted into the feeding tube during insertion, but it is possible to insert the wire into the tube after its release from the forceps, before removal of the endoscope. Inadvertent removal of the feeding tube when the endoscope is withdrawn will be avoided by this technique.

After inserting the tube into the stomach or beyond, a small quantity of air should be introduced using a syringe as the patient's abdomen is auscultated with a stethoscope. The familiar burbling sound should be heard. The proximal end of the tube may produce intestinal fluid. The proximal end of the tube should then be fastened securely to the skin of the face using tape. It is usual to pass the tape round the tube and to fasten it either to the nose or to the cheek. As an additional safeguard a loop of the tube should be passed around the ear and fastened to the cheek. Although the auscultation of insufflated air and the aspiration of intestinal contents makes infusion into the lungs or pleural, mediastinal or peritoneal cavities most unlikely, most doctors prefer to confirm the position of a radio–opaque tube by radiology before beginning an infusion.

If it is considered likely that naso–enteric feeding will be required after operation, the surgeon can help the anaesthetist to advance a feeding tube introduced during operation into the jejunum. If a narrow gauge tube is used it is possible to insert it and a nasogastric tube for aspiration through the same nostril. It is inadvisable to insert naso–enteric tubes through both nostrils as this may impair air entry. If a tube of larger diameter is inserted at operation, it may be brought out through the oropharynx just below the angle of the jaw (Graham & Royster, 1967). Patients find this method of feeding through a pharyngostomy to be very comfortable. The tube may be fixed to the skin using a purse–string suture (Fig. 6.1) making the technique ideal for patients such as those with oesophageal anastomoses in whom the re–insertion of a feeding tube may be hazardous.

An alternative method of introducing the feeding tube to the gastro–intestinal tract at operation is to create a gastrostomy or preferably a jejunostomy may be a particularly appropriate site for enteral feeding distal to the anastomoses of major resections in the upper gastro–intestinal tract. However, a gastrostomy or jejunostomy requires the creation of an unnatural opening in the gastro–intestinal tract and the abdominal wall and the presence of a tube in the peritoneal cavity. Ideally, the site of insertion into the stomach or the jejunum should be sutured to the opening in the abdominal wall so that the length of the tube in the peritoneal cavity may be reduced to an absolute minimum. In spite of this precaution, the incidence of complications following the creation of a jejunostomy is greater than is often appreciated (Delaney et al 1977). The most dangerous complication that may follow the creation of a gastrostomy or jejunostomy is leakage of gastric or jejunal contents into the peritoneal cavity and subsequent peritonitis. Other complications include volvulus of the gut, intestinal obstruction, haemorrhage and failure of the jejunostomy to close spontaneously when the tube is removed. Because of these complications, gastrostomy or jejunostomy should be used only when particularly appropriate following major upper gastro–intestinal operations or in patients in whom the feeding tube cannot be introduced naturally through the nose or the oropharynx.

INFUSION

If the gastro–intestinal tract has not been in use because of peritonitis or following operation, it is advisable to start the infusion with water at a slow rate (50 ml/ h for example). If this infusion is tolerated without unexpected complication for 3–4 hours, the infusion of nutrients can be started. The nutrients should be diluted to one–quarter strength on the first day, one–half strength on the second day and full–strength nutrient should not be infused until the third day. These infusions should be at the rate of 50 ml/h for these three days and may be increased to the required intake over the next five days. If full–strength nutrients are infused at the rate of required intake on the first day, the majority of patients will suffer from diarrhoea. The incidence of this complication will be reduced if the above regimen is used which corresponds to the normal restitution of oral intake following operation. Few patients can tolerate the infusion of nutrients in volumes sufficient to supply more than 8.36 MJ/d (2000 kcal/d). If greater quantities of energy are required it may be necessary to supply these intravenously and severely malnourished patients may benefit from feeding by both routes. The nutrients should be infused constantly during day and night. The incidence of diarrhoea and other complications is greatly reduced when compared with that observed during bolus infusion (Woolfson et al 1976, Tweedle et al 1979). These complications may be further reduced if the rate of infusion is controlled by an infusion pump.

Many clinicians use infusion pumps for enteral infusions (Dobbie & Hoffmeister 1976), but it has been observed that the majority of patients may be given continuous infusion without the need for this added sophistication (Jones et al 1980). As might have been expected this study also demonstrated that although diarrhoea and abdominal pain and distension due to osmolar overload may respond to improved regulation of infusion with a pump, regurgitation and aspiration persist. Fluctuations in the rate of infusion of nutrients containing large quantities of carbohydrate may also produce hyperglycaemia and the incidence of this complication is likely to be reduced by the use of an infusion pump. Blockage of the feeding tube is very uncommon when an infusion pump is being used.

Table 10.1 Enteral infusion pumps

Manufacturer	Infusion range (ml/h)	Battery life (h)	Weight (kg)	Dimensions (cm)
Viomedex®	25–200	70	0.8	20.0 × 8.5 × 7.0
Vygon®	0–300	4	3.	21.6 × 17.6 × 11.3
Roussel®	25–250	7	1.4	11.6 × 11.3 × 7.7

Infusion pumps for enteral feeding require less sophistication than those used for intravenous feeding and, consequently, they are usually less bulky (Table 10.1). The control of the rate of infusion does not need to be as accurate and the very low rates of infusion required for the intravenous infusion of drugs are unnecessary. Consequently, the pumps do not monitor the rate of their infusion as occurs with intravenous infusion. Their accuracy varies by up to 10% of the selected rate, which is sufficient for enteral infusion. Some pumps are built with audible and visual alarms that are activated if the infusion system becomes blocked. The range of infusion varies from 25–300 ml/h. The pumps work by compressing a tubular insert and the rate of flow may be different to that selected if a tubular insert is used that differs from that designed for the pump. The power may be obtained from the mains or from rechargeable batteries. The life of these batteries varies from 4–70 hours depending upon the rate of infusion. The shorter–lived batteries may limit the time that the patient is ambulant. A warning light indicates when the battery requires recharging and this can be achieved from the mains supply during use. The weight and size of the pumps may also restrict ambulation. Using a compact, light pump and a convenient infusion system it is possible to construct a small carrying frame so that the entire system may be sus-

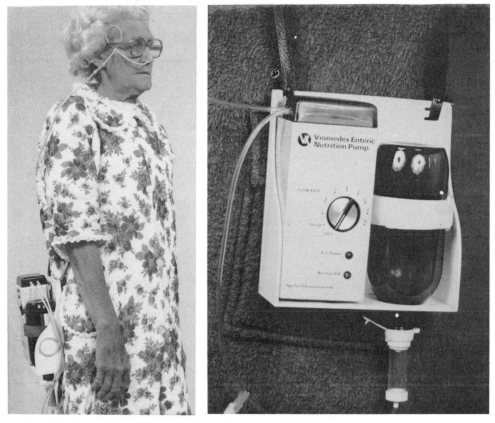

Fig. 10.5 Carrying frame for pump–assisted naso–enteral infusion

pended from the shoulder (Fig. 10.5) allowing the patient to use both arms (Gallagher et al 1981). If such a system is unavailable or the patient is unable to bear the weight, the pump and the infusion system should be fixed to a mobile stand and the patient encouraged to push the stand. Most patients can be taught how to use an infusion pump and, if necessary, they can be used at home.

COMPLICATIONS

Although the incidence of complications produced by the use of a rigid Ryle's tube have been considerably reduced by the introduction of pliable tubes of smaller diameter, a few patients may still complain of a dry mouth or sore throat and nurses should pay particular attention to the oral hygiene of patients with naso–enteral tubes. This problem is more likely to occur in patients who also require endotracheal intubation. Oesophagitis, ulceration and stricture are also less likely to occur when these tubes are used, but the physical attributes of the tube do not produce the inflammation, which is caused by reflux of acid from the stomach through the incompetent lower oesophageal sphincter. Aspiration following reflux is a dangerous complication that is more likely to occur in the unconscious patient.

In addition to aspiration of refluxed nutrient, the very narrow tubes may be regurgitated into the pharynx with comparative ease and continued infusion in an unconscious patient would be extremely dangerous. Infusion of nutrients directly into the lung may occur if the tube is passed into the trachea. This may occur in the conscious patient but is more likely to follow intubation of an unconscious individual. Although radiological examination may confirm that the distal end of the tube is in the required part of the gastro–intestinal tract, infusion into the peritoneal cavity may occur if there is leakage from an adjacent suture line. When this occurs, the signs and symptoms of peritoneal irritation may be less evident than might be expected and most patients develop a localised abscess that requires surgical drainage. If leakage is suspected from the nature of the fluid being drained from the abdomen, this may be confirmed by infusing a small volume of a dilute solution of methylene blue. If this appears in the drainage, enteral infusion and any oral intake should be stopped and intravenous feeding begun. The fistula frequently heals without the need for surgical intervention (Tweedle 1980a).

In the past, the use of homogenised food or mixtures of nutrients prepared in the diet kitchen often produced nausea, belching of foul–smelling gas and even vomiting. The incidence of these complications is far lower when commercial preparations containing whole protein are used. However, elemental diets may provoke reflex vomiting or gastric stasis even in unconscious patients (Jones et al 1980). The incidence of these complications is reduced to a very low level if the nutrients are infused distal to the pylorus, but even then an occasional patient will complain of tasting the feed (Gallagher et al 1981). In some patients, these symptoms may be alleviated by metoclopramide.

Intestinal colic and abdominal distension are more likely to occur in patients who have not received enteral nutrients for a few days, particularly when undiluted solutions are infused into the small intestine. The incidence of these complications is reduced if infusion is begun with dilute solutions and they may also be alleviated by metaclopramide. Although in one study enteral infusion on the first day after major gastro–intestinal operations produced few complications (Sagar et al 1979) in another study the incidence of colic and abdominal distension on the first two days after operation severely restricted the quantity of nutrients that could be infused (Gallagher et al 1981).

Hyperglycaemia during enteral feeding may be more common than has previously been suspected and the blood glucose concentration should be measured regularly. Patients who have not received enteral carbohydrate may be intolerant of glucose (Himsworth & Kerr 1939) and glucose tolerance is impaired after injury (see Ch. 3). Hyperosmolar, hyperglycaemic non–ketotic dehydration may occur during enteral feeding (Kaminski 1976). This complication was observed by Engel & Jaeger (1954) and was formerly known as the 'tube feeding syndrome'. It is produced by the rapid absorption of excessive quantities of glucose from the gastro–intestinal tract with subsequent hyperglycaemia and glycosuria. It is less likely to occur if the nutrients are infused continuously throughout the day and night and if the initial infusions are diluted. A few patients require exogenous insulin during enteral infusion. If an excessive quantity of glucose is infused enterally but not absorbed, the patient may suffer from the classical symptoms of the early dumping syndrome.

Diarrhoea is the most frequent complication of enteral feeding. It is less likely to occur when whole protein is used and may be particularly evident following infusion of mixtures of amino acids which are hypertonic. Hypertonicity may also be due to the concentration of glucose in the feed. As it is increasingly recognised that the initial infusions should be of diluted nutrients and that infusion should be continuous throughout the day and night, the incidence of osmolar diarrhoea should be reduced to a minimum, particularly when the rate of infusion is regulated by a pump. Another common cause of diarrhoea is antibiotics. This is particularly likely to occur if the antibiotics are given orally when the change in the bacterial flora of the gastro–intestinal tract may be considerable. However, it may also occur when antibiotics are given parenterally. If antibiotics are suspected as a cause of diarrhoea, careful consideration should be given to changing the method of administration, changing the type of antibiotics or stopping treatment with antibiotics. Ampillicin given by mouth is particularly likely to cause diarrhoea. The possibility that the diarrhoea is infective in origin should always be borne in mind. Disaccharidase deficiency is uncommon in Europe, but lactose intolerance may cause diarrhoea in Asians receiving nutrients containing milk products (see above). Although medium chain triglycerides should be absorbed without digestion, they may produce diarrhoea if infused in excessive quantities. Tablets and capsules containing iron usually cause constipation, but some patients may suffer from diarrhoea when given liquid forms of iron.

As there may be many causes of diarrhoea, treatment of this complication may differ according to the cause. However, if it is due to enteral feeding, diarrhoea may often be controlled by a temporary reduction in the rate of infusion combined with the giving of 30 mg of codeine phosphate syrup every four hours as a bolus down the tube (Tweedle et al 1979).

11

Paediatrics

The infant and child differ from the adult in many respects. It is evident that size and body proportions are different and in health changes in body size and proportion take place by growth at a remarkable pace. The younger the child the more rapid and evident are such changes. Growth in different tissues and organs takes place mainly by cell division and the rate of cell division within a particular tissue is dependent upon the genetic control of the cell nucleus, the provision of a well–balanced and adequate supply of nutrients and freedom from insult and injury. A deficient or inappropriate supply of nutrients or a disease process can interrupt the genetic potential for a particular tissue and result in a permanent cellular and functional deficit in that tissue. Although many organs in the developing child have a remarkable capability for compensatory growth at a later stage, the risk of permanent deficit increases the earlier in life that cell division is inhibited and the greater the duration of the inhibition. Intellectual as well as physical stature may be stunted by starvation, insult and injury.

BODY COMPOSITION

Infants are not all born nutritionally equal. Some have starved in utero because of maternal or placental dysfunction and some venture from the uterus prematurely and do not carry the reserves of nutrient which normal term infants possess. Table 11.1 shows the body compositions of two representative preterm infants who have grown appropriately in utero but were delivered at 28 and 34 weeks respectively and of a normal term (40 weeks) infant. The relative excess of water in the more immature infant is related to the larger ratio of extracellular to intracellular fluid. As cell division proceeds, so the relative amount of extracellular water diminishes. In the 28–week infant water constitutes 85% of the body weight and 50% of this is extracellular. At term, water comprises 69% of total body weight and about 40% of the total body weight is extracellular water. A relative excess of water in the preterm infant confers no protection against dehydration since that infant's surface area is relatively greater than the mature infant and the obligatory daily turnover of water is equal to 15–20% of the total body water pool. The relatively large surface area in younger infants is shown by the decrease in surface area/body weight ratio in Table 11.2

The relative mineral contents of the preterm and term infant are shown in Table 11.1 which demonstrates that for most minerals there is a considerable in-

Table 11.1 Body composition in preterm and term infants at birth (BW = body weight)

Gestation (weeks):	28	34	40
Body weight (g)	1000	2500	3500
Fat (g)	10	170	530
Fat–free body weight (g)	990	2330	2970
Extracellular water (g)	520	1088	1400
Total water (g)	850	1875	2400
Total water (g/kg fat–free BW)	859	805	808
Total water (g/kg total BW)	850	750	686
Carbohydrate (g)	5	14	34
Protein (g)	85	250	390
Minerals[a]			
Sodium (mmol)	94	200	286
Potassium (mmol)	42	108	185
Chloride (mmol)	68	139	192
Calcium (g)	6.3	19	33.6
Phosphorus (g)	3.9	11.9	19.6
Magnesium (g)	0.2	0.58	0.91
Iron (mg)	65	200	229
Copper (mg)	3.4	8.8	16.4
Zinc (mg)	20	40	70

[a] Expressed in terms of fat–free body tissue and adapted from data of Widdowson & Dickerson (1964)

crease, relative as well as absolute, in the mineral content in the six week period between 28 and 34 weeks and again between 34 and 40 weeks gestation. The distribution of minerals is changing as the ratio between intracellular and extracellular fluid compartments alter and different tissues have differing contents of minerals; high concentrations of calcium, phosphorus and sodium are found in bone and high concentrations of iron and copper in liver. Minerals not shown include suphur, chromium, selenium, molybdenum, manganese, cobalt, iodine and fluorine which increase with maturation. These are elements known to be involved in essential metabolic processes.

Water–soluble vitamins B and C transfer readily from mother to fetus so that term tissue concentrations of these vitamins exceed maternal. Fat–soluble vitamin concentrations (vitamins A — retinol, D — cholecalciferol, E — tocopherol, and K — phytylmenaquinone) are not as great as those found in adults and because of their high rates of utilisation and low initial values, the infant can quickly run into deficit unless an adequate intake is assured.

Perhaps the most striking feature in the body composition of the preterm compared to the term infant is the total energy content. Of the total energy in the

Table 11.2 Relationships between surface area (SA) and body weight (BW) in infant, child and adult

Bodyweight (kg)	SA (M^2)	SA:BW
2	0.15	0.075
3	0.20	0.067
5	0.25	0.050
10	0.45	0.045
20	0.80	0.040
50	1.50	0.030
70	1.75	0.025

1 kg preterm infant, 350 kcal (1.47 MJ) are contained in protein and 110 kcal (0.46 MJ) in fat and carbohydrate. In term infants the total non–protein energy reserves are approximately 5000 kcal (21 MJ) or 1430 kcal (6 MJ)/kg. The fat and carbohydrate in the preterm infant are almost entirely structural and in the absence of fresh nutrient supply tissue breakdown must commence within hours and growth must cease. There is also virtually no reserve of free amino acids in the infant's tissues and tissue protein breakdown must commence very quickly. In term infants delay in feeding is less critical because of the larger non–protein energy reserves but again as there is little reserve of free amino acid in body, new functional peptides and proteins such as hormones and enzymes can only be obtained through the destruction of structural proteins in organs such as muscle and liver.

After oxygen requirements have been met the next immediate need for survival in the newborn infant is an adequate supply of water. It has been calculated that the 28–week gestation infant might survive for three to four days, the 40–week infant 30 days, and a well–nourished adult 90 days if supplied with water alone. Growth cannot take place until a minimum balanced fluid and nutrient intake supplying at least 110 kcal (0.46 MJ)/kg per day is achieved. In starvation a minimal catabolic energy release of 76 kcal (0.32 MJ)/kg per day is necessary to maintain life. Once growth is established there is a gradual change in body water and mineral distribution and the composition of carbohydrate, fat and protein towards the final adult structure.

Blood volume

The blood volume in the infant and child is relatively greater than in the adult. During the first year of life this is about 85 ml/kg, between 2 and 5 years 80 ml/kg, and 75 ml/kg between 6 and 12 years. The 1 kg preterm infant has a plasma volume of only 40 ml; which volume, although relatively large in terms of body weight, in absolute terms is a small fluid compartment easily depleted and overloaded by fluid loss and infusion.

IMMATURITY OF TISSUE AND ORGAN FUNCTION

When the functions of individual organs of the term human infant are compared with those of the adult it is easy to demonstrate that the infant organs are usually less able to deal with extraordinary environmental stresses, particularly those which induce tissue catabolism. Whereas ingestion or infusion of excess quantities of sodium can overload the kidneys and cause hypernatraemia in term infants, the normal breast–fed infant adequately fed and protected from adverse environmental conditions has no such problem. Indeed, in terms of heat production from brown adipose tissue the term newborn may be considered more efficient than the adult (Hull 1976).

The skin

The skin is a large and important organ in the young infant and is particularly liable to damage from minor trauma, hypoxia, hypothermia and infection. Losses of water from skin and lungs account for the greater part of fluid requirement in the unstressed infant (30–70 ml/kg per day) but may double when the environmental temperature is increased (Levine et al 1929, Darrow et al 1954). In the first three years of life evaporative water loss accounts for approximately two–thirds of the total water requirement. Because of a large surface area relative to weight and skin immaturity, the preterm infant is particularly liable to excessive fluid loss.

Kidneys

Water tolerance is reduced because of renal immaturity and is also markedly influenced by the accompanying osmotic load, either exogeous in the form of sodium, glucose, amino acids and electrolytes or endogenous from urea production. During the first three days of life the newborn infant has very little response to a water load but usually by the fifth day can dilute to about 50 mosmol/kg. Hypoxia, hypotension or other stress conditions will reduce renal efficiency. Urinary concentrations of 400 mosmol/kg are achieved in the newborn and by three months about 750 to 1000 mosmol/kg can be reached. Early exposure to high osmolality feeds will result in earlier maturation of renal concentrating mechanisms. Together with the lungs, the kidneys play an essential part in the maintenance of acid–base balance. Respiratory disorders in young infants commonly produce hypercarbia with respiratory acidosis and hypoxia with metabolic acidosis which interfere with cell membrane function and tissue metabolism. Renal threshold for bicarbonate is at a slightly lower level than in the adult (21.5–22.5 mmol/l) and the threshold may be further reduced by increases in the extracellular volume associated with infusions of saline and increased by potassium deficiency. The mature kidney excretes hydrogen ions in combination with ammonia (produced in the kidney from glutamine) as ammonium ions (NH_4^+) and the principal urinary buffer is the phosphate buffer, disodium monohydrogen phosphate (Na_2HPO_4). Unless phosphate intake is adequate the infant's capacity to excrete titratable acid is limited. Renal mechanisms control potassium, sodium and chloride balance and the extracellular fluid volume, under the influence of antidiuretic hormone and aldosterone. Infants may have gross distortions of fluid and electrolyte when infused with imbalanced quantities of electrolyte or when there is tissue breakdown from injury and infections, particularly when the kidneys are poorly perfused or poorly oxygenated. Maintenance of good renal, gut and hepatic perfusion and oxygenation is a vital factor in promoting anabolism and growth. Hyperoxygenation may be as hazardous as hypoxia for it will decrease renal flow and aggravate a catabolic state.

Glucose, freely filtered at the glomerulus, is actively reabsorbed at the proximal tubule. Infusions of concentrated solutions of glucose may exceed the tubular threshold but even in infancy tubules have a remarkable capacity to adapt when the total quantities of glucose infused are increased slowly. Amino acids are efficiently reabsorbed at the proximal renal tubule even in immature infants and account normally for less than 2% of total urinary nitrogen. Phosphate concentrations are controlled by reabsorption in the proximal tubule by an active carrier process linked with glucose. Phosphate reabsorption is inhibited by parathyroid hormone. When excessive quantities of amino acids are infused and there is, for example, urinary overflow of glycine, tryptophan, leucine and phenylalanine, phosphate reabsorption can be inhibited.

Endocrine system

Endocrine function may be absent, poor, or even inappropriate in the stress situations likely to be associated with the need for parenteral feeding. This inadequacy may be aggravated by immaturity of hypothalamic, brain stem and autonomic nervous system function with failure of homeostatic mechanisms controlling the distribution of blood and blood volume, body temperature, plasma osmolality and sodium, calcium and glucose concentrations. In states of asphyxia, hypotension and septicaemia, haemorrhage into the adrenal gland can occur and adrenocortical control of mineral metabolism can be lost resulting in hyperkalaemia, hyponatraemia and circulatory failure. These same pathological conditions can further adversely influence the hypothalamic and pituitary control of the endocrine glands and the functions which they subserve.

Diabetes mellitus and hyperglycaemia are the commonest of the pancreatic endocrine disorders and can cause major fluid, electrolyte and metabolic disturbance in the child. Hyperinsulinism can produce severe hypoglycaemia in the newborn infant born to the diabetic mother and can occur in association with islet cell tumours. In young infants hypoglycaemia is more commonly associated with lack of nutritional reserve and an inadequate supply of nutrients. Unless adequately fed before surgical procedures, young infants can have considerable metabolic disturbance from hypoglycaemia (Morrice et al 1974).

The role of enteric hormones such as glucagon is uncertain. Mature infants fed normally with breast milk show an increase in blood sugar, a rise in plasma insulin, growth hormone, gastrin and enteroglucagon. These changes are not seen in similarly fed preterm infants (Lucas et al 1978). The importance of gut–associated hormones in enterally and parenterally fed infants is unknown but they might well be important determinants in the recovery of a damaged gastro–intestinal tract and of nutritional homeostasis.

Gastro–intestinal tract, liver and exocrine pancreas

The function of the gastro–intestinal tract may be insufficient to sustain anabolism in the newborn infant. Even when an adequate supply of human milk is available a diminished ability to digest and absorb together with abnormalities of gut hormone and enzymatic activity can delay or prevent the synthesis of new peptides and proteins. Deficient hepatic glucuronyl transferase activity results in unconjugated hyperbilirubinaemia which can cause cellular damage probably by inhibition of oxidative phosphorylation at the mitochondria. Deficiencies of p-hydroxyphenylpyruvic acid oxidase and cystathionine synthetase result in hypertyrosinaemia and hypermethioninaemia which in turn may inhibit protein synthesis or cause cellular damage. Poor hepatic function can reduce the production of fibrinogen and prothrombin, required for effective haemostasis, and of plasma albumin necessary for the maintenance of plasma osmotic pressure and the transport of lipids, vitamins, hormones and drugs. The half–lives of plasma proteins vary considerably (e.g. fibrinogen 3–4 days, liver and plasma proteins 7–28 days) but unless synthesis is established quickly deficits will soon arise. Preterm infants and infants subjected to hypoxia during or before birth may have severe hepatic insufficiency as may children with viral or toxic hepatic damage so that any or all of these functions can be significantly impaired. A low plasma albumin in association with leaking immature capillaries or capillaries damaged by hypoxia can result in gross fluid shifts and oedema.

FLUID AND NUTRIENT REQUIREMENTS

Table 11.3 gives the requirements for water, energy, carbohydrate, fat, amino acids, minerals and vitamins in infants and children. These allowances are sufficient for growth in all but severe stress conditions but there is considerable individual variation depending upon the underlying disorder. The infant and child are normally anabolic and grow. Failure to achieve an adequate intake of nutrients results in catabolic states for which the infant is poorly equipped. If possible catabolism should be prevented by providing adequate nutrition, preferably

Table 11.3 Allowances per kg bodyweight per day for total parenteral nutrition in infants and children (sufficient for growth in all but severe stress conditions). After Cockburn (1978)

Age (years):	0–1	1–6	6–12	12–18
Water (ml)	120–150	90–120	60–90	30–60
Energy (MJ)	0.38–0.50	0.31–0.38	0.25–0.31	0.13–0.25
Energy (kcal)	90–120	75–90	60–75	30–60
Glucose (g)	12–20	6.0–12.0	3.0–6.0	2.0–4.0
Fat (g)	2.5–4.0	2.0–3.0	2.0–3.0	2.0–2.5
Amino acids (g)	2.0–3.0	1.5–2.5	1.3–2.0	1.0–1.3
Sodium (mmol)	1.0–2.5	1.0–2.0	1.0–2.0	1.0–1.5
Potassium (mmol)	2.0–2.5	1.0–2.0	0.9–2.0	0.7–1.2
Calcium (mmol)	0.5–1.0	0.3–0.7	0.2–0.7	0.11–0.20
Magnesium (mmol)	0.15–0.40	0.08–0.20	0.06–0.20	0.04–0.08
Phosphorus (mmol)	0.4–0.8	0.20–0.50	0.18–0.50	0.15–0.25
Iron (μmol)	2.0–3.0	1.5–2.5	1.5–2.5	1.0–1.5
Copper (μmol)	0.2–0.4	0.1–0.3	0.1–0.3	0.07–0.12
Zinc (μmol)	0.5–0.7	0.4–0.5	0.4–0.5	0.2–0.4
Manganese (μmol)	0.8–1.0	0.7–0.9	0.7–0.9	0.6–0.8
Chlorine (mmol)	1.8–4.3	1.5–2.5	1.5–2.5	1.3–2.3
Iodine (μmol)	0.03–0.05	0.02–0.04	0.02–0.04	0.015–0.03
Vitamins (water–soluble)				
Thiamine (mg)	0.05	–	–	0.02–0.04
Riboflavine (mg)	0.10	–	–	0.03–0.05
Nicotinamide (mg)	1.00	–	–	0.20–0.50
Pyridoxine (mg)	0.10	–	–	0.03–0.05
Folic acid (μg)	20.00	–	–	3.00–6.00
Cyanocobalamin (μg)	0.20	–	–	0.03–0.10
Pantothenic acid (mg)	1.00	–	–	0.20–0.50
Biotin (μg)	30.00	–	–	5.00–10.00
Ascorbic acid (mg)	3.00	–	–	0.50–1.00
Vitamins (fat–soluble)				
Retinol (μg)	100.00	–	–	10.00–25.00
Cholecalciferol (μg)	2.50	–	–	0.04–1.00
Phytylmenaquinone (μg)	50.00	–	–	2.00–10.00
α–Tocopherol (mg)	3.00	–	–	1.50–2.00

by the gastro–intestinal tract, but where this is not possible the parenteral route must be used.

Water

Requirements are dependent upon evaporative losses from skin and lungs, faecal losses, water necessary for renal excretion of solutes and water required for growth. Assuming normal growth, a thermoneutral environment, a diet of low renal solute load (human milk) and an ability to concentrate urine to 1000 mosmol/kg water, Bergmann et al (1974) calculated the sources of water loss in infants (Table 11.4). Any increase in environmental temperature, solute intake, or fluid loss from gut, kidney, lung or skin can quickly produce a change in these requirements.

Table 11.4 Estimated water expenditure (ml/day) in infants. Adapted from Foman (1974) — assumes an average rate of growth, thermoneutral environment, low solute (breast milk) diet and an ability to concentrate urine to 1000 mosmol/kg water

Age (months)	1	4	12	36
Body weight (kg)	4.2	7.0	10.5	15
Growth (ml/day)	18	9	6	5
Insensible loss, skin and lung (ml/day)	210	350	500	600
Faecal loss (ml/day)	42	70	105	140
Urine (ml/day)	56	105	182	203

Rates of water loss from skin depend on the surface area of the skin, movement of air over the surface and the vapour pressure of the water on the skin and in the adjacent air. Respiratory loss depends on the rate and tidal volume of respiration and the difference in humidity between inspired and expired air. High rates of loss can occur in children ventilated with unhumidified gas, nursed in dry environments or when there is extensive skin damage from infection, trauma and burns. For every gram of water vapourised 0.6 kcal of heat is released so that prevention of evaporative loss helps preserve heat and energy as well as fluid. Additional volumes of water are required to compensate for any additional losses or to excrete an endogenous or exogenous solute load as well as to make up any pre–existing deficit.

Carbohydrate

Requirements, like most of the other nutrient requirements given in Table 11.3, are based on the average intakes of a breast–fed infant during the first six months of life and thereafter on the mixed diet of a well–nourished growing infant and child allowing for the very rapid rates of growth in the first year of life and at puberty. Specialised carbohydrates such as the oligosaccharides of human milk required to sustain the bifidus bacillus in the infant gut can be obtained only from that source. Adequate nutrition can be achieved even in the most immature by supplying glucose as the sole source of carbohydrate. Glucose is the carbohydrate of choice for parenteral use because it is immediately available for use by the brain, prevents excessive sodium and water loss and causes insulin secretion which in turn has an anabolic effect. Fructose, alcohol and the polyalcohols, sorbitol and xylitol, have little to commend themselves as energy sources particularly in the child under the age of two years. At high rates of infusion fructose may cause greater osmotic diuresis because of its lower renal threshold and in the immature infant it tends to produce severe metabolic acidosis as does ethyl alcohol and the polyalcohols.

Fats

Isotonic preparations of vegetable oils in water with an emulsifier to stabilise the mixture contain a concentrated energy supply in a small volume and can at the same time provide essential fatty acids and phosphate while acting as a vehicle for the infusion of fat–soluble vitamins. Deficiencies of essential fatty acids occur very quickly in infants and although the commercially available fat emulsions are relatively deficient in unsaturated fatty acids and have a relative excess of oleic (C18:1) and linoleic (C18:2) acids they appear adequate in practice. It would seem rational to provide both essential and non–essential fatty acids for surfactant and prostaglandin synthesis, as well as for structural lipid synthesis and a source of energy. High plasma concentrations of free fatty acids can displace bilirubin from albumin and might increase the risk of kernicterus in the low birth–weight, hypo–albuminaemic, jaundiced infant. In the absence of metabolic acidaemia and circulatory failure most young infants can utilise between 2 and 4 g fat per kg per day (Borreson et al 1970, Grotte 1971).

Amino acids

Mixtures of crystalline L–amino acids available for parenteral use have a ratio of essential to non-essential amino acids (E/T ratio) of about 3.2 which corresponds to that found in the proteins of human milk. This ratio is higher than that for infant body proteins which is nearer 2.8 but in practice it seems that any excess essential amino acids are transaminated effectively with little loss of nitrogen as urea. Table 11.5 shows the estimated essential amino acid requirements per kg/day which will promote growth and prevent tissue catabolism in infants and children. In addition to the eight so–called essential amino acids, histidine and prob-

Table11.5 Estimated* requirements per kg per day for parenteral essential amino acids** in infants and children. After Cockburn (1978)

Age (years):	0–1		1–12		12–18	
Threonine (mg) (mmol)	45–92	(0.38–0.77)	20–40	(0.17–0.34)	6–34	(0.05–0.29)
Valine	85–140	(0.73–1.19)	20–48	(0.17–0.41)	11–33	(0.09–0.28)
Cystine	15–55	(0.06–0.23)	17–35	(0.10–0.20)	11–27	(0.06–0.15)
Methionine	35–52	(0.23–0.35)				
Isoleucine	100–130	(0.76–0.99)	18–36	(0.14–0.27)	10–28	(0.08–0.21)
Leucine	75–230	(0.57–1.75)	38–60	(0.29–0.46)	11–49	(0.08–0.37)
Tyrosine	?					
Phenylalanine	50–100	(0.30–0.61)	17–35	(0.10–0.20)	13–27	(0.08–0.16)
Tryptophane	15–30	(0.07–0.15)	3–7	(0.01–0.03)	26–37	(0.01–0.02)
Lysine	110–160	(0.75–1.09)	41–74	(0.28–0.51)	9–59	(0.06–0.40)
Histidine	15–48	(0.10–0.31)	–		–	
Total	545–1037 mg		174–335 mg		74–261 mg	

* Values are based on average oral intakes and can only provide guidelines for parenteral use
** In addition to the 8 accepted essential amino acids, cystine, tyrosine and histidine are indispensable in the immature infant

ably, taurine are essential for infants. Arginine is also necessary, particulary when glycine forms a large part of the non−essential amino acid component. Cystine and tyrosine are essential for the infant with immature hepatic cystathionase and phenylalanine hydroxylase activities. If non−essential amino acids are not provided in the correct proportion the body can synthesize them, but optimal utilisation of essential amino acids is promoted when non−essential amino acids are provided in balanced quantities. When imbalanced amino acid solutions with an excess or deficiency of one essential amino acid are infused, protein synthesis will cease and severe tissue damage can result.

Routine requirements in the infant lie somewhere between 1.2 and 2.2 g/kg per day. In practice, 2.5 g/kg per day of a well balanced crystalline L−amino acid solution will promote growth in infants on total parenteral nutrition where metabolic stress is not too severe. As the child grows older lesser amounts suffice (Table 11.5).

Minerals

The values quoted in Table 11.3 are based on the data of Wretlind (1972) for growth in healthy children. In catabolic states children are unable to tolerate high intakes of sodium and potassium but as soon as an anabolic state is achieved the quantities of sodium and potassium given can be increased. Individual requirements vary so much that in the event of failure to grow during apparently adequate parenteral nutrition, plasma analyses should be made to detect specific deficiencies. Increased quantities of calcium, phosphorus, magnesium, copper, zinc and iron are required during periods of rapid growth in the first months of life and at puberty. The preterm infant is particularly liable to develop deficiencies of sodium and of the aforementioned minerals.

Zinc is a component of the enzymes carboxypeptidase and carbonic anhydrase and of the hormone insulin. In the early days of life there is a nett negative balance of zinc even when 1 μmol/kg per day of parenteral zinc is given. Intakes of zinc can fluctuate markedly for it is frequently a contaminant of solutions from tubing, taps and bottle stopper. The optimal rates of infusion of zinc, copper, iron and manganese are as−yet unknown but careful studies are beginning to allow tentative recommendations to be made (James & MacMahon 1976). Copper is an essential element for the function of many enzyme systems including cytochrome oxidase, ascorbic acid oxidase, catalase, monoamine oxidase, tyrosinase and urease. It is also essential for normal haemoglobin synthesis and is found in plasma bound to caeruloplasmin, in the red cell to the protein erythrocuprein and in the brain to cerebrocuprein. Iron, an integral part of porphyrin, is necessary for cytochrome, haemoglobin and myoglobin functions. It is also present in catalase and peroxidase. Manganese is necessary for normal activity of the enzyme pyruvic decarboxylase, arginase, leucine aminopeptidase, alkaline phosphatase and of the enzymes of oxidative phosphorylation. When manganese is infused parenterally into young infants it is avidly retained and there is a strong positive balance unlike copper, iron and zinc. Approximately 91% of infused manganese is retained by preterm infants during intravenous feeding and this during a time when serum manganese concentrations are falling (James & MacMahon 1976). The present estimate of manganese requirements is 10 μg/kg per day for preterm infants reducing to 6 μg/kg per day because intravenous infusion of larger doses of manganese have been shown to produce cholestasis in rats (Witzelben et al 1968). Phosphorus is necessary for growth and bone and teeth structure in the infant and deficiencies can reduce erythrocyte 2,3–diphosphoglycerate and adenosine triphosphate which in turn increase the red cell's affinity for oxygen (Travis et al 1971).

Chloride is the major anion in extracellular fluid and its requirement varies according to the amounts of anion given in the form of amino acid, phosphorus and sulphur. Iodide, necessary for normal thyroid function, must be provided in an amount adequate to allow normal growth and normal brain development. Fluorine may not be an essential element although it appears to assist the maintenance of bone and teeth structure. Sulphur is obtained from the sulpur–containing amino acids methionine and cystine and cobalt is present in vitamin B_{12}.

The safe ranges of long–term infusion of trace elements for children are unknown and may be narrow. Failure to supply individual trace elements must, however, inhibit normal growth and development.

Vitamins

Vitamins given parenterally may not be utilised or function in precisely the same manner as internally absorbed vitamins and there is therefore some empiricism about the amounts of vitamins given parenterally in order to maintain the metabolic processes for which they are necessary. It is likely that thiamine, which is necessary for carbohydrate metabolism and which is absorbed almost completely from the intestine, is required in an amount equal to the recommended oral intake of 0.05 mg thiamine/kg body weight per day. Riboflavin, an active component of oxidative enzymatic activities, is required in an amount of approximately 0.1 mg/kg per day. Nicotinamide can be formed from the amino acid tryptophane and when there is an adequate amount of tryptophane in the parenteral infusions the daily requirement of nicotinamide is approximately 1 mg/kg per day. It is a component of NAD and NADPH and is essential for glycolysis.

Pyridoxine (vitamin B_6) is involved in protein, carbohydrate and fat metabolism. Deficiencies interfere with tryptophane metabolism and can produce seizures, particularly in young infants. The recommended parenteral intake for infants is approximately 0.1 mg/kg per day. Folic acid and its metabolites, e.g. tetrahydrofolic acid, is essential for normal phenylalanine metabolism and for synthesis of purines and pyrimidines as well as for the synthesis of normal red cells. Young growing infants require approximately 10 μg/kg per day parenterally. Cyanocobalamin, an essential vitamin for normal central nervous system function and red cell production, has an approximate requirement of 0.2 μg/kg per day. Pantothenic acid requirements are estimated at 1 mg/kg per day and this vitamin is involved in carbohydrate and fatty acid metabolism, steroid hormone and porphyrin synthesis as well as being essential for normal acetylcholine function. Biotin, an essential nutrient material for the urea cycle and for carboxylation, maintains an anabolic state in young infants when given at 30 μg/kg per day.

Ascorbic acid (vitamin C) is essential for normal collagen structure and for normal proline/hydroxyproline metabolism. It is also involved in the metabolism of phenylanlanine, tyrosine and tryptophane, particularly in preterm infants. It is essential for adequate p-HPPA oxidase activity and helps prevent the transient hypertyrosinaemia seen in the parenterally nourished preterm infant. Approximately 3 mg/kg per day is required for infants having complete parenteral nutrition.

Choline has not been demonstrated to be an essential nutrient in man although animals do not thrive well without it. As it is present in fairly large quantities in fat emulsions containing phosphatides and acts as a source of labile methyl groups, it is unlikely that a deficiency would arise when lipid emulsions are used as a source of energy. A reasonable estimate of requirement in the active growing infant is 150 mg choline chloride per day.

Carnitine (α–trimethylamino–β–hydroxybutyric acid) is necessary for the mitochondrial oxidation of fatty acids. In general, the rate of fatty acid oxidation in young actively growing infants is high during the postnatal period. The requirement of this material is unknown. In starvation states free carnitine falls but acetyl carnitine increases and there is a negative correlation between free carnitine and β–hydroxybutyrate (Hahn 1979). Human milk contains fairly large quantities of carnitine but at present parenteral nutrient solutions contain very little. Sufficient carnitine should probably be given to actively growing infants and children to maintain a plasma concentration of greater than 20 μmol/l.

Fat–soluble vitamins A, D, E and K are absorbed from the gastro–intestinal tract with fats and the amounts absorbed vary with the type of dietary lipid. For this and other reasons it is difficult to assess just how much fat–soluble vitamin is absorbed from the gastro–intestinal tract. Vitamin A, which is necessary for normal retinal and skin function, has to be given in the form of retinol at a dose of 0.1 mg/kg. The provitamin A, carotenoid, cannot be used for intravenous nutrition. The infant and child in hospital is unlikely to synthesise much vitamin D from 7–dihydrocholesterol in the skin and a daily intake of 2.5μg cholecalciferol or ergocholecalciferol per kg should be given. Omission of this vitamin from prolonged parenteral nutrition in infancy can result in severe demineralisation of bone and hypocalcaemic tetany.

Haemolytic disease of the newborn with anaemia and red cell breakdown can develop acutely in preterm newborn infants lacking vitamin E. α–Tocopherol requirements vary with the amount of polyunsaturated fatty acid infused and it is estimated that about 1 mg of α–tocopherol per gram of polyunsaturated fatty acids is sufficient to prevent haemolysis (Harris & Embree 1963). Approximately 65% of the fat in Intralipid® is polyunsaturated so that 0.65 mg of α–tocopherol per gram of fat should be supplied. There is about 1.0 mg of tocopherol per gram of fat in this emulsion.

Vitamin K_1 (phytylmenaquinone) is essential for the maintenance of normal prothrombin values and for the maintenance and production of coagulation factors V, VII, IX and X. Requirements are uncertain but is estimated that approximately 50 μg of phytylmenaquinone/kg body weight per day should be given with intravenous therapy or by intramuscular injections of 1–3 mg twice weekly. Infants and children on broad–spectrum antibiotics will produce little endogenous vitamin K from bacterial action in the gut. Estimation of thrombotest and, where necessary, concentrations of individual factors will determine whether vitamin K intake is adequate.

CORRECTION OF CIRCULATORY, FLUID AND ELECTROLYTE DISTURBANCES

Before adequate nutrition and growth can be achieved, adequate tissue perfusion with oxygenated blood must be ensured. Correction of hypovolaemia, dehydration, anaemia, acidaemia (respiratory and metabolic), hypoglycaemia and electrolyte disorder is a first priority. When blood is required for infants in the first weeks of life it may be given partially packed (packed cell volume of 60%). In conditions of gross metabolic disturbance and anaemia, exchange transfusion with fresh whole blood may be life–saving. Fresh frozen plasma can be given to expand the circulating volume but a drawback to its use in young infants is its high sodium content. In this situation the best available plasma expander is low–salt albumin which can be used in circulatory failure without anaemia and can be given to any infant with a plasma albumin concentration of less than 2.8 g/ 100 ml. In acute hypotension 5% low–salt albumin may be infused at a rate of 15 mg/kg over one hour. If more albumin is required then great care must be taken because of the risk of circulatory overload. Each gram of albumin retains 12 ml water in the vascular compartment. In immature infants with jaundice there may be a rapid increase in the plasma bilirubin concentration because bilirubin as well as water and other materials are attracted back into the vascular compartment from adjacent tissue. This increase in plasma bilirubin will be associated with a reduced risk of kernicterus as free unconjugated bilirubin is withdrawn from extravascular tissues.

Aetiology

The varying aetiologies of fluid and electrolyte disturbances although important are not critical, in that survival depends on re–establishment of circulation and tissue perfusion with reversal of tissue catabolism. Survival of an infant with infective gastro–enteritis depends more on the correction of the fluid and electrolyte disturbances rather than on eliminating the offending organisms.

Gastro–intestinal obstructions from the congenital malformations oesophageal atresia, duodenal atresia, reduplication, volvulus, pyloric stenosis and Hirschsprung's disease can all result in isotonic dehydration with some degree of chloride loss where the lesion is below the pylorus. Infective gastro–enteritis probably accounts for the majority of fluid and electrolyte disturbances in the total childhood population and in most instances this is an isotonic dehydration. When infants have a high solute intake, hypertonic (hypernatraemic) dehydration can occur and if low solute replacement is used as a form of treatment, hypotonic (hyponatraemic) dehydration can result. There are rare gastro–intestinal abnormalities in which a chloride–losing state can occur. In the inherited disaccharidase defects and the disaccharidase defects secondary to gastro–enteritis, isotonic dehydration with a loss of potassium and bicarbonate can occur. Fluid loss from enteral fistulae can produce severe dehydration and potassium deficiency.

Most anomalies in the renal tract produce an isotonic dehydration but occasionally there can be a variable potassium and bicarbonate loss.

Congenital malformations of the central nervous system such as hydrocephalus and hydranencaphalus can result in hyponatraemia due to loss of homeostasis.

Fluid loss from large meningocoeles can cause hyponatraemic dehydration with chloride loss. Hyponatraemia may be observed in infants suffering from meningitis, encephalitis, hypoxia, severe haemorrhage or trauma and following the use of opiate drugs due to loss of homeostasis and excessive production of antidiuretic hormone.

When large areas of skin are damaged by infection (as in Ritter's disease) or extensive scalding and burning there can be isotonic dehydration with variable protein loss. In cystic fibrosis the skin defect can result in sodium loss and hyponatraemic dehydration.

When severe respiratory disorders cause hyperventilation, hypertonic dehydration may occur, particularly if the inspired gases are dry. Rarely saturation of the inspired gases with water can result in hyponatraemia.

Endocrine disorders have a variable influence on the fluid and electrolyte condition of a child. In diabetes insipidus dehydration of the isotonic type occurs, whereas in adrenocortical defect or damage hyponatraemic dehydration with potassium retention and sodium loss may occur. Parathyroid disorders can severely disturb the concentration of calcium, phosphorus and magnesium in the plasma and the cells. Disorders of glucose homeostasis may be produced by disorders of pancreatic endocrine function. In diabetes mellitus, hyperglycaemia with potassium loss is associated with isotonic dehydration and glycosuria.

Inborn errors of carbohydrate metabolism such as galactosaemia, fructose intolerance, glycogenosis type 1, ketotic hypoglycaemia and xylosidase deficiency can result in isotonic dehydration with vomiting and metabolic acidosis. Inborn errors of amino acid metabolism such as maple syrup urine disease, hypervalinaemia, methylmalonic aciduria, propionic acidaemia, hyperglycinaemia and hyperammonaemia from urea cycle defects are all associated with vomiting and isotonic dehydration.

Severe infections in infancy and childhood are associated with hyponatraemia but hyponatraemia is perhaps most commonly seen in association with infusions of low electrolyte solutions (e.g. in the treatment of hypoglycaemia). Hypernatraemia is most commonly seen in association with high solute artificial milk feeding and when excessive quantities of sodium bicarbonate are given for the treatment of metabolic acidaemia.

Clinical features
Normal infants may lose up to 15% of their extracellular fluid, equivalent to 10% of body weight loss, in the first three to four days after birth. Usually there are no abnormal signs apart from a low–grade pyrexia (sometimes called dehydration fever) and a reduced urinary output. Generally no treatment is necessary other than improving the feeding or giving a complement of 5% dextrose/water or plain water.

Diarrhoea with or without vomiting, apathy and diminished oral intake are features common to the large majority of infants with disordered fluid and electrolyte metabolism. The primary problem is that of rapid extracellular fluid loss. Diarrhoea and vomiting, producing up to 5% body weight loss within 24 hours, causes loss of skin turgor in addition to reduced urinary output and low–grade fever. When 5–10% of body weight is lost in 24 hours a state of dehydration is reached which is critical to the infant. Skin turgor is then markedly reduced and the skin is slow to unwrinkle when released from a gentle pinch; the fontanelle is sunken in young infants where this is patent and the eyes are sunken with low tension on palpation. Reduced urinary output, dry mucous membranes and variable temperature control is usual and there is tachycardia with low pulse pressure but a normal pink colour and capillary refill. When 10–15% of body weight is lost within 24 hours, signs of peripheral circulatory failure are added to these findings. Skin pallor and mottling is marked, the skin feels cool and capillaries fill very slowly after being blanched by fingertip pressure. Superficial veins are flattened and empty and tachycardia may be extreme with poor peripheral pulses. Tachypnoea, a response to severe metabolic acidosis, can be marked and the infant is usually hypothermic. When the loss of body weight exceeds 15% within 24 hours the infant is moribund.

In the vast majority of instances dehydrated infants have isotonic dehydration where there is a proportionate loss of extracellular water and electrolyte. Plasma sodium and osmolality are normal. Where losses are disproportionate there are differences in clinical findings associated with the same absolute water loss. In states of hypertonic dehydration more water than extracellular electrolyte is lost. As sodium is the major extracellular electrolyte, in this condition there is an increase in plasma osmolality and sodium concentration (greater than 150 mmol/l). Hypertonic (hypernatraemic) dehydration, for a given absolute loss of extracellular fluid and body weight, is associated with less than the expected degree of circulatory failure and subcutaneous tissue change. This is because the high extracellular and plasma sodium concentrations cause cellular desiccation which preserves for a time the extracellular and circulating plasma volumes. Although dehydration is clinically less apparent (a 10% weight loss may cause no circulatory disturbance), signs of disordered central nervous function do appear and are probably directly related to loss of central nervous intracellular fluid and disordered cell membrane activity. Increased blood viscosity and a high haematocrit diminish effective cerebral blood flow and predispose to a vascular thrombosis. This in the infant will involve the sagittal and other cerebral venous sinuses as well as renal veins. When the disorder progresses to a stage of circulatory failure, plasma sodium may exceed 180 mmol/l and cerebral signs become obvious. Coexistent metabolic acidaemia, hypoglycaemia or hyperglycaemia, increased blood urea and hypocalcaemia complicate the clinical picture. The infant appears sleepy and drowsy but when roused is irritable and jittery. Intracellular dehydration gives the skin, subcutaneous tissue and muscles a characteristic waxy, doughy feel. Muscle tone is generally increased in the roused infant and there may be marked extensor hypertonus progressing to clonic and tonic convulsions. If a stage of muscular hypotonia is reached prognosis for undamaged survival is poor.

Hypotonic dehydration is less common than the other forms of dehydration and there is almost always hyponatraemia (plasma sodium less than 132 mmol/l). Hyponatraemic dehydration causes severe circulatory disturbance with signs of peripheral circulatory failure and coma when there are lesser degrees of dehydration than in either isotonic or hypertonic dehydration states.

Since the introduction of modified milk feeds for children there has been a reduction in the incidence of hypertonic dehydration. High solute artificial feeds, particularly when given to infants nursed in high ambient temperatures and dry environments, was a major cause of the hypernatraemic type of dehydration. The use of unmodified cow's milk in the feeding of young infants carries with it a risk of this damaging form of fluid and electrolyte disorder.

Assessments of fluid deficits

Change in body weight within any 24–hour period may for practical purposes be considered a measure of change in body water content. When measured weights are unavailable a rough clinical assessment of dehydration is required. The previously mentioned 5, 10 or 15% categories are clinically valuable. Thus, a 3.5 kg infant with signs of dehydration and severe circulatory failure probably has a 10% loss of body weight as fluid and a fluid deficit of 350 g, equivalent to about 350 ml of fluid. Although this would mean that the infant's true weight before dehydration was 3.85 kg, for practical purposes 350 ml can be accepted as the fluid deficit which must be replaced.

Maintenance requirements

Tables 11.3 and 11.4 give the estimated water expenditure and requirements for normal maintenance. This volume should be given in addition to the previously determined body volume fluid deficit. Where there is continuing abnormal fluid loss this can usually be measured in the hospital by collecting urine, stool and vomit and weighing or measuring volumes.

The laboratory estimations of dehydration and bicarbonate and electrolyte loss are related to the average composition of fluids in the different body compartments. These compositions are shown in Table 11.6. In practice the plasma or serum electrolyte concentrations and plasma osmolality are measured and used as a basis for rational therapy. The plasma osmolality is largely dependent on its sodium content. Sodium and the anions required to maintain electro-neutrality (mainly chloride) contribute 270–280 mosmol out of a total plasma osmolality of

Table 11.6 Composition of fluids in the body compartments. After Harris (1972)

	Plasma	Interstitial fluid	Intracellular fluid
Cation (mEq/l)			
Na^+	140	138	9
K^+	5	8	155
Ca^{2+}	5	8	4
Mg^{2+}	4	6	32
	154	160	200
Anion (mEq/l)			
Cl^-	100	119	5
HCO_3^-	26	26	10
Protein	19	7	65
Organic acid	6	6	–
HPO_4^{2-}	2	1	95
SO_4^{2-}	1	1	25
	154	160	200

280–300 mosmol. Glucose (5 mmol/l) and urea (5 mmol/l) normally contribute little to total plasma osmolality but under pathological conditions may exert a considerable osmotic effect if they increase suddenly. Gradual increases in plasma glucose or urea concentrations do not cause shifts of water because both substances equilibrate across cell membranes, unlike sodium which is effectively confined to the extracellular space. Comparisons of plasma and urinary osmolalities can indicate inappropriate secretion of antidiuretic hormone when the plasma osmolality is decreased and urinary osmolality increased. When plasma solids are in high concentrations (e.g. during intravenous infusions of lipids) plasma water is reduced. Measurements of plasma osmolality by freezing–point depression are little altered by lipid and a discrepancy between normal plasma osmolality and low sodium should prevent misinterpretations during lipid infusion.

Plasma hydrogen ion concentration is frequently increased in dehydrated infants because of loss of bicarbonate in the diarrhoeal stool, production of keto acids from tissue catabolism and renal retention of hydrogen ion because of diminished renal perfusion and function. Metabolic acidosis can also occur in association with primary renal insufficiency, renal tubular acidosis, hypoxia with secondary lactic acidosis, primary lactic acidosis, diabetes mellitus, septicaemia, starvation and other metabolic disturbances. When carbohydrates, fats and organic acids are incompletely catabolised plasma hydrogen ion concentration increases. A major source of hydrogen ion, particularly in artificially fed infants or infants infused with currently available amino acid solutions, is sulphuric acid from oxidation of sulphur–containing amino acids. Phosphoric acid produced by oxidation and hydrolysis of milk phosphoproteins also contributes hydrogen ion. The presence of metabolic acid in the plasma produces a fall in bicarbonate concentration while chloride concentration usually remains constant. Occasionally in renal tubular disorders with bicarbonate loss, where the plasma chloride concentration increases to match the fall in bicarbonate, states of hyperchloraemic acidosis can occur. Hypochloraemic alkalosis can occur when there is loss of hydrogen ion and chloride ion from persistent vomiting of gastric hydrochloric acid or after prolonged gastric aspiration without adequate chloride replacement.

Sodium is the major cation and chloride the major anion of extracellular fluid. The young infant with a large extracellular volume has, therefore, relatively more sodium per unit body weight (infant 75 mmol/kg: adult 50 mmol/kg) and more chloride (infant 52 mmol/kg: adult 29 mmol/kg). About 10% of the infant's total sodium is combined in bone compared with 33% in the adult. Bone sodium is readily available to the infant, particularly in catabolic states associated with metabolic acidaemia. There are substantial quantities of chloride in collagen and erythrocytes.

Potassium is chiefly an intracellular ion and as most cell water is contained in muscle, the potassium content of the body is essentially determined by muscle mass. Potassium intake in milk–fed infants exceeds daily requirements. In the large bowel potassium is withdrawn from the extracellular fluid to the gut lumen and an equivalent amount of sodium moves in the reverse direction. Excessive losses of lower gut content in diarrhoea can thus produce severe potassium deficit. Relatively slow and incomplete renal conservation of potassium, compared with the effective sodium–retaining capability of the infant renal tubules make him liable to severe degrees of hypokalaemia. Potassium deficiency states reduce aldosterone secretion so that renal tubular and intestinal loss of potassium ion is decreased. In catabolic states arising from anoxia, septicaemia, starvation or metabolic defect associated with metabolic acidosis, cell membrane activity is disrupted and large quantities of potassium ion are released into the extracellular fluid while sodium enters the intracellular fluid. This can mask a critical potassium ion shortage if only plasma potassium ion concentrations are considered. The deficiency may not become apparent until the child is rehydrated and the acidaemia corrected when low potassium ion concentrations are evident. This potassium deficiency may present clinically as weakness, muscular hypotonia, abdominal distension, paralytic ileus and with characteristic electrocardiographic changes.

Isotonic dehydration

Dehydration from gastro–enteritis can be severe before diarrhoea becomes evident as loss of fluid can occur into the bowel lumen and affect fluid distribution within the body. When the degree of dehydration is mild (less than 5%) oral glucose/electrolyte solutions can be given at a rate of 180 ml/kg body weight during the first 24 hours. The optimum solution is one which replaces the losses of water and electrolytes and stimulates the absorption of substrate by the gut. Absorption is also facilitated if the fluid is approximately isotonic (about 300 mmol/l) so that preliminary osmotic exchanges in the gut are unnecessary. Diarrhoeal stools contain variable concentrations of electrolytes. For example, in cholera the stool may contain over 100 mmol of sodium per litre. Most children with acute diarrhoea lose 50 mmol of sodium per litre. A commercial preparation Dioralyte® (Armour Pharmaceutical Company Ltd) contains sodium 35 mmol/l, potassium 20 mmol/l, chloride 37 mmol/l, bicarbonate 18 mmol/l, glucose 200 mmol/l and has a total osmolality of 310 mosmol/kg when prepared according to instructions. Each packet then provides 200 ml of solution. Oral rehydration should be started early in the course of diarrhoea because the child's homeostatic mechanisms are still effective. The 4–5 kg infant with moderate dehydration would require about 150 ml/h, the 10 kg infant about 300 ml/h and the older child (20 kg) about 600 ml/h. During the recovery phases these volumes would be reduced to 30 ml, 60 ml and 120 ml respectively. Occasionally the mixture may have to be given by nasogastric tube when the child is having difficulty in retaining the materials taken by mouth.

When dehydration is moderate to severe (7–15% reduction in body weight) intravenous rehydration is necessary. If there are signs of circulatory failure, blood is taken for biochemical analysis and an immediate infusion of 20 ml/kg of a 10% glucose solution containing sodium 75 mmol/l, bicarbonate 20 mmol/l, and chloride 55 mmol/l should be given over the first 15 minutes. This can be followed by 5% low–salt albumin, or whole blood if the patient is anaemic, at a rate of 15 ml/kg during the next 60–90 minutes. If low–salt albumin is unavailable and the infant is not anaemic, plasma may be used in the same volume.

Replacement therapy is then organised by assessing the fluid volume required for deficit and maintenance. If the example of a 3.5 kg infant with a 10% deficit is considered then 350 ml of fluid would be given to replace this deficit and an additional 350 ml (100 ml/kg per day) would be required for maintenance, i.e. a total

Table 11.7 Electrolyte solutions

	Na	K	Ca	Mg mmol/l	Cl	HCO₃⁻	Lactate	Dextrose g/l	kcal/l	Osmolality mosmol/kg	pH
0.9% Sodium chloride (isotonic saline)	154				154					286	6.7
0.9% Sodium chloride in 5% dextrose	154				154			50	200	564	5.8
Darrow's	121	35			103	53				286	5.8
Half–strength Darrow's in 2.5% dextrose	60	17.5			52	26		25	100	290	5.6
Hartmann's	131	5	2		111		29			278	6.2
Ringer lactate	130	4	1.5	3	109		28			273	6.2
Brück's	57	25			50			100	400	NK	NK
Vamin	50	20	2.5	1.5	55				650	1400	5.2
Cockburn's	59	15	0.9	3.3	49		16	95	380	714	4.8

(Sulphate 3.3 mmol/l and phosphate 6.0 mmol/l)

of 700 ml. If emergency treatment had been given the infant would have received 70 ml of a 10% glucose/electrolyte mixture and 52.5 ml low–salt albumin. This would leave a deficit of about 230 ml plus 350 ml = 580 ml still to be replaced. Infants with isotonic dehydration could be given a solution such as half–strength Darrow's solution in 2.5% glucose according to Table 11.7. The replacement of deficit usually takes up to 8 hours and during the remaining 16 hours maintenance requirements are met together with a provision for any excessive continuing loss (Table 11.8). After 24 hours' therapy the patient is again assessed clinically and ideally should have regained at least 7% of the estimated 10% weight loss. If there is still a deficit of greater than 5%, recalculation of deficit, maintenance and continuing abnormal losses must be made and fluid management replanned. Plasma calcium and magnesium concentrations should be measured in addition to electrolytes, glucose, urea and bicarbonate. Deficiencies of the divalent ions should be corrected by infusions of magnesium sulphate and/or calcium gluconate. Oral feeding is introduced gradually with a preparation such as Dioralyte® and intravenous therapy appropriately reduced. Infants with severe continuing fluid losses from gastro–intestinal fistulae should be given more complete parenteral nutrition within 48 hours. Failure to provide amino acids and other essential nutrients only prolongs the catabolic process and aggravates the fluid and electrolyte disturbances.

Table 11.8 Treatment of isotonic dehydration

Therapy	Time	Solution	Volume
Emergency	0–15 min	10% glucose; Na^+ 75 mmol/l HCO_3 20 mmol/l; Cl^- 55 mmol/l	20 ml/kg
	15–90 min	5% low salt albumin, or whole blood, or plasma	15 ml/kg
Deficit replacement	1½–8 h	If 10% loss of body weight, deficit is 100 ml/kg minus emergency 35 ml/kg = 65 ml/kg of a solution like half-strength Darrow's in 2.5% glucose	65 ml/kg
Maintenance+ excessive losses	8–24 h	Same solution as for deficit replacement with added K^+, Na^+ and bicarbonate as decided by type of excess fluid lost and plasma biochemistry	100 ml/kg + vol. of fluid loss

Hypernatraemic dehydration

Children with hypernatraemic dehydration have very small deficits (2–4 mmol/kg) of sodium with moderate to severe degrees of dehydration. In some the high plasma osmolalities cannot be accounted for entirely in terms of plasma sodium, glucose and urea concentrations. If the extracellular deficit is rapidly replaced, water will enter the cells with virtually no hindrance and this can produce cell distension which in the brain, for example, may produce increased intracranial pressure and convulsions. Convulsions occur more frequently during therapy than in the dehydrated state.

If circulatory failure is present in the hypernatraemic state this is corrected as for isotonic dehydration. Low–salt albumin is particularly useful and the use of plasma, which has a high sodium concentration, should be avoided if possible. Deficit and maintenance requirements for two days are calculated. The aim is to give this total volume at a slow constant rate over a 48–hour period. There must be no attempt at rapid correction of deficit. In the 3.5 kg infant with a 10% hypernatraemic dehydration 350 ml of fluid would be given to replace the deficit, less 120 ml emergency replacement fluid, and 350 ml for each day's maintenance. The total 930 ml volume would be given at about 19 ml per hour over the subsequent 48 hours. A suitable fluid to use for hypernatraemic dehydration would be 0.5% sodium chloride (77 mmol sodium/l) and 2.5 dextrose until urine flow is established. Once urine flow is established half–strength Darrow's solution in 2.5% dextrose can be used. This solution contains potassium and after about one hour calcium gluconate can be given to correct coexistent hypocalcaemia.

Hyponatraemic dehydration

Infants with this form of dehydration may have sodium deficits of up to 20 mmol/kg. Circulatory failure is likely to occur early and be severe and the same emergency treatment as that used to correct isotonic dehydration is given. This can be followed by full–strength Darrow's solution at 40 ml/kg during the next 3–4 hours when half–strength Darrow's/2.5% dextrose solution is given to complete the estimated deficit and maintenance requirements for the remainder of the first 24 hours. Although dehydration states produced by diarrhoea have been considered, all forms of dehydration require a similar type of therapy, no matter what the aetiology. Particular consideration must be given to the management of fluid and electrolyte problems in infants with burns, scalds and skin damage. Not only must the large surface area be considered but the different body proportions must be remembered, particularly in relation to heat loss and in the management of neonates with scalds or burns. The head and neck of the newborn infant account for 19% of the surface area, compared with 9% in the adult, while the lower limbs each comprise 9% in the newborn infant and 18% in the adult. The rule of nines can be used in calculating the surface area involved on the trunk and upper limbs (Young 1973). In scalds, burns, dermal sepsis and epidermolysis bullosa there can be considerable protein loss. Although some of this can be replaced

Table 11.9 Some indications for parenteral feeding

---

1. Extensive resection of small intestine (gastro – intestinal anomalies)
2. After cardiac and lung surgery or after repair of oesophageal atresia, diaphragmatic defect or gastroschisis
3. Multiple trauma and burns
4. Infections (meningitis and septicaemia)
5. Intractable diarrhoea (enteritis or disaccharide intolerance)
6. Ileus (gut infarction, peritonitis, necrotising enterocolitis or severe metabolic upset producing electrolyte disorder)
7. Acute renal failure
8. Ulcerative colitis and Crohn's disease
9. Acute hepatic disease
10. Immature infants intolerant of gastro – intestinal feeding
11. Infants with severe respiratory difficulty (recurrent apnoeic attacks, idiopathic respiratory distress syndrome, aspiration and bronchopneumonia, pneumothorax and pneumomediastinum)
12. During and after removal of an endotracheal tube to reduce the risks of aspiration
13. To complement enteral feeding in very immature infants

---

with albumin it is most important to ensure an adequate intake of amino acids or protein to ensure new protein synthesis.

PARENTERAL NUTRITION

In some hypercatabolic states such as extensive burns, enteral and parenteral feeding can be combined. Table 11.9 shows examples of conditions in which parenteral nutrition may be used with benefit.

Management

Table 11.10 gives a guide to the management of complete parenteral nutrition in infancy and childhood. It is based on the Stockholm regimen (Wretlind 1974a). After correction of hypovolaemia, acidaemia, dehydration and electrolyte disorders, the three solutions are infused continuously at the appropriate constant rate. The solutions are allowed to mix through a three–way junction or tap system as near to the indwelling catheter as possible. If bicarbonate or other alkaline solutions require to be given, the infusions should be stopped, otherwise there is a risk of precipitation of calcium phosphate and other nutrient materials. Lipid emulsions should never be given to the infant when the plasma pH is less than 7.28 as lipid is not cleared from the blood below this value. It is a good practice to maintain the simultaneous continuous infusion of amino acids, glucose and mineral solutions and lipid emulsion for optimal utilisation. The infusion of lipid emulsion is discontinued at 0500 h, blood being taken for biochemical estimations at 0900 h when the lipid emulsion infusion is recommenced. This allows one to check that lipid is being removed from the plasma and prevents errors in biochem-

Table 11.10 Examples of solutions for complete parenteral nutrition (volume in ml per kg bodyweight per day). After Cockburn (1978)

Age (years):	0–1	1–6	6–18
Solution 1			
a. Solution of L-amino acids (7%) with glucose (10%) Vamin® with	25–45	22–30	14–30
b. Electrolyte solution containing: 0.6 mmol Ca, 0.1 mmol Mg, 2 μmol Fe, 0.6 μmol Zn, 1.0 μmol Mn, 0.3 μmol Cu, 1.26 μmol Cl, 0.3 μmol P,3 μmol F and 0.04 μmol I in 4 ml 10% Dextrose	4.0	3.0	2.0
Solution 2			
a. Fat emulsion 20% Intralipid® 20% with	15–20	10–15	10–15
b. Emulsion of fat-soluble vitamins containing: 0.1 mg vitamin A, 2.5 μg vitamin D and 0.05 mg vitamin K_1	1.0	0.2	0.1
Solution 3			
a. Glucose 10% with 0.1 mmol Na, 1.4 mmol K, 0.2 mmol Ca, 1.61 mmol Cl and 0.16 mmol P with	75–100	70–90	15–60
b. Lyophilised water-soluble vitamins containing: 0.12 mg thiamine, 0.18 mg riboflavine, 1.0 mg niacin, 0.2 mg vitamin B_6, 0.02 mg folic acid, 0.2 μg vitamin B_{12}, 1.0 mg pantothenic acid, 0.03 mg biotin and 3.0 mg ascorbic acid dissolved in 5 ml 10% dextrose solution	5	3	1–2

ical estimations which can result when measurements are made on plasma with a high lipid content. A variety of syringe and peristaltic pumps is available for infusion at the low rates which are required. Ideally, each solution should be infused by an individual pump and an almost obsessive regard for the accuracy and maintenance of the pumps is essential.

Catheters

Scalp and other peripheral veins can be used to give nutrients where isotonic fat emulsions provide up to 40% of the non–protein energy supplied. During the first week of life the umbilical artery route can be used to infuse the fat emulsion and other solutions into the aorta. Great care must be exercised in the insertion of the catheter and in its supervision. Percutaneous catheterisation of the vena cavae using silastic tubing of 0.025 inch (0.64 mm) external diameter inserted into peripheral veins provides a most convenient access route for young infants.

Complications of parenteral nutrition often relate not so much to the solutions employed but to neglect or inadequate care and selection of the catheter. All infants and young children with indwelling catheters should be kept under close supervision. Infants can be attached to electrocardiographic or arterial pressure monitors. Major hazards of intravascular catherisation are septicaemia, formation of clots and vascular thrombosis, air emboli, exsanguination and electrocution. It is best not to use infusion catheters for blood sampling but if this is necessary, a quantity of heparinised saline (10 iu/ml) equivalent to three times the catheter capacity should be injected to clear blood from the catheter. Heparinised saline must be prepared freshly each day and three–way taps and giving sets changed at least every 24 hours. The volumes of blood withdrawn and fluid given during these procedures must be measured accurately and the volumes recorded on the fluid balance chart. Blocked catheters must be removed and replaced and no attempts should be made to force flush a catheter. When a catheter is removed the tip should be cut off and sent for bacteriological culture. There is disagreement about the best position for the tip of an aortic catheter but the author's preference is to have the catheter tip at the level of the third or fourth lumbar vertebra (confirmed radiologically) below the origin of intestinal and renal arteries. Bacterial infections and infections with *Candida albicans* are particular hazards and may necessitate removal of indwelling catheters and systemic treatment with the appropriate antibiotic and 5–fluocytosine respectively. No catheter should remain in situ longer than is necessary. Arterial thrombi occur in less than 2–3% of infants with long–term indwelling arterial catheters. Transient ischaemic episodes producing discolouration of the toes of one foot are more common than this but permanent damage rarely results.

The practice of using bacterial filters between the catheter and infusion pump is debatable because of doubt about their value and their inability to transmit lipid emulsions. It has been the author's policy to use a broad–spectrum antibiotic routinely in any infant with an indwelling catheter. Usually cephalothin or cephalexin, or ampicillin combined with cloxacillin, has been used. The effects of different antibiotics, particularly broad–spectrum antibiotics, on the metabolism of growing infants and children has not been ascertained but tissue utilisation of individual amino acids may be altered.

Clinical assessment

It is essential to know the initial weight of the infant and thereafter to weigh daily. Occasionally this is difficult in the infant connected to a ventilator but such difficulties can be overcome. Adequate and prompt refilling of skin capillaries after blanching with fingertip pressure and the presence of warm fingers and toes are indices of good peripheral circulation. It is not possible to achieve adequate nutrition in the presence of circulatory failure, which must be promptly and efficiently treated. Skin and core temperatures can be maintained by careful control of environmental temperature and humidity. Clinically detectable oedema is not uncommon, particularly in preferm infants, and depending on aetiology, the intakes of sodium and water may have to be reduced, albumin infused and a diuretic (frusemide) given. In the ventilated child measurements of arterial oxygen, carbon dioxide and hydrogen ion concentration will be required in most instances as a guide to appropriate ventilatory assistance. Tachycardia, bradycardia or arrhythmia can indicate circulatory failure, hypoxaemia and severe electrolyte disturbance. Most infants requiring parenteral nutrition should have continuous electrocardiographic monitoring. Measurements of arterial and venous pressures are helpful but if unavailable frequent observation of the position of the liver edge, the distension of scalp veins, the presence of peripheral and pulmonary oedema, tachypnoea, tachycardia and cardiac arrhythmias may indicate cardiac failure and circulatory overload. Urinary volume should be measured and the urine tested for osmolality and glucose concentrations.

Biochemical assessment

Daily estimations of plasma pH, bicarbonate, sodium, potassium, chloride, glucose and urea concentrations and osmolality are necessary in the first two to three days of treatment and the mineral composition of the infusion altered accordingly. Plasma calcium, phosphorus, magnesium, ammonia and amino acid concentrations may be estimated twice in the first week. Thereafter the biochemical assessment need be less frequent if the clinical status is judged reasonable. Serum triglyceride concentration during the infusion should not exceed 200 mg/100 ml and should be less than 100 mg/100 ml 4 hours after the discontinuation of the lipid infusion. According to progress and the child's ability to tolerate oral or gavage feeding, the volumes infused parenterally are reduced stepwise as oral intake is increased.

Total parenteral nutrition in very low birth–weight infants is an effective way of maintaining life. A recent controlled trial (Yu et al 1979) showed that total parenteral nutrition in very low birth–weight infants resulted in a greater mean daily weight gain and a reduced time to regain birth weight and maintain growth. Metabolic complications during parenteral nutrition were no greater than those observed in an enterally fed group who were less severely ill. Long–term survival and effective rehabilitation of children with nearly total absence of small bowel has been made possible by a programme of total parenteral nutrition (Goldberger et al 1979).

Parenteral feeding has a definite mortality and morbidity and its use should be restricted to infants and children in whom it is likely to be beneficial. Used sensibly, it can be vital in securing undamaged survival in the sick infant and child.

REFERENCES

Abbott, W.E., Levey, S., Krieger, H. Benson, J.W. & Rayburn, C.J. (1956) *Surg. Forum*, 7, 80.
Abel, R.M., Shih, V.E., Abbott, W.M., Beck, C.H. & Fischer, J.E. (1973a) *Ann. Surg.*, 180, 350.
Abel, R.M., Beck, C.H., Abbott, W.M., Ryan, J.A., Barnett, G.O. & Fischer, J.E. (1973b) *N. Engl. J. Med.*, 288, 695.
Abel, R.M., Fischer, J.E., Buckley, M.J., Barnett, O. & Austen, W.G. (1976) *Arch. Surg.*, 111, 45.
Albright, F., (1943) *Harvey Lect.*, 38, 123.
Allardyce, B., Hamit, H.F., Matsumoto, T. & Mosely, R.V. (1969) *J. Trauma*, 9, 403.
Allison, S.P., Prowse.K, & Chamberlain, M.J. (1967) *Lancet*, 1, 478.
Allison, S.P., Hinton, P & Chamberlain, M.J. (1968) *Lancet*, 2, 1113.
Amris, C.J., Brockner, J., Larsen, V. (1964) *Acta. Chir. Scand.*, (Suppl) 325, 70.
Andersson, B., & McCann, S.M. (1955) *Acta. Physiol. Scand.*, 33, 333.
Appel, W. (1971) *Med. Klin.*, 66, 484.
Armstrong, R.F., Peters, J.L. & Cohen, S.L. (1977) *Lancet*, 1, 954.
Ashmore, J. & Weber, G. (1968) In: *Carbohydrate Metabolism and Its Disorders*. Academic Press. London, New York: vol. 1, p. 335.
Askanazi, J., Elwyn D.H., Silverbert, P.A., Rosenbaum, S H & Kinney, J M (1980a) *Surgery*, 87, 596.
Askanazi, J., Carpentier, Y.A., Elwyn, D.H., Nordenstrom, J., Jeevanandam, M., Rosenbaum, S.H., Gump, F.E., & Kinney, J.M. (1980b) *Ann. Surg.*, 191, 40.
Atkinson, M., Walford, S. & Allison, S.P. (1979) *Lancet*, 2, 829.
Atwater, W.O. & Benedict, F.G. (1896) *Mem. Natn. Acad. Sci.*, 8, 235.
Aubaniac, R. (1952) *Presse Med.*, 60, 1456.
Baker, D.R., Schrader, W.H. & Hitchcock, C.R. (1964) *JAMA*, 190, 586.
Bark, S., Holm, I., Hakansson, I. & Wretlind, A.(1976) *Acta. Chir. Scand.*, 142, 423.
Barr, P.O., Birke, G., Liljedahl, S.O. & Plantin, L.O. (1968) *Lancet*, 1, 164.
Barson, A.J., Chiswick, M.L. & Doig, C.M. (1978) *Arch. Dis. Child.*, 53, 218.
Baxter, C.R. & Shires, T. (1968) *Ann. N.Y. Acad. Sci.*, 150, 874.
Becker, R., Johnson, D.W., Woeber, K.A. & Wilmore, D.W. (1976) *Fed. Proc.*, 35, 216.
Behnke, A.R. (1942) *Harvey Lect.*, 37, 198
Benatar, S.R., Hewlett, A.M. & Nunn, J.F. (1973) *Br. J. Anaesth.*, 45, 711.
Benedict, F.G. (1915) *A Study of Prolonged Fasting*. Washington: Carnegie Institute of Washington.
Bergmann, K.E., Ziegler, E.E. & Fomon, S.J. (1974) Water and renal solute load. In: *Infant Nutrition*, ed. Fomon, S.J. p. 246. Philadelphia: W.B. Saunders.
Bergstrom, J., Furst, P., Josephson, B. & Noree, L.O. (1970) *Life Sci.*, 9, 787.
Bergstrom, J., Bucht, H., Furst, P., Hultman, E., Josephson, B., Noree, L.O. & and Vinnars, E. (1972) *Acia. Med. Scand.*, 191, 359.
Bernard, C. (1949) *Introduction to the Study of Experimental Medicine* New York.
Berne, T.V. & Barbour, B.H. (1971) *Arch. Surg.*, 102, 594.
Beverley, S., Hambleton, R. & Allwood, M.C. (1973) *Pharm. J.*, 211, 321.
Bewley, T.H. (1964) *Br. Med. J.*, 2, 861.
Birch, G.G. (1971) *Lancet*, 2, 1419.
Bircher, J., Muller, J., Guggenheim, P. & Haemmerli, U.P. (1966) *Lancet*, 1, 890.
Birkhahn, R.H., Long, C.L. & Blakemore, W.S. (1979) *J. Parent & Ent. Nutr.*, 3, 346.
Bistrian, B.R. & Blackburn, G.L. (1974) *Fed. Proc.*, 33, 691.
Bistrian, B.R. Blackburn, G., Hallowell, E. & Heddle, R. (1974) *JAMA*, 230, 858.

Bistrian, B.R., Blackburn, G.L., Scrimshaw, N.S. & Platt, J.P. (1975) *Am. J. Clin. Nutr.*, **28**, 1147.
Bivins, B.A., Rapp, R.P., DeLuca, P.P., McKean, H. & Griffen, W.O. (1979) *Surgery*, **85**, 388.
Blackburn, G.L., Flatt, J.P., Clowes, G.H.A., O'Donnell, T.F. (1973a) *Am. J. Surg.*, **125**, 447.
Blackburn, G.L., Flatt, J.P., Clowes, G.H.A., O'Donnell, T.F., & Hensle, T.E. (1973b) *Ann. Surg.*, **177**, 588.
Blaisdell, F.W.(1974) *Arch. Surg.* **177**, 588.
Blaisdell, F.W., Lim, R.C. & Stallone, R.J. (1970) *Surg. Gynecol. Obstet.*, 130, 15.
Blalock, A. (1939) *Arch. Surg.*, **20**, 959.
Blennow, G. (1975) *Am. J. Dis. Child.*, **129**, 1456.
Bone, R.C. (1978) *Crit. Care Med.*, **6**, 136.
Bonnar, J. (1965) *Br. Med. J.*, **2**, 1030.
Booth, C.C., Hanna, S. Barbouris, N. & McIntyre, I. (1963) *Br. Med. J.*, **2**, 141.
Borresen, H.C., Coran, A.G. & Knutrud, O. (1970) *Ann. Surg.*, **172**, 291.
Borst, J.G.G. (1948) *Lancet*, **1**, 824.
Boston Collaborative Drug Surveance Programme (1973) *JAMA*, **224**, 613.
Bradley, J.A., King, R.F.J.G., Schorah, C.J. & Hill, G.L. (1978) *Br. J. Surg.*, **65**, 492.
Brennan, M.F. & Moore, F.D. (1973) *J. Surg. Res.*, **14**, 501.
Brennan, M.F., Fitzpatrick, G.F., Cohen, K.H. & Moore, F.D. (1975) *Ann. Surg.*, **182**, 386.
Brennan, M.F., Goldman. M.H, O'Connell, R.C., Kundsin, R.B. & Moore, F.D. (1972) *Ann. Surg.*, **176**, 271.
Br. Med. J. (1979) Leading article, *Br. Med. J.* **4**, 1529.
Brocks, A., Reid, H. & Glazer, G. (1977) *Br. Med. J.*, **1**, 1390.
Brocklehurst, G., Gleave, J.R.W., Millar, R.A. & Adams, A.K. (1967) *Arch. Dis. Child.*, **42**, 166.
Broviac, J.W., Cole, J.J. & Scribner, B.H. (1973) *Surg. Gynecol. Obstet.*, **136**, 602.
Brown, H., Trey, C. & McDermott, W.V. (1971) *Arch. Surg.*, **102**, 25.
Brucke, P., Kucher, K., Steinbereithner, K. & Wagner, O. (1966) *Z. Prakt. Anaesth.*, **1**, 319.
Bull, G.M., Joekes, A.M. & Lowe, K.G. (1949) *Lancet.*, **2**, 229.
Bull, G.M., Jaekes, A.M. & Lowe, K.G. (1950) *Clin. Sci.*, **4**, 379.
Burr, G.O. & Burr, M.M. (1930) *J. Biol. Chem.*, **86**, 587.
Burr, W.A., Griffiths, R.S., Black, E.G. & Hoffenberg, R. (1975) *Lancet*, **2**, 1277.
Burri, C. & Ahnefeld, F.W. (1978) *The Caval Catheter.* p. 39. Berlin: Springer-Verlag.
Bursztein, S., Taitelman, U., Myttenaeve, S., Michelson, M., Dahan, E., Gepstein, R., Edelman, D. & Melamed, Y. (1978) *Crit. Care. Med.*, **6**, 162.
Bury, K.D., Stephens, R.V. & Randall, H.T. (1971) *Am. J. Surg.*, **121**, 174.
Cahill, G.F. (1970) *N. Eng. J. Med.*, **282**, 668.
Cahill, G.F. & Aoki, T.T. (1970) *Med. Times*, **98**, 106.
Cahill, G.F., Herrera, M.G., Morgan, A.P., Soeldner, J.S., Steinke, J., Levy, P.L., Reichard, G.A. & Kipris, D.M. (1966) *J. Clin. Invest.*, **45**, 1751.
Caldwell, M.D., Jonsson, H.T. & Othersen, H.B. (1972) *J. Pediat.*, **81**, 849.
Cameron, J.S., Ogg, C. & Trounce, J.R. (1967) Lancet, **1**, 1188.
Cannon, P.R. (1945) *Protein Metabolism*, **128**, 360.
Cannon, W.B. (1918) *JAMA.*, **70**, 611.
Carpentier, Y.A., Askanazi, J., Elwyn, D.H., Jeevanandam, M., Gump, F.E., Hyman, A.I., Burr, R. & Kinney, J.M. (1979) *J. Trauma.*, **19**, 649.
Carstensen, H., Terner, N., Thoren, L. & Wide, L. (1972) *Acta. Chir. Scand.*, **138**, 1.
Casewell, M.W. & Philips, I. (1978) *J.Clin. Pathol.*, **31**, 845.
Cason, J.S. (1966) In: *Research in Burns* ed. Wallace, A.B. Wilkinson, A. W., p.l. Edinburgh: Livingstone.
Chakmakjian, Z.H. & Bethune, J.E. (1966) *N. Engl. J. Med.*, **275**, 862.
Chart, J.J., Gordon, E.S., Helmer, P. & LeSher, M. (1956) *J. Clin. Invest.*, **35**, 254.
Charters, A., Odell, W. & Thompson, J. (1969) *J. Clin. Endocrinol. Metab.*, **29**, 63.
Christensen, H.N. & Lynch, E.L. (1946) *J. Biol. Chem.*, **166**, 652.
Clarke, A.M., Hill, G.L. & Macbeth, W.A.A.G. (1967) *Gastroenterology.*, **53**, 444.
Clarke, R., Topley, E., Fisher, M. & Davies, J.W. (1961) *Lancet*, **2**, 381.
Clothier Report (1972) Report to the Committee appointed to inquire into the circumstances, including the production, which led to the use of contaminated infusion fluids in the Devonpart Section of Plymouth General Hospital. London: H.M.S.O.
Coats, D.A. (1972) The place of ethanol in parenteral nutrition. In *Parenteral Nutrition.* ed. Wilkinson, A.W. Edinburgh: Churchill Livingstone.
Cobb, C.A., Le Quire, V.S., Gray, M.E. & Hillman, J.W. (1959) *Surg. Forum*, **9**, 751.
Cockburn, F. (1978) Parenteral nutrition in infants and children. In: *Textbook of Paediatrics.* ed. Forfar, J.O. & Arneil, G.A. Edinburgh: Churchil-Livingstone.

Coleman, W. & Dubois, E. (1915) *Arch. Intern Med.*, **15**, 887.

Coller, F.A., Iob, V., Vaughan, H.H., Kalder, N.B. & Moyer, C.A. (1945) *Ann. Surg.*, **122**, 663.

Collin, J., Tweedle, D.E.F., Venables, C.W., Constable, F.L. & Johnston, I.D.A. (1973) *Br. Med. J.*, **4**, 456.

Collins, F.D., Sinclair, A.J., Royle, J.P., Coats, D.A., Maynard, A.T. & Leonard, R.F. (1971) *Nutr. Metab.*, **13**, 150.

Conn, J.N. (1967) *Ann. Intern. Med.*, **66**, 1283.

Conn, J.W. & Louis, L.H. (1956) *Ann. Intern. Med.*, **44**, 1.

Connell, R.S. & Swank, R.L. (1973) *Ann. Surg.*, **177**, 40.

Cook, G.C. (1973) *Clin. Sci.*, **44**, 425.

Cori, C.F. (1931) *Phys. Rev.*, **11**, 143.

Craig, R.P., Davidson, H.A., Tweedle, D.E.F. & Johnson, I.D.A. (1977) *Lancet*, **2**, 8.

Crane, C. (1960) *N. Engl. J. Med.*, **262**, 947.

Crawford, M.A. & Hassam, A.G. (1976) *Lancet*, **2**, 94.

Crile, G.W. (1899) *An Experimental Research into Surgical Shock*. Philadelphia: Lippincott.

Cronberg, S. & Nilsson, I.M. (1967) *Thromb. Diath. Haemorrh.*, **18**, 664.

Cuthbertson, D.P. (1930) *Biochem. J.*, **24**, 1244.

Cuthbertson, D.P. (1932) *Q.J. Med.*, **25**, 233.

Cuthbertson, D.P. (1942) *Lancet*, **1**, 433.

Daily, P.O., Griepp, R.B. & Shumway, N.E. (1969) *Arch. Surg.*, **101**, 534.

Dale, G., Young, G., Latner, A.L., Goode, A.W., Tweedle, D.E.F. & Johnston, I.D.A. (1977) *Surgery*, **81**, 295.

D'Arcy, P.F. (1976) Additives — an additional hazard? In *Microbiological Hazards of Infusion Therapy*. ed. Philips, I., Meers, P.D. & D'Arcy, P.F. Lancaster: MTP Press.

D'Arcy, P.F. & Griffin, J.P. (1974) *Prescribers J.*, **14**, 38.

Darrow, D.C., Cooke, R.E. & Segar, W.E. (1954) *Pediatrics*, **14**, 602.

Davidson, E.C. (1926) *Arch. Surg.*, **13**, 262.

Davidson, S. & Passmore, R. (1969) In *Human Nutrition and Dietetics*, 4th edn. Edinburgh: Livingstone.

Davies, J.W.L. (1970) *J. Clin. pathol.*, 23, Suppl. (Roy. Coll. Path.) 4, 56.

Davies, J.W.L. (1975a) *Burns*, **1**, 319.

Davies, J.W.L. (1975b) *Burns*, **1**, 331.

Davies, J.W. & Topley, E. (1956) *Clin. Sci.*, **15**, 135.

Davies, J.W.L., Lamke, L.O. & Liljedahl, S.O. (1977a) *Acta. Chir. Scand.*, Suppl. 468, 1.

Davies, J.W.L., Lamke, L.O. & Liljedahl, S.O. (1977b) *Acta. Chir. Scand.*, Suppl. 468, 25.

Delany, H.M., Carnevale, N., Garvey, J.W. & Moss, C.M. (1977) *Ann. Surg.*, **186**, 165.

DeLuca, P.P., Rapp, R.P., McKean, H.E. & Griffen, W.D. (1975) *Am. J. Hosp. Pharm.*, **32**, 1001.

Department of Health and Social Security (1969) *Rep. Health Soc. Subj. Lond.* No. 120.

DeVisser, J. & Overbeek, G.A. (1960) *Acta Endocrinol.*, **35**, 405.

De Weese, M.S. & Hunter, D.C. (1963) *Arch. Surg.*, **86**, 852.

De Wys, W.D. (1977) *Cancer Res.*, **37**, 2354.

De Wys, W.D. & Walters, K. (1975) *Cancer*, **36**, 1888.

Dinley, R.J. (1976) *Curr. Med. Res. Opin.*, **3**, 607.

Dobbie, R.P. & Hoffmeister, J.A. (1976) *Surg. Gynecol. Obstet.*, **143**, 273.

Donahoe, J.F. & Powers, R.J. (1970) *N. Engl. J. Med.*, **282**, 690.

Dowling, R.H., Bell, G.D. & White, J. (1972) *Gut*, **13**, 415.

Dubois, E. (1924) *Basal Metabolism in Health and Disease*. New York. Lea and Febiger.

Dudley, H.A.F., Robson, J.S., Smith, M. & Stewart, C.P. (1959) *Metabolism*, **8**, 895

Dudrick, S.J., Steiger, E. & Long, J.M. (1970) *Surgery*, **68**, 180.

Dudrick, S.J., Steiger, E., Long, J.M. & Rhoads, J.E. (1970) *Surg. Clin. N. Amer.*, **50**, 1031.

Dudrick, S.J., Steiger, E., Long, J.M., Ruberg, R.L., Allen, T.R., Vars, H.M. & Rhoads, J.E. (1972) General principles and technique of administration in complete parenteral nutrition. In *Parenteral Nutrition*. ed. Wilkinson, A.W. Edinburgh: Churchill Livingstone.

Duma, R.J., Warner, J.F. & Dalton, H.P. (1971) *N. Engl. J. Med.*, **284**, 257.

Dunlap, W.M., James, G.W. & Hume, D.M. (1974) *Ann. Intern. Med.*, **80**, 470.

Durnin, J.V.G.A. & Womersley, J. (1974) *Br. J. Nutr.*, **32**, 77–97.

Eckart, J., Tempel, G.,Kaul, A., Witzke, G., Schurnbrand, P. & Schaaf, H. (1973) *Am. J. Clin. Nutr.*, **26**, 578.

Eckart, J., Tempel, G., Kaul, A. & Witzke, P.D. (1974) *Eur. Surg. Res.*, (suppl. 1), 110.

Eckart, J., Adolph, M. & Wolfram. G. (1980) *Elimination of parenterally administered medium chain* 2nd European Congress of Parenteral and Enteral Nutrition (Abstract), Newcastle-upon-Tyne.

Edmunds, L.H.Jr., Williams, G.M. & Welch, C.E. (1960) *Ann. Surg.*, **152**, 445.

Eisenberg, H.L., Kolb, L.H. & Yam, L.T. (1964) *Ann. Surg.*, **159**, 604.
Elman, R. (1939) *Proc. Soc. Exp. Biol. Med.*, **40**, 484.
El'Ode, J.E., Dornseifer, T.P. Keith, T. & Powes, J.J. (1966) *J. Food Sci.*, **31**, 351.
Elwyn, D. (1970) In *Mammalian Protein Metabolism*, vol. IV. ed. Munro, H.N. New York: Academic Press.
Engel, F.L. & Jaeger, C. (1954) *Am. J. Med.*, **17**, 196.
England, P.C., Duari, M., Tweedle, D.E.F., Jones, R.A. & Gowland, E. (1979) *Br. J. Surg.*, **66**, 340.
Espiner, E.A. (1966) *J. Endocrinol.*, **35**, 29.
Fahey, J.L. (1957) *J. Clin. Invest.*, **36**, 1647.
Fantus, B. & Schirmer, E.H. (1938) *JAMA*, **111**, 317.
Feldman, E.J., MacNaughton, J. & Dowling, R.H. (1973) *Gut*, **14**, 831.
Ferrer, J.M. (1970) *N. Engl. J. Med.*, **282**, 688.
Fischer, J.E. & Baldessarini, R.J. (1971) *Lancet*, **2**, 75.
Fischer, J.E., Funovics, J.M., Aguirre, A., James, J.H., Keane, J.M., Wesdorp, R.I.C., Yoshirmura, N. & Westman, T. (1975) *Surgery*, **78**, 276.
Fischer, J.E., Rosen, H.M., Ebeid, A.M., James, J.H., Keane, J.M. & Soeters, P.B. (1976) *Surgery*, **80**, 77.
Fisher, M. (1977) *Br. J. Anaesth.*, **49**, 1023.
Fisher, R.B. (1954) In *Protein Metabolism* London: Methuen.
Fishman, L.S., Griffin, J.R., Sapico, F.L. & Hecht, R. (1972) *N. Engl. J. Med.*, **286**, 675.
Flack, F.C. & Whyte, T.D. (1974) *Br. med. J.*, **3**, 439.
Flink, E.B. (1956) *JAMA*, **160**, 1406.
Forman, J.V. & Powell, D. (1969) *Br. J. Hosp. Med. Equip.*, Suppl. **2**, 37.
Fossard, D.P., Kakkar, V.V. & Elsey, P.A. (1974) *Br. Med. J.*, **2**, 465.
Franksson, C., Hastad, K. & Larsson, L.G. (1959) *Acta. Chir. Scand.*, **118**, 264.
Freeman, J.B. (1978) *Can. J. Surg.*, **21**, 489.
Freeman, J.B. & Maclean, L.D. (1971) *Can. J. Surg.* **14**, 180.
Freeman, J.B. & Litton, A.A. (1974) *Surg. Gynecol. Obstet.*, **139**, 905.
Freeman, J.B., Lemire, A. & MacLean, L.D. (1972) *Surg. Gynecol. Obstet.*, **135**, 708.
Friedman, E., Grable, E. & Fine, J. (1966) *Lancet*, **2**, 609.
Friedman, L. & Kline, O.L. (1950) *J. Nutr.*, **40**, 295.
Froesch, E.R. (1974) The metabolism of Glucose, its endocrine control and comparative aspects with Fructose, Sorbitol and Xylitol metabolism. In *Parenteral Nutrition in Acute Metabolic Illness.* ed. Lee, H.A. London: Academic Press.
Fujita, T., Samaya, T. & Yokoyama, K. (1971) *Eur. Surg. Res.*, **3**, 436.
Furber, T.H., Hambleton, R. & Scobie, S.D. (1978) *Pharm. J.*, **221**, 458.
Furst, P., Bergstrom, J., Vinnars, E., Schildt, B., & Holmstrom (1978) Intracellular amino acids and energy metabolism in catabolic patients with regard to muscle tissue. In *Advances in Parenteral Nutrition.* ed. I.D.A. Johnson. Lancaster: MTP Press.
Gallagher, P. & Tweedle, D.E.F. (1981) In press.
Gallagher, P., Schofield, P.F. & Tweedle, D.E.F. (1981) In press.
Gamble, J.L. (1947) *Harvey Lect.*, **42**, 247.
Gamble, J.L. (1954) *Chemical Anatomy, Physiology and Pathology of Extracellular Fluid*, 6th edn. London: Geoffrey Cumberlege.
Gamble, J.L. & Ross, S.G. (1925) *J. Clin. Invest.*, **1**, 403.
Garvan, J.M. & Gunner, B.W. (1971) *Br. J. Clin. Pract.*, **25**, 119.
Gazzaniga, A.B., Bartlett, R.H. & Shobe, J.B. (1975) *Ann. Surg.*, **182**, 163.
Geyer, R.P. (1970) *Fed. Proc.*, **29**, 1758.
Geyer, R.P. (1973) *N. Eng. J. Med.*, **289**, 1077.
Ghadimi, H., Kumar, S. & Abaci, F. (1971) *Biochem. Med.*, **5**, 447.
Gilder, H., Cornell, G.N., Johnson, G. Jr., Craver, W.L. & Beal, J.M. (1957) *Surg. Forum.*, **8**, 58.
Giordano, C. (1963) *J. Lab. Clin. Med.*, **62**, 231.
Giovannetti, S. & Maggiore, Q. (1964) *Lancet*, **1**, 1000.
Glick, S.M., Roth, J., Yalow, R.S. & Berson, S.A. (1965) *Rec. Prog. Horm. Res.*, **21**, 241.
Goldberg, M. (1963) *Am. J. Med.*, **35**, 293.
Goldberger, E. (1957) *Acta Med. Scand.*, **157**, 417.
Goldberger, J.H., De Luca, F.G., Wesselhoeft, C.W. & Randall, H.T. (1979) *J. Pediat.*, **94**, 325.
Goldsmith, R.S. & Ingbar, S.H. (1966) *N. Engl. J. Med.*, **274**, 1.
Goodman, M.J. & Truelove, S.C. (1976) *Br. Med. J.*, **3**, 354.
Gouillou, P.J., Morgan, D.B. & Hill, G.L. (1976) *Lancet*, **2**, 710.
Gove, L., Walls, A.D.F. & Scott, W. (1979) *Pharm. J.*, **223**, 6051, p. 587.

Graham, W.P. & Royster, H.P. (1967) *Surg. Gynecol. Obstet.*, **125**, 127.

Grant, J.P., Cox, C.E. & Kleinman, L.M. (1977) *Surg. Gynecol. Obstet.*, **145**, 573.

Grant, R.T. & Reeve, E.B. (1941) *Br. Med. J.*, **2**, 293.

Greene, H.L. (1976) Effect on Intralipid on Pulmonary function. In *Fat Emulsions in Parenteral Nutrition.* ed. Meng, H.C. & Wilmore, D.W. Chicago: American Medical Association.

Griepp, R.B. (1977) *J. Thor. Cardiovasc. Surg.* **73**, 489.

Grotte, G. (1971) Atrémie digestive et nutrition parentérale du nourrison. In: *Les Solutes de Substitution Re équilibration Métabolique.* ed. Nahas, G.H. & Viars, P. p. 509. Paris: Librairie Annette.

Groves, A.C., Woolf, L.I. & Allardyce, D.B. (1974) *Surg. Forum.*, **25**, 54.

Gruber, U.F. (1969) *Blood replacement.* Heidelberg: Springer.

Guignier, M., Hernandex, J.L., Pircher, C., Muller, J.M., Morena, H., Guidicelli, H. & Banon, F. (1975) *Nouv Presse Med*, **4**, 973.

Guyton, A.C. (1969) *Interstitial Fluid Pressure — volume relationships and their regulation.* CIBA Found. Symp. London: Churchill.

Haffejee, A.A., Anghorn, I.B., Brain, P.P., Duursma, J. & Baker, L.W. (1978) *Br. J. Surg.*, **65**, 480.

Hahn, P. (1979) The perinatal role of carnitine. Abstract — *The 1st Samuel Z. Levine Conference*, ed. A. Minkowski, p. 62. Paris.

Hakansson, I. (1968) *Nutr. Diet.*, **10**: 54.

Hallberg, D. (1965) *Acta Physiol. Scand.*, **65**, 153.

Hallberg, D., Schuberth, O. & Wretlind, A. (1966) *Nutr. Diet.*, **8**, 245.

Halmagyi, D.F.J. & Kinney, J.M. (1975) *Surgery*, **77**, 492.

Hambidge, K.M., Hambidge, C., Jacobs, M. & Baum, J.D. (1972) *Pediatr. Res.* **6**, 868.

Hansen, A.E., Wiese, H.F., Boelsche, A.N., Haggard, M.E., Adam, D.J.D. & Davis, H. (1963) *Pediatrics*, **31** (Suppl.), 171.

Harper, A.E. & Rogers, O.E. (1965) *Proc. Nutr. Soc*, **24**, 173.

Harries, J.T., Peisowicz, A.T., Seakins, J.W. T., Francis, D.E.M. & Wolff, O.H. (1971) *Arch. Dis. Child.*, **46**. 72.

Harris, P.L. & Embree, N.D. (1963) *Am. J. Clin. Nutr*, **13**, 385

Havill, J.H. & Faracs, F. (1975) *N.Z. Med. J.*, **81**, 420.

Haynes, B.W., Martin, M M & Purnell, O.J. (1955) *Ann. Surg.*, **142**, 674.

Heatley, R.V., Williams, R.H.P. & Lewis, M.H. (1979) *Postgrad. Med. J.*, **55**, 541.

Heaton, F.W., Clark, C.C. & Goligher, J.C. (1967) *Br. J. Surg.*, **54**, 41.

Heaton, K.W., & Read, A.E. (1969) *Br. Med. J.*, **3**, 494.

Hegsted, D.M. (1964) In *Mammalian Protein Metabolism*, vol. 2. ed. Munro, H.N. & Allison, J.B. New York: Academic Press.

Heird, W.C., Dell, R.B., Driscoll, J.M., Grebin, B. & Winters, R.W. (1972a) *N. Engl. J. Med.*, **287**, 943.

Heird, W.C., Nicholson, J.F., Driscoll, J.M., Schullinger, J.N. & Winters, R.W. (1972b) *J. Pediat.*, **81**, 162.

Helmkamp, G.M.Jr., Wilmore, D.W. & Johnson, A.A. (1973) *Am. J. Clin. Nutr.*, **26**, 1331.

Henkin, R.I., Patten, B.M., Re, P.K. & Bronzert, D.A. (1975) *Arch. Neurol.*, **32**, 745.

Henzel, J.II. & De Weeze, U.S. (1971) *Am. J. Surg.*, **121**, 600.

Hers, H.G. (1955) *J. Biol. Chem.*, **214**, 273.

Hershberger, L.G., Shipley, E.G. & Meyer, R.K. (1953) *Proc. Soc. exp. Biol.*, **83**, 175.

Hill, G.L., Mair, W.S.J. & Goligher, J.C. (1975a) *Br. J. Surg.*, **62**, 720.

Hill, G.L., Goligher, J.C., Smith, A.H. & Mair, W.S.J. (1975b) *Br. J. Surg.*, **62**, 524.

Hill, G.L., Mair, W.S.J. & Goligher, J.C. (1975c) *Gut*, **16**, 932.

Hill, G.L., Main, W.S.T., Edwards, J.P. & Goligher, J.C. (1976) *Br. J. Surg.*, **63**, 133.

Hill, J.D., Osborn, J.J. & Swank, R.L. (1970) *Arch. Surg.*, **101**, 649.

Hill, J.D., O'Brien, T.G. & Murray, J.J. (1972) *N. Engl. J. Med.*, **286**, 629.

Himsworth, H.P. & Kerr, R.B. (1939) *Clin. Sci.*, **4**, 1.

Hint, H. (1968) *Acta Anaesth. Belg.*, **19**, 119.

Hinton, P., Allison, S.P., Littlejohn, S. & Lloyd, J. (1971) *Lancet*, **1**, 767.

Hirsch, E.F., Fletcher, R. & Lucas, S. (1971) *Ann. Surg.*, **174**, 211.

Hodges, J.E., Fisher, B.E. & Nelson, E.C. (1963) *Am. Soc. Brew. Chem. Proc.*, **84**.

Hogan, J.F. (1915) *JAMA*, **54**, 1342.

Holdsworth, C.D. (1972) In *Transport Across the Intestine.* ed. Burland, W.L. & Samuel, P.D. Edinburgh: Churchill Livingstone.

Holman, R. T. (1975) Function and biologic activities of essential fatty acids in man. In *Fat Emulsions in Parenteral Nutrition* ed. Meng, H.C. & Wilmore, D.W. Chicago: American Medical Association.

Holt, L.E. (1967) *Curr. Ther. Appr.*, **9**, 149.
Holter, A.R. & Fisher, J.E. (1977) *J. Surg. Res.*, **23**, 31.
Hoshal, V.L., Ause, R.G. & Hoskins, P.A. (1971) *Arch. Surg.*, **102**, 353.
Howard, J.M. & Brown, R.B. (1970) Military Surgery. In *Surgery, Principles and Practice*. 4th edn. Philadelphia: Lippincott.
Hull, D. (1976) Temperature regulation and disturbance in the newborn infant *Clin. Endocrinol. Metab.*, **5**, 1, 39.
Hunter, J. (1791a) *A treatise on the Blood, Inflammation and Gunshot Wounds*. Part II, p. 239. London: G. Nichol.
Hunter, J. (1791b) *A treatise on the Blood Inflammation and Gunshot Wounds*. Part II, p. 411. London: G. Nichol.
Ibbotson, R.M., Colvin, B.T. & Colvin, M.P. (1975) *Br. Med. J.*, **4**, 522.
Ingle, D.J., (1954) *J. Clin. Endocr.*, **14**, 1272.
Jacob, H.S. & Amsden, T. (1971) *N. Engl. J. Med.*, **285**, 1446.
Jacobson, S. (1969) Complete parenteral nutrition in man for seven months. In *Advances in Parenteral Nutrition*. ed. Berg, G. Stuttgart: Georg Thieme Verlag.
Jacobson, S., Wretlind, A. (1970) The use of fat emulsions for complete intravenous nutrition. In *Body Fluid Replacement in the Surgical Patient*. ed. Fox,C.L.Jr. & Nahas, G.G. New York: Grune & Stratton.
Jaeger, R.J. & Rubin, R.J. (1972) *N. Engl. J. Med.*, **287**, 1114.
James, B.E. & MacMahon, R.A. (1976) *Aust. Paediatr. J.*, **12**, 154.
Jansen, H. (1972) *Acta, Chir. Scand.*, Suppl. 427.
Jeejeebhoy, K.N., Zohrab, W.J., Langer, B., Philips, M.J., Kuksis, A. & Anderson, G.H. (1973) *Gastroenterology*, **65**, 811.
Jeejeebhoy, K.N., Anderson, G.H., Nakhooda, A.F. Greenberg, G.R., Sanderson, I and Marlis, E.B. (1976) *J. Clin. Invest.*, **57**, 125.
Jeejeebhoy, K.N., Chu, R., Marliss, E.B., Greenberg, G.R. & Bruce-Robertson, A. (1977) *Am. J. Clin. Nutr.*, **30**, 531.
Jelenko, C., Wheeler, M.L., Anderson, A.P., Calaway, B.D. & MacKinley, J.C. (1975) *Ann. Surg.*, **182**, 562.
Jernigan, W.R., Gardner, W.C., Mahr, M.N. & Milburn, J.L. (1970) *Surg. Gynecol. Obstet.*, **130**, 520.
John, G.E. (1972) DHSS, DS (Supply), 6/72.
Johnson, J.D., Albritton, W.L. & Sunshine, P. (1972) *J. Pediat.*, **81**, 154.
Johnston, A.O.B. & Clark, R.G. (1972) *Br. J. Surg.*, **59**, 897.
Johnston, I.D.A. & Chenneour, R. (1963) *Br. J. Surg.*, **227**, 924.
Johnston, I.D.A. & Hadden, D.R. (1963) *Lancet*, **1**, 584.
Johnston, I.D.A., Marino, J.D. & Stevens, J.Z. (1966) *Br. J. Surg.*, **54**, 438.
Jones, B·J.M., Payne, S. & Silk, D.B.A. (1980) *Lancet*, **1**, 1057.
Jones, H.V. & Craig, D.B. (1972) *Can. Anaesth. Soc. J.*, **19**, 491.
Jones, R., Thomas, W.A. & Scott, R.F. (1962) *Exp. Mol. Path.*, **1**, 65.
Jurgens, P. & Dolip, D (1968) *Klin. Wochenschr.*, **46**, 131.
Kaminski, M.V. (1976) *Surg. Gynecol. Obstet.*, **143**, 12.
Kaminski, D.L., Adams, A. & Jellinek, M. (1980) *Surgery*, **88**, 93.
Kapp, J.P., Duckert, F. & Hartmann, G. (1971) *Nutr. Metab.*, **13**, 92.
Karpel, J.T. & Peden, V.H. (1972) *J. Paediatr.*, **80**, 32.
Kay, D. & Robinson, D.S. (1962) *Q. J. Exp. Physiol.*, **47**, 258.
Kay, R.G., Tasman-Jones, C., Pybus, J., Whiting, R. & Block, H. (1976) *Ann. Surg.*, **183**, 331.
Kennedy, J.H., Peters, H.A. & Serif, G.S. (1959) *Surg. Forum*, **9**, 364.
Keys, A., Brozek, J., Henschel, A., Mickelsen, O. & Taylor, H.L. (1950) *The Biology of Human Starvation*, vol. 1, p. 329. Minneapolis: University of Minnesota Press.
Kinney, J.M. & Moore. F.D. (1956) *Surgery*, **40**, 16.
Kinney, J.M., Duke, J.H., Long, C.L. & Gump, F.E. (1970) *J. Clin. Pathol.* **23**, Suppl. (Roy, Coli. Path.) 4, 65.
Kirby, R. & Johnston, I.D.A. (1971) *Br. J. Surg.*, **58**, 305.
Klim, R. & Hardy, G. (1980) Personal communication.
Knowles, H.C. Jr. & Kaplan, S.A. (1953) *Arch. Intern. Med.*, **92**, 189.
Krebs, H.A. (1978) Some general considerations concerning the use of carbohydrates in parenteral nutrition. In *Advances in Parenteral Nutrition*. ed. Johnston, I.D.A. Lancaster: MTP Press.
Krebs, H.A. & Perkins, J.R. (1970) *Biochem. J.*, **118**, 635.
Kwaan, H.M. & Weil, M.H. (1969) *Surg. Gynecol. Obstet.*, **128**, 37.
Lancet (1959) Editorial, *Lancet*, **1**, 559.

Lancet (1963) Editorial, *Lancet*, 2, 1265.

Lancet (1973) Editorial, *Lancet*, 2, 366.

Lancet (1975) Editorial, *Lancet*, 2, 263.

Larrey, D.J. (1829) *Clinique Chirurgicale*, vol. 1, p. 182. Paris: Imprimerie de Cosson.

Lavagh, J.H. (1962) *Circulation*, 25, 1015.

Lavender, J.P. (1979) Radio Isotopic Lung Scanning and the Chest X-ray in Pulmonary Disease. In *Recent Advances in Radiology and Medical Imaging*.Sixth Ed. Ed. Lodge & Steiner. Edinburgh: Churchill-Livingstone.

Law, D.K., Dudrick, S.J. & Abdou, N.I. (1973) *Ann. Intern. Med.*, 79, 545.

Lawson, L.J. (1965) *Br. J. Surg.*, 52, 795.

Ledingham, I. MCA. & McArdle, C.S. (1978) *Lancet*, 1, 1194.

Ledingham, I. MCA, McArdle, C.S. & Macdonald, R.C. (1980) Septic Shock. In *Recent Advances in Surgery*. ed. Taylor, S. Edinburgh: Churchill Livingstone.

Le Drau, H.F. (1743) *A Treatise or Reflections, Drawn from Practice on Gun-shot wounds*. London: Clarke.

Lee, H.A., Sharpstone, P. & Ames, A.C. (1967) *Postgrad. Med. J.*, 43, 81.

Lee, H.A., Hill, L.F., Ginks, W.R. & Pohl, J.E.F. (1968) Some aspects of parenteral nutrition in the treatment of renal failure. In *Nutrition in Renal Disease*. ed. Berlyne, G.M. Edinburgh: Livingstone.

Lee, H.A., Morgan, A.G., Waldram, R. & Bennett, J. (1972) Sorbitol: some aspects of its metabolism and role as an intravenous nutrient. In *Parenteral Nutrition*. ed. Wilkinson, A.W. Edinburgh: Churchill Livingstone.

Lee, J. Bisset, G.W. (1958) *Proc. Roy. Soc. Med.*, 51, 361.

Le Quesne, L.P. (1954) *Lancet*, 1, 172.

Le Quesne, L.P. (1961) *Surg. Gynecol. Obst.*, 113, 1.

Lemd, N. (1973) *Br. J. Anaesth.*, 45, 929.

Levene, M.I., Wigglesworth, J.S. & Desai, R. (1980) *Lancet*, 2, 815.

Levenson, S.M., Howard, J.M. & Rosen, H. (1955) *Surg. Gynecol. Obstet.*, 101, 35.

Levine, S.Z., Wilson, J.R. & Kelley, M. (1929) *Am. J. Dis. Child.*, 37, 791.

Liljedahl, S.O., Gemzell, C.A., Plantin, L.O. & Birke, G. (1961) *Acta Chir. Scand.*, 122, 1.

Lillehei, R.C. & Dietzman (1974) Circulatory Collapse and Schock. In *Principles of Surgery*. ch. 4. ed. Schwartz, S.I. McGraw HIll.

Lind J. (1753) *A Treatise of the Scurvy*, Reprinted by Edinburgh University Press 1953.

Ljungqvist, U. (1973) *J. Surg. Res.*, 15, 132.

Loirat, Ph., Rohan, J.E., Chapman, A., Beaufils, F., David, R & Nedey, R. (1975) *Europ. J. Int. Care Med.*, 1, 11.

Long, C.L., Crosby, F., Geiger, J.W. & Kinney, J.M. (1976) *Am. J. Clin. Nutr.*, 29, 380.

Long, J.M., Wilmore, D.W., Mason, A.D. & Pruitt, B.A. (1977) *Ann. Surg.*, 185, 417.

Lordon, R.E. & Burton, J.R. (1972) *Am. J. Med.*, 53, 137.

Lowry, S.F., Goodgame, J.T., Smith, J.C., Maher, M.M., Makuch, R.W., Henkin, R.I. & Brennan, MF. (1979) *Ann. Surg.*, 189, 120.

Lucas, A., Bloom, S.R. & Aynsley-Green. A. (1978) *Arch Dis. Child.*, 53, 731.

McArthur, B., Hargiss, C. & Schoenknecht, F.D. (1975) *Am. J. Nurs.*, 75, 96.

McDonald, A. (1974) *J. Hosp. Pharm.*, Sept, 80.

MacFadyen, B.V. Jr. & Dudrick, S.J. (1976) *Acta Chir. Scand.*, Suppl, 466, 90.

MacFarlane, D.A. & Thomas, L.P. (1977) *Textbook of Surgery*, 4th edn. Edinburgh: Churchill Livingstone.

McMichael, H.B., Webb, J. & Dawson, A.M. (1967) *Br. Med. J.*, 2, 1037.

Madden, S.C., Woods, R.R., Shull, S.W., Remington, J.H. & Whipple, G.H. (1945) *J. Exp. Med.*, 81, 439.

Maddox, R.R., Rush, D.R., Rapp, R.P., Foster, T.S., Mazella, V. & McKean, H.E. (1977) *Am. J. Hosp. Pharm.*, 34, 29.

Maki, D.G. (1976a) Sepsis arising from extrinsic contamination of the infusion and measures for control. In *Microbiological Hazards of Infusion Therapy*. ed. Phillips, I., Meers, P.D. & D'Arcy, P.F.

Maki, D.G. (1976b) *Hosp. Inf. Control.*, 3, 22.

Maki, D.G., Goldmann, D.A. & Rhame, R.S. (1973) *Ann. Intern. Med.*, 79, 867.

Maki, D.G., Rhame, F.S., Mackel, D.C. & Bennett, J.V. (1976) *Am. J. Med.*, 60, 471.

Mallette, L.E., Exton, J.H. & Park, C.R. (1969) *J. Biol. Chem.*, 244, 5713.

Manchester, K.L. (1968) Hormonal control of protein biosynthesis. In *Biological Basis of Medicine*. ed. Bittar, E.E. & Bittar, N. vol. 2, p. 221. New York and London: Academic Press.

Manchester, K.L. (1970) *Biochem. J.*, 117, 457.

Marshall, B.E., Wurzel, H.A., Neufeld, G.R. & Klinebery, P.L. (1976) *Anaesthesia*, 44, 525.

Marx, G.F., Koenig, J.W. & Orkin, L.R. (1960) *JAMA*, **174**, 1834.
Masterton, J.P., Macrae, S. & Dudley, H.A.F. (1963) *Br. Med. J.*, **2**, 909.
Matsumoto, K., Takeyasu, K., Mizutani, S., Hamanaka, Y. & Uozumi, T. (1970) *Acta Endocrinol.*, **65**, 11.
Medicines Commision (1972) *Interim Report on Heat Sterilised Fluids for Parenteral Administration.* London: H.M.S.O.
Meguid, M.M. & Brennan, M.F. (1974) *Lancet*, **1**, 319.
Meng, H.C., Law, D.H. & Sandstead, H.H. (1969) Some clinical experiences in parenteral nutrition. In *Advances in Parenteral Nutrition.* ed. Berg, G. Stuttgart: Georg Thieme Verlag.
Messmer, K. (1975) *Surg. Clin. N. Amer.*, **55**, 627.
Michelson, E. (1968) *N. Engl. J. Med.*, **278**, 552.
Miller, R.C. & Grogan, J.B. (1973) *J. Paediatr. Surg.*, **8**, 185.
Milligan, G.F., MacDonald, J.A.E., Mellon, A. & Ledingham, I. McA. (1974) *Surg. Gynecol. Obstet.*, **138**, 43.
Mitra, K. (1942) *Indian J. Med. Res.*, **30**, 91.
Moghissi, K. (1979) Personal communication.
Moghissi, K., Hornshaw, J. Teasdale. P.R. & Dawes, E.A. (1977) *Br. J. Surg.*, **64**, 125.
Monafo, W.W. (1970) *J. Trauma*, **10**, 575.
Moore, F.D. (1959) In *Metabolic Care of the Surgical Patient.* p. 44. Philadelphia: Saunders.
Moore, F.D. (1970) Surg. Clin. N. Amer., **50**, 1249.
Moore, F.D. & Ball, M.R. (1952) *The Metabolic Response to Surgery.* Springfield: Thomas.
Moore, F.D., Oleson, K.H., McMurrey, J.D., Parker, H.V., Ball, M.R. & Boyden, C.M. (1963) *The Body Cell Mass and its Supporting Environment.* Philadelphia: Saunders.
Moore, F.D., Lyons, J.H., Pierce, E.C., Morgan, A.P., Drinker, P.A., MacArthur, J.D. & Dammin, G.J. (1969) *Post-Traumatic Pulmonary Insufficiency.* Philadelphia: Saunders.
Moretz, W.H., Rhode, C.M. & Shepherd, M.H. (1959) *Arch. Surg.*, **25**, 617.
Morgan, A.P. (1968) *Anaesthesiology*, **29**, 570.
Morgan, M.Y., Milsom, J.P. & Sherlock, S. (1978) *Gut*, **19**, 1068.
Morrice, J.J., Taylor, K.M., Blair, J.I. & Young, D.G. (1974) *Arch. Dis. Child.*, **49**, 898.
Arch. Dis. Child., **49**, 898.
Myers, J.A. (1972) *Pharm. J.*, **208**, 547.
Myers, J.A. (1974) *Pharm. J.*, **212**, 308.
Najarian, J.S. & Harper, H.A. (1952) *Am. J. Med.*, **21**: 832.
Nash, G., Blennerhassett, J.B. & Pontoppidan, H. (1966) *N. Engl. J. Med.*, **276**, 368.
National Academy of Scientists (1979) *Recommended dietary allowances*, 9th edn. Washington D.C.: National Academy of Scientists.
Neale, G. (1968) *Proc. Roy. Soc. Med.*, **61**, 1099.
Neely, W.A., Berry, D.W., Rushton, F.W. & Hardy, J.D. (1971) *Ann. Surg.*, **173**, 657.
Newey, H. & Smyth, D.H. (1962) *J. Physiol.*, **164**, 527.
Newsome, H.H. & Rose, J.C. (1971) *J. Clin. Endocrinol.*, **33**, 481.
Newton, C.R. (1978) *Gut*, **19**, 377.
Newton, D., Connor, H. & Woods, H.F. (1978) Metabolic pathways for carbohydrates in parenteral nutrition. In *Advances in Parenteral Nutrition.* ed. Johnson, I.D.A. Lancaster: MTP Press.
Nuguid, T.P., Bacon, H.E. & Boutwell, J. (1961) *Surg. Gynecol. Obstet.*, **113**, 733.
Oberhammer, E.P. (1980) *Lancet*, **2**, 1028.
O'Keefe, S.J.P., Sender, P.M. & James, W.P.T. (1974) *Lancet*, **2**, 1035.
Orlowski, M., Sessa, G., & Green, J.P. (1974) *Science*, **184**, 66.
O'Shaughnessy, W.B. (1831) *Lancet*, **2**, 225.
Owen, O.E., Morgan, A.P., Kemp, H.G., Sullivan, J.M., Herrera, M.G. & Cahill, G.F. Jr. (1967) *J. Clin. Invest.*, **46**, 1589.
Page, D.L., Caulfield, J.B., Kastor, J.A., De Sanctis, R.W. & Sanders, C. (1971) *N. Engl. J. Med.*, **285**, 133.
Patterson, R.H. Jr. & Twichell, J.B. (1971) *JAMA*, **215**, 76.
Peaston, M.J.T. (1968) *Br. J. Hosp. Med.*, 708.
Phillips, I., Eykyn, S. & Laker, M. (1972) *Lancet*, **1**, 1258.
Pittman, J.A. & Cohen, P. (1964) *N. Engl. J. Med.*, **271**, 403.
Polak, J. & Bloom, S.R. (1979) The hormones of the gastrointestinal tract. In *Scientific Basis of Gastroenterology.* ed. Duthie, H.L. & Wormsley, K.G. Edinburgh: Churchill Livingstone.
Porte, D., Jr. & Robertson, R.P. (1973) *Fed. Proc.*, **32**, 1792.
Portnoy, J., Wolf, P.L., Webb, M. & Remington, J.S. (1971) *N. Engl. J. Med.*, **285**, 1010.
Powell-Tuck, J. (1980) Long-term intravenous feeding. In *Practical Nutritional Support.* ed. Karran, S.J. & Alberti, K.G.M.M. Bath: Pitman Medical.

Powers, S.R., Jr., Mannal, R. & Neclerio, M. (1973) *Ann. Surg.*, **178**, 265.
Pozefsky, T., Felig, P. & Tobin, J.D. (1969) *J. Clin. Invest.*, **48**, 2273.
Prentice, T.C., Olney, J.M., Artz, C.P. & Howard, J.M. (1954) *Surg. Gynecol. Obstet.*, **99**, 542.
Press, M., Hartop, P.J. & Prottey, C. (1974) *Lancet*, **1**, 597.
Preston, F.W., Barnes, A.U., Staley, C.J. & Trippel, O.H. (1957) *Metabolism*, **6**, 758.
Proctor, H.J., Ballantine, T.V.N. & Broussard, N.D. (1970) *Ann. Surg.*, **172**, 2.
Prout, W.G. (1968) *Lancet*, **1**, 1108.
Prys-Roberts, C., Greenbaum, R., Nunn, J.F. & Kelman, G.R. (1970) *J. Clin. Pathol.*, **23**, Suppl. (Roy. Coll. Path.) 4, 143.
Pullan, J.M. (1959) *Proc. Roy. Soc. Med.*, **52**, 31.
Quie, P.G. & Curry, C.R. (1971) *N. Engl. J. Med.*, **285**, 1221.
Randall, R.E., Cohen, E.D., Spray, C.C., Jr. & Rossmeisl, E.C. (1964) *Ann. Intern. Med.*, **61**, 73.
Rechigl, M., Loosli, J.K. & Williams, H.H. (1957) *J. Nutr.*, **63**, 177.
Reid, D.J. (1967) *Br. J. Surg.*, 54, 198.
Reid, D.J., & Ingram, G.I.C. (1967) *Clin. Sci.*, **33**, 399.
Reilly, J., Ryan, J., Strole, W. & Fischer, J. (1976) *Acta Chir. Scand.*, Suppl. **466**, 92.
Reul, G.J., Jr., Beall, A.C., Jr. & Greenberg, S.D. (1974) *Chest*, **66**, 4.
Riella, M.C. & Scribner, B.H. (1976) *Surg. Gynecol., Obstet.*, **143**, 205.
Riella, M.C., Broviac, J.W., Wells, M. & Scribner, B.H. (1975) *Ann. Intern. Med.*, **83**, 786.
Riordan, J.F. & Walters, G. (1968) *Lancet*, **1**, 719.
Rithalia, S.J. & Tinker, J. (1978) *Brit. J. Clin. Equip.*, **3**, 163.
Rose, W.C. (1949) *Fed. Proc.*, **8**, 546.
Rose, W.C. & Dekker, E.E. (1956) *J. Biol. Chem.*, **223**, 107.
Root, H.D., Hanser, C.W., McKinley, C.R., La Fane, J.W. & Mendiola, R.P. (1965) *Surgery*, **57**, 633.
Rush, B.F. (1974) *Surg. Gynecol. Obstet.*, **138**, 515.
Rusmin, S., Althauser, M.B. & DeLuca, P.P. (1975) *Ann. Intern. Med.*, **83**, 786.
Russell, R.C.G., Walker, C.J. & Bloom, S.R. (1975) *Br. Med. J.*, **1**, 10.
Ryan, J.A., Abel, R.M., Abbott, W.M., Hopkins, C.C., Chesney, T. McC., Colley, R., Phillips, K., & Fischer, J. (1974) *N. Engl. J. Med.*, **290**, 757.
Sagar, B., Harland, P. & Shields, R. (1979) *Br. Med. J.*, **1**, 293.
Sahebjamil, H. & Scalettar, R. (1971) *Lancet*, **1**, 366
Sailer, D. & Muller, M. (1980) *Middle Chain Triglycerides in Parenteral Nutrition.* 2nd European Congress of Parenteral and Enteral Nutrition (Abstract), Newcastle-upon-Tyne.
Sanders, R. & Sheldon, G. (1976) *Am. J. Surg.*, **132**, 214.
Scheig, R. (1968) Hepatic metabolism of medium chain fatty acids. In *Medium Chain Triglycerides.* ed. Senior, J.R. Philadelphia: University of Pennsylvania Press.
Schier, J., Gryszkiewicz, A., Moscicka, M., Rudowski, W. & Koscielak, J. (1974) *Acta Haematol. Pol.*, **5**, 313.
Schulte, H.D. (1969) *Dtsch. Med. Wochenschr.*, **94**, 1793.
Schumer, W. (1976) *Ann. Surg.*, **184**, 333.
Schumer, W. & Nyhus, L.M. (1970) *Corticosteroids in the treatment of shock.* University of Illinois Press.
Schwartz, A.E. & Roberts, K.E. (1957) *Surgery*, **42**, 814.
Seldinger, S.L. (1953) *Acta radiol.*, **39**, 368.
Sevitt, S. (1962) *Fat Embolism.* London: Butterworth Scientific Publications.
Shepherd, J.A. (1975) In *A Concise Surgery of the Abdomen*, p. 186. Edinburgh: Livingstone.
Sherlock, S. (1962) *Br. Med. J.*, **1**, 1359.
Sherlock, S. (1968) In *Diseases of the Liver and Biliary System.* Oxford: Blackwell Sci. Pub.
Sherlock, S. (1969) *Br. J. hosp. Med.*, **2**, 1257.
Shields, R. (1965) *Br. J. Surg.*, **52**, 774.
Shimoda, S.S., Saunders, R.D., Schuffler, M.D. & Leinbach, G.L. (1974) *Gastroenterology*, **67**, 19.
Shires, T., Williams, J. & Brown, J. (1961) *Ann. Surg.*, **41**, 803.
Shires, T. & Carrico, C.J. (1966) *Curr. Probl. Surg.*, **3**, 67.
Silk, D.B.A. (1979) *Res. Clin. For.*, **1**, 29.
Silva, H., Pomeroy, J., Rae, A.I., Rosen, S.M. & Shaldon, S. (1964) *Br. med. J.*, **2**, 407.
Silvis, E.S. & Paragas, P.D. (1972) *Gastroenterology*, **63**, 4.
Simoons, F.J. (1969) *Am. J. Dig. Dis.*, 14, 819.
Sitges-Creus, A., Canadas, E. & Vilar, L. (1977) Cholestatic Jaundice during parenteral alimentation in adults. In *Advances in Parenteral Nutrition.* ed. Johnston, I.D.A. Lancaster: MTP Press.
Sitges-Serra, A., Puig, P., Jaurrieta, E., Garau, J., Alastrue, A. & Sitges-Creus, A. (1980) *Surg. Gynecol. Obstet.*, **151**, 481.

Sloviter, H.A. (1958) *J. Clin. Invest.*, **37**, 619.
Soeters, P.B. & Fischer, J.E. (1976) *Lancet*, **2**, 880.
Solassol, C. & Joyeux, H. (1976) *Acta. Chir. Scand.*, Suppl. 466, 85.
Solis, R.T., Goldfinger, D., Gibbs, M.B. & Zeller, J.A. (1974) *Transfusion*, **14**, 538.
Soutter, R.D., Myers, W.O. & Wenzel, F.J. (1972) *J. Thorac. Cardiovasc. Surg.*, **63**, 54.
Starling, E.H. (1896) *J. Physiol.*, **19**, 312.
Stoner, H.R. (1979) *J. Clin. Pathol*, **23**, Supplement (Roy. Coll. Path.) 4, 47.
Studley, H.O. (1936) *JAMA*, **106**, 458.
Sturman, J.A., Gaull, G. & Raiha, N.C.R. (1970) *Science*, **169**, 74.
Susuki, F., & Shoemaker, W.C. (1964) *Surgery*, **55**, 304.
Swan, H.J.C. & Ganz, W. (1975) *Surg. Clin. N. Amer.*, **55**, 501.
Swan, H.J.C., Ganz, W., Forrester, J., Marcus, H., Diamond, G. & Chohette, D. (1970) *N. Eng. J. Med.*, **283**, 447.
Swendseid, M.E., Harris, C.L. & Tuttle, S.G. (1960) *J. Nutr.*, **71**, 105.
Swendseid, M.E., Feeley, R.J., Harris, C.L. & Tuttle, S.G. (1959) *J. Nutr.*, **68**, 203.
Tanaka, H., Manabe, H., Koshiyama, K., Hamanaka, Y., Matsumoto, K. & Uozumi, T. (1970) *Acta Endocrinol.*, **65**, 1.
Taylor, R.H., Barnardo, D.E., Polanska, N. & Misiewicz, J.J. (1979) *Gut*, **20**, A450.
Thomas, C.S. (1969) *Arch. Surg.*, **98**, 217.
Thomas, D.W., Edwards, J.B. & Edwards, R.G. (1970) *N. Engl. J. Med.*, **283**, 437.
Thompson, S.W. (1976) Hepatic Toxicity of Intravenous Fat Emulsions. In *Fat Emulsions in Parenteral Nutrition*. ed. Meng, H.C. & Wilmore, D.W. Chicago: American Medical Association.
Thoren, L. (1962) *Acta Chir. Scand.*, **325**, 75.
Threlfall, C.J. (1970) Intermediary carbohydrate metabolism in injured rat liver in relation to heat production. In *Energy Metabolism in Trauma*. CIBA Found. Syrup. London: Churchill.
Tinckler, L.F. (1966) *Br. Med. J.*, **1**, 1263.
Travis, S.F., Sugarman, H.J., Ruberg, R.L., Dudrick, S.J., Delivoria-Papadopoulus, M., Miller, L.D. & Oski, F.A. (1971). *N. Engl. F. Med.*, **285**, 763.
Truelove, S.C. & Jewell, D.P. (1974) *Lancet*, **1**, 1067.
Turner-Warwick, R.T. (1969) Urinary Diversion. In *Recent Advances in Surgery*, ch. 21. ed. Taylor, S. London: Churchill.
Tweedle, D.E.F. (1974) *Energy Balance in the Surgical Patient*. Ch. M. Thesis, University of Dundee.
Tweedle, D.E.F. (1980a) *Z. Gastroenterol.*, **16**, 68.
Tweedle, D.E.F. (1980b) *J. Parent. & Ent. Nutr.*, **4**, 165.
Tweedle, D.E.F. (1981) *Acta Chir. Scand.*, Suppl. **507**, 292.
Tweedle, D.E.F. & Johnston, I.D.A. (1971) *Br. J. Surg.*, **58**, 771.
Tweedle, D.E.F., Spivey, J & Johnston, I.D.A. (1972) *Metabolism*, **22**, 173.
Tweedle, D.E.F., Walton, C. & Johnston, I.D.A. (1973) *Br. J. Clin. Pract.*, 27, 130.
Tweedle, D.E.F., Fitzpatrick, G.F., Brennan, M.F., Culebras, J.M., Wolfe, B.M., Ball, M.B. & Moore, F.D. (1977) *Ann. Surg.*, **186**, 60.
Tweedle, D.E.F., Skidmore, F.D., Gleave, E.N., Knass, D.A. & Gowland, E. (1979) *Res. Clin. Forums*, **1**, 59.
Underwood, E.J. (1977) *Trace Elements in Human and Animal Nutriton*, 4th edn. New York: Academic Press.
Upjohn, H.C., Creditor, M.C. & Levenson, J.M. (1957) *Metabolism*, **6**, 607.
Venables, C.W., Ellis, H. & Smith, A.D.M. (1966) *Lancet*, **2**, 1390.
Venning, E.H., McCorriston, J.R., Dryenfurth, I. & Beck, J.C. (1958) *Metabolism*, **7**, 293.
Walker, W.F. (1965) *Proc. Roy. Soc. Med.*, **58**, 1015.
Walker, W.F., Zileil, M.S., Reutter, F.W., Shoemaker, W.C. & Moore, F.D. (1959) *Am. J. Physiol.*, **197**, 773.
Wannemacher, R.W., Pekarek, R.S. & Bartelloni, P.J. (1972) *Metabolism*, **21**, 67.
Wardrop, C.A.J., Heatley, R.V., Tennant, G.B. & Hughes, L.E. (1975) *Lancet*, **2**, 640.
Watkin, D.M. (1957) *Metabolism* **6**, 785.
Watson, A.J. (1970) *J. Clin. Pathol.*, **23**, Suppl. (Roy. Coll. Path.) 4, 132.
Webb, D.J., Lovesay, J.M., Ellis, A. & Knight, A.H. (1980) *Br. Med. J.*, **1**, 362.
Webb, W.R., Doyle, R.S. & Howard, H.S. (1960) *Metabolism*, **9**, 1047.
Welch, G.W., McKeel, D.W., Silverstein, P. & Walker, H.L. (1974) *Surg. Gynecol. Obstet.*, **138**, 421.
Wellman, K.F., Rheinhard, A. & Salazar, E.P. (1968) *Circulation*, **37**, 380.
Wells, F.E. & Smits, B.J. (1978) *Am. J. Clin. Nutr.*, **31**, 442.
Wene, J.D., Connor, W.E. & Denbesten, L. (1975) *J. Clin. Invest.*, **56**, 127.
Wenzel, M. (1972) *Med. Ernahr*, **13**, 100.
Widdowson, E.M., Dickerson, J.W.T. (1964) Chemical composition of the body. In: *Mineral*

Metabolism ed. Comar C.L., Bronner, F., 11A, New York: Academic Press.

Widmark, E.M.P. (1952) *Fortschr. naturw. Forsch.*, **11**, 1.

Wilkinson, A.W. (1955) In *Body Fluids in Surgery*, p. 75. Edinburgh: Livingstone.

Wilkinson, A.W. (1956) *Lancet*, **1**, 184.

Wilkinson, A.W. (1958) *Br. J. Plast. Surg.*, **10**, 275.

Wilkinson, P. & Sherlock, S. (1962) *Lancet*, **2**, 1125.

Williams, J.R., Wilcox, W.C., Andrews, G.J. & Burns, R.R. (1963) *JAMA*, **184**, 473.

Wilmore, D.W., Moylan, J.A., Helcamp, G.M. & Pruitt, B.A. (1973) *Ann. Surg.*, **178**, 503.

Wilmore, D.W., Long, J.M., Mason, A.D. Jr., Skreen, R.W. & Pruitt, B.A., Jr. (1974a) *Ann. Surg.*, **180**, 653.

Wilmore, D.W., Lindsey, C.A., Moylan, J.A., Faloona, G.R., Pruitt, B.A. Jr. & Unger, R.H. (1974b) *Lancet*, **1**, 73.

Wilmore, D.W., Moylan, J.A., Jr., Bristow, B.F., Mason, A.D., Jr. & Pruitt, B.A., Jr. (1974c) *Surg. Gynecol. Obst.*, **138**, 875.

Wilson, G.M., Edelman, I.S., Brooks, L., Myrden, J.A., Harken, D.E. & Moore, F.D. (1954) *Circulation*, **9**, 199.

Winitz, M., Du Ruisseau, J.P., Otey, M.C., Birnbaum, S.M. & Greenstein, J.P. (1956) *Arch. Biochem.*, **4**, 368.

Witzelben, C.L., Pitlick, P., Bergmeyer, J. & Benoit, R. (1968) *Am. J. Pathol.*, **53**, 409.

Wolfe, R.R., Allsop, J.R. & Burke, J.F. (1979) *Metabolism*, **28**, 210.

Wolfe, R.R., O'Donnell, T.F., Stone, M.D., Richmand, D.A. & Burke, J.F. (1980) *Metabolism*, **29**, 892.

Wolfram, G. & Zollner, N. (1971) *Wiss. Veroff. Dt. Ges. Ernahr.*, **22**, 51–60.

Wolfram, G., Eckart, J., Walther, B. & Zollner, N. (1978) *J. Parent, & Ent. Nutr.*, **2**, 634.

Woods, H.F., Eggleston, L.V. & Krebs, H.A. (1970) *Biochem. J.*, **119**, 501.

Woolfson, A.M.J. (1980) *Int. Care. Med.*, **7**, 11.

Woolfson, A.M.J., Heatley, R.V. & Allison, S.P. (1977) Significance of insulin in the metabolic response to injury. In *Nutritional aspects of care in the critically ill.* ed. Richards, J.R. & Kinney, J.M. Edinburgh: Churchill Livingstone.

Woolfson, A.M.J., Ricketts, C.R., Hardy, S.M., Saour, J.N., Pollard, B.J. & Allison, S.P. (1976) *Postgrad. Med. J.*, **52**, 678

Wretlind, A. (1972) Complete intravenous nutrition: theoretical and experimental background. *Nutr. Metab.*, **14**, (Supplement 1), 57.

Wretlind, A. (1974a) Assessment of patient requirements. In: *Parenteral Nutrition in Acute Metabolic Illness.* ed. Lee, H.A. London: Academic Press.

Wretlind, A. (1974b) Fat Emulsions. In *Parenteral Nutrition in Acute Metabolic Illness.* ed. Lee, H.A. London: Academic Press.

Wretlind, K.A.J. (1972) *Nutr. Metab.*, **14**, suppl 1, 1.

Wright, H.K. & Tilson, M.D. (1971) The Short Gut Syndrome: Pathophysiology and Treatment. In *Current Problems in Surgery.* Chicago: Year Book Medical Publishers.

Wright, P.D., Henderson, K. & Johnston, I.D.A. (1974) *Br. J. Surg.*, **61**, 5.

Yoffa, D. (1965) *Lancet*, **2**, 614.

Young, D.G. (1973) Fluid balance in paediatric surgery. *Br. J. Anaesth.*, **45**, 953.

Young, L.S., Martin, W.J., Meyer, R.D., Weinstein, R.J. & Anderson, E.T. (1977) *Ann. Intern. Med.*, **86**, 456.

Yu, V.Y.H., James, P., Hendry, P. & MacMahon, R.A. (1979) *Arch Dis. Child.*, **54**, 653.

Zimmerman, B. (1945) *Science*, **101**, 566.

Zimmerman, B. & Wangensteen, O.H. (1954) *Surgery*, **31**, 654.

Zimmermann, B., Casey, J.H. & Black, H.S. (1955) *Surg. Forum*, **6**, 3.

Zohnan, L.R. & Williams, M.H. (1959) *Am. J. Cardiol.*, **4**, 373.

Zollner, N. (1978) Evaluation of non-glucose carbohydrates in parenteral nutrition. In *Advances in Parenteral Nutrition.* ed. Johnston, I.D.A. Lancaster: MTP Press.

Index